Occupational Medicine

Occupational Epidemiology

Guest Editor:

Ki Moon Bang, PhD, MPH
National Institute for Occupational Safety and Health
Morgantown, West Virginia

STATE OF THE ART REVIEWS

Volume 11/Number 3
HANLEY & BELFUS, INC.

July–September 1996
Philadelphia

Publisher: HANLEY & BELFUS, INC.
210 South 13th Street
Philadelphia, PA 19107
(215) 546-4995
Fax (215) 790-9330

OCCUPATIONAL MEDICINE: State of the Art Reviews is included in *Index Medicus, MEDLINE, BioSciences Information Service, Current Contents* and *ISI/BIOMED.*

OCCUPATIONAL MEDICINE: State of the Art Reviews   (ISSN 0885-114X)
July-September 1996   Volume 11, Number 3   (ISBN 1-56053-226-2)

OCCUPATIONAL MEDICINE: State of the Art Reviews is published quarterly by Hanley & Belfus, Inc., 210 South 13th Street, Philadelphia, Pennsylvania 19107. Periodical postage paid at Philadelphia, PA, and at additional mailing offices.

POSTMASTER: Send address changes to OCCUPATIONAL MEDICINE: State of the Art Reviews, Hanley & Belfus, Inc., 210 South 13th Street, Philadelphia, PA 19107.

The 1996 subscription price is $88.00 per year U.S., $98.00 outside U.S. (add $40.00 for air mail).

Occupational Medicine: State of the Art Reviews
Vol. 11, No. 3, July–September 1996

OCCUPATIONAL EPIDEMIOLOGY
Ki Moon Bang, PhD, MPH, Editor

CONTENTS

The development of occupational epidemiology has been steadily accelerating, both with regard to methodology and the number of studies being conducted. This chapter reviews the general applications of occupational epidemiology and illustrates some of the various studies reported in the literature in order to assist in the practical application of the epidemiologic approach.

When information about subjects in a study is unavailable from other sources, surrogate respondents, such as family members, have provided information about the subject. This chapter focuses on the quality of occupational histories provided by surrogates. The author addresses the issues of (1) nonresponse of the surrogate, (2) surrogate-subject and surrogate-record agreement, and (3) the impact of misclassification on estimates of relative risk.

The optimal study design to evaluate potential occupational hazards varies according to research objectives, disease, understanding of etiology, and location of the study populations. This chapter provides a description of the application of the most frequently used epidemiologic designs for occupational studies and focuses on issues especially important in hypothesis-testing investigations of chronic diseases.

This chapter focuses on the "response" side of the exposure-response relationship and summarizes some of the measures of effect that are commonly used in occupational epidemiologic research. The author covers some basic statistical standardization procedures that are used to help compare these measures among groups that differ with respect to age or other factors.

One of the most important roles for occupational epidemiology is to provide a scientific basis for assessing causation. This chapter discusses the criteria for causation considered by the U.S. Surgeon General, the International Agency for Research on Cancer, and others to place the evidence in historical context. As a case study, the criteria for judging the evidence for potential carcinogenicity of silica dust are examined. The importance of communication with workers and management about causal concerns from workplace exposures is also discussed.

The authors discuss various methodologic issues pertinent to the epidemiologic study of chronic occupational lung disease. Examples to illustrate problems inherent in chronic occupational lung disease epidemiology and approaches to surmounting them are presented from the extensive literature on coal miners' lung diseases.

This chapter provides an up-to-date review of the occurrence and causes of occupational cancer based on epidemiologic studies in humans and discusses the characteristics of occupational cancer, research, priorities, and cancer surveillance.

The author outlines the methods by which the International Agency for Research on Cancer evaluates study design and results when it reviews epidemiologic studies to determine carcinogenicity and mutagenicity. The chapter concludes with an extensive series of tables summarizing (1) the tests relevant to mutagenicity and (2) the IARC rating system for carcinogens, categorizing industrial and agricultural chemicals according to evidence of mutagenicity.

The rise in reports of occupational disorders of the upper extremity has been meteoric. This chapter examines the frequency and prevalence of upper extremity disorders, reviews the active surveys of upper extremity disorders in selected occupations, examines current surveillance systems, and discusses the problem of effective case definition.

Ergonomics is the study of people at work. This chapter outlines ergonomic principles, describes low back pain and upper extremity cumulative trauma disorders from an ergonomic perspective, and discusses control and prevention approaches for selected scenarios.

PUBLISHED ISSUES
(available from the publisher)

CONTRIBUTORS

Michael Attfield, PhD
Acting Section Chief, Epidemiology Section, Division of Respiratory Disease Studies, National Institute for Occupational Safety and Health, Morgantown, West Virginia

Ki Moon Bang, PhD, MPH
Chief, Surveillance Section, Division of Respiratory Disease Studies, National Institute for Occupational Safety and Health, Morgantown, West Virginia; Adjunct Professor, Department of Community Medicine, West Virginia University School of Medicine, Morgantown, West Virginia

Aaron Blair, PhD
Chief, Occupational Studies Section, Environmental Epidemiology Branch, National Cancer Institute, Bethesda, Maryland

Martin G. Cherniack, MD, MPH
Associate Professor of Medicine, Division of Occupational and Environmental Medicine, University of Connecticut Health Center, Farmington, Connecticut

David F. Goldsmith, MSPH, PhD
Senior Scientist, California Public Health Foundation, University of San Francisco, Berkeley, California

Richard B. Hayes, DDS, PhD
Epidemiologist, Occupational Studies Section, National Cancer Institute, Bethesda, Maryland

Paul K. Henneberger, MPH, ScD
Visiting Scientist, Epidemiological Investigations Branch, National Institute for Occupational Safety and Health, Morgantown, West Virginia

Paul Hewett, PhD, CIH
Industrial Hygienist, Division of Respiratory Disease Studies, National Institute for Occupational Safety and Health, Morgantown, West Virginia

Grace Kawas Lemasters, PhD
Professor, Department of Occupational and Environmental Health, University of Cincinnati College of Medicine, Cincinnati, Ohio

Gary M. Marsh, PhD
Professor, Department of Biostatistics, University of Pittsburgh, Graduate School of Public Health, Pittsburgh, Pennsylvania

Avima M. Ruder, PhD
Chief, Epidemiology 2 Section, Industrywide Studies Branch, National Institute for Occupational Safety and Health, Cincinnati, Ohio

Patricia Ann Stewart, PhD
Industrial Hygienist, Occupational Studies Section, National Cancer Institute, Bethesda, Maryland

Terrence J. Stobbe, PhD
Professor, Department of Industrial Engineering and Mineral Resources, College of Engineering, West Virginia University, Morgantown, West Virginia

Gregory R. Wagner, MD
Division of Respiratory Disease Studies, National Institute for Occupational Safety and Health, Morgantown, West Virginia

Shelia Hoar Zahm, ScD
Epidemiologist, Occupational Studies Section, Division of Cancer Epidemiology and Genetics, National Cancer Institute, Rockville, Maryland

1996 ISSUES

Law and the Workplace
Edited by Jack W. Snyder, MD, JD, PhD
Thomas Jefferson University Hospital
Philadelphia, Pennsylvania
and Julia E. Klees, MD, MPH
BASF Corporation
Mount Olive, New Jersey

Violence in the Workplace
Edited by Robert Harrison, MD, MPH
California Department of Health Services
Berkeley, California

Occupational Epidemiology
Edited by Ki Moon Bang, PhD, MPH
National Institute for Occupational Safety
and Health
Morgantown, West Virginia

Impact of Psychiatric Conditions in the Workplace
Edited by Ibrahim Farid, MD
United States Postal Service
San Bruno, California
and Carroll Brodsky, MD, PhD
University of California School of Medicine
San Francisco, California

1995 ISSUES

Effects of the Indoor Environment on Health
Edited by James M. Seltzer, MD
University of California School of Medicine
San Diego, California

Construction Safety and Health
Edited by Knut Ringen, DrPH,
Laura Welch, MD, James L. Weeks, ScD, CIH,
and Jane L. Seegal, MS
Washington, DC
and Anders Englund, MD
Solna, Sweden

Occupational Hearing Loss
Edited by Thais C. Morata, PhD,
and Derek E. Dunn, PhD
National Institute for Occupational Safety
and Health
Cincinnati, Ohio

Firefighters' Safety and Health
Edited by Peter Orris, MD
Cook County Hospital
Chicago, Illinois
and Richard M. Duffy, MSc
International Association of Fire Fighters
Washington, DC
and James Melius, MD, DrPH
Center to Protect Workers' Rights
Washington, DC

1994 ISSUES

Occupational Skin Disease
Edited by James R. Nethercott, MD
University of Maryland
Baltimore, Maryland

Occupational Safety and Health Training
Edited by Michael J. Colligan, PhD
National Institute for Occupational
Safety and Health
Cincinnati, Ohio

Reproductive Hazards
Edited by Ellen B. Gold, PhD, B. L. Lasley,
PhD, and Marc B. Schenker, MD, MPH
University of California
Davis, California

Tuberculosis in the Workplace
Edited by Steven Markowitz, MD
Mount Sinai School of Medicine
New York, New York

Ordering Information:
Subscriptions for full year and single issues are available from the publishers—
Hanley & Belfus, Inc., 210 South 13th Street, Philadelphia, PA 19107
Telephone (215) 546-7293; (800) 962-1892. Fax (215) 790-9330.

PREFACE

Occupational epidemiology has become an important and integral part of occupational health and safety. The primary goal of occupational epidemiology is to determine what kinds of exposure in the workplace are associated with certain diseases or injuries in order to present the best disease-prevention strategy.

The field of occupational health is rapidly evolving. Interest in this field has grown because of serious implications associated with recognized diseases and injuries that have occurred in the workplace. In 1993, 6.7 million injuries and illnesses were reported in private industry workplaces, resulting in a rate of 8.5 cases for every 100 full-time workers. Most of these cases are preventable. Workers in many industries face occupational hazards due to chemical, physical, and biological exposures, ergonomics, and psychosocial factors. Occupational epidemiology can be applied to identify the causes of work-related diseases and injuries, evaluate the hazards, create ways to control hazards so that workers are protected, and make recommendations for occupational health and safety issues.

The chapters in this book deal with a variety of occupational epidemiologic issues and provide useful information for designing and conducting epidemiologic studies in the workplace. It is my hope that this book will be of practical benefit to health professionals, both as a textbook and as a handy source of reference to prevent and control the potential diseases of the occupational environment. In addition, I believe that students in occupational epidemiology and health may also benefit from a widening of their horizons for investigation in occupational medicine.

The chapters discuss basic principles and applications of occupational epidemiologic studies and review study results of common occupational diseases in the workplace. This volume is organized into 12 chapters. The first five chapters discuss applications of occupational epidemiology and provide guidelines for data collection, study design, epidemiologic measures, and interpretation of epidemiologic study. The second six chapters offer concise discussions of selected common occupational diseases and injuries: chronic occupational respiratory diseases, occupational cancers in humans, occupational carcinogens and mutagens, occupational disorders of the upper extremity, ergonomics and injury prevention, and reproductive hazards. The last chapter addresses interpretation and use of occupational exposure limits for chronic disease agents in the workplace.

Developing this text has been a challenging experience in my occupational epidemiology career. I was fortunate to have distinguished authors who have contributed to this text. I am indebted to the efforts of the contributing authors who persevered through drafts and revisions, and I wish to thank them for these efforts. I also thank Dr. Kenneth C. Weber, Dr. Jesse Monestersky, Dr. Paul Henneberger, Mr. Sam S. Bang, and Mr. Lou Fintor for reviewing several chapters. I would like to acknowledge Dr. Gregory R. Wagner and Dr. John E. Parker for their support and encouragement. Finally, I would like to dedicate this book to my wife, Hanok, and my two sons, Sam and David, who saw several months of weekends disappear into this effort.

Ki Moon Bang, PhD, MPH
GUEST EDITOR

KI MOON BANG, PhD, MPH

APPLICATIONS OF OCCUPATIONAL EPIDEMIOLOGY

From the Division of Respiratory
  Disease Studies
National Institute for Occupational
  Safety and Health
Morgantown, West Virginia

Reprint requests to:
Ki Moon Bang, PhD, MPH
Division of Respiratory Disease
  Studies
NIOSH-Room 234
1095 Willowdale Road
Morgantown, WV 26505-2888

Occupational epidemiology is the study of the distribution and determinants of work-related disease and injuries in the workplace. Occupational epidemiologic studies have become an important and integral part of occupational health. Occupational epidemiology has grown rapidly since the late 1970s. Recent developments in occupational epidemiology include the integration of epidemiologic courses into occupational health training, methodologic development, and access to computers and statistical software packages. A primary goal of occupational epidemiology is to determine what kinds of exposures in the workplace are associated with certain diseases or injuries in order to present the best disease-prevention strategy.

Employment in the United States is projected to increase from 121.1 million in 1992 to 147.5 million in 2005, according to a projection by the Bureau of Labor Statistics.[31] In 1993, 6.7 million injuries and illnesses were reported in private industry workplaces, resulting in a rate of 8.5 cases for every 100 full-time workers.[38] Costs of occupational injuries and illnesses in 1992 were estimated to be $173.9 billion, or 3% of the gross domestic product.[19] These changes in occupational workforces and health statistics have recently led to increased attention to occupational health in the United States.

The occupational epidemiologic approach to a particular disease is intended to identify high-risk subgroups within the population and determine the effectiveness of subsequent preventive measures. In principle, the epidemiologic study of work-related disease does not differ from other aspects of epidemiologic research. This chapter reviews the general application of occupational epidemiology and illustrates some studies reported in the literature. It is intended to assist in the practical application of the epidemiologic approach.

USE OF EPIDEMIOLOGY IN OCCUPATIONAL HEALTH

It was the science of epidemiology that demonstrated the serious health risks associated with asbestos, radiation, coal dusts, and other occupational exposures. The rapid growth in the use of potentially hazardous materials has been accompanied by numerous observations of serious health effects in humans as a result of occupational exposures. An example of early occupational epidemiology came from the observations in 1879 of an increased occurrence of lung cancer among miners in Schneeberg.[11] Some decades later an excess of bladder cancer among German aniline workers was reported.[26] An example of modern epidemiologic study is workers at plastic manufacturing plants who handled the gas vinyl chlorine and were discovered in 1974 to be developing hepatic angiosarcoma, an unusual cancer.[39] At about the same time, infertility and an extreme decrease in spermatogenesis were discovered in workers at a California plant producing dibromochloropropane.[41] Some advances have occurred in improving the work environment and avoiding dangerously uncontrolled industrial plant emissions. However, there are still many reported occupational diseases and injuries that could be prevented in the workplace.

Epidemiologic principles can be readily applied to occupational studies. Occupational studies are designed according to the study objectives. In general, there are three major types of epidemiologic studies: descriptive, analytic, and experimental.[28] Most studies in occupational epidemiology are analytic rather than descriptive.

Descriptive studies are used to characterize person, place, and time. What are the age, sex, race, occupation, industry, socioeconomic status, and other personal characteristics of people who get a particular disease? Where does the disease occur? When does the disease occur? Does temporal variation or seasonal fluctuation exist?

Analytic studies determine the etiologic factors associated with a disease by calculating estimates of risk. What exposures do people with the disease have in common? What is the degree of the increased risk by exposure? Analytic methods are available to control for known confounders, but unknown ones are free to distort risk estimates.

Experimental studies involve a search for strategies to alter the natural history of disease. Examples are intervention trials to reduce risk factors, screening studies aimed at identifying the early stages of disease, and clinical trials of different treatment modalities to improve prognosis. Experimental studies have the advantage of randomization, a procedure that distributes both known and unknown confounders equally between the test and control groups.[23]

Occupational epidemiologic studies include observational studies and experimental studies. Observational studies are the most common. The major types of observational studies in epidemiology are the cohort, case-control, and cross-sectional designs. Other types of study designs are ecologic studies, meta-analysis, occupational surveillance, and the recently developed molecular epidemiologic studies.

Occupational epidemiology has been used for testing specific hypotheses. The specific hypothesis means in principle that "a causes b" can be tested through either a follow-up or a case-control study.[13] If the disease is rare, a case-control study is appropriate. If the exposure is rare, a follow-up study is more efficient. If both the exposure and the disease are common, both designs are feasible, and the decision depends on the availability of data, possibility of tracing records, financial resources, length of study periods, and other factors. Methods of study design and measure are described in the next two chapters.

For establishing causal relationships, several criteria have been proposed to evaluate whether a positive association in epidemiologic studies indicates causality. The most important criteria are strength, consistency, biologic gradient, biologic plausibility, and temporality.[10] The strength of an association is the magnitude of the relative risk in the exposed group compared to that of the control group. Consistency of an association is the extent to which it is reported from multiple studies conducted. The biologic gradient of an association is its dose-response validity. The biologic plausibility of the study is based on the assessment that it makes sense in light of what is known about the mechanism of production of the adverse effect. Temporality of the study is a test on the conclusion or observation that the cause preceded the effect in time. Fulfillment of some of the criteria may occur when the association is due to chance or bias. If most of the criteria are met, the likelihood of an association being causal rather than due to chance is high.

TYPES OF STUDIES AND EXAMPLES

Various types of occupational epidemiologic studies are described below with examples.

Cohort Studies

A cohort study is the follow-up (prospective) study in which a group or groups of individuals are defined on the basis or absence of exposure to a suspected risk factor for a disease over time. The disease rate among those exposed to a particular factor is compared with the rate among the nonexposed in the cohort to assess if an association exists between the study factor and disease.

Cohort studies are useful and effective in occupational epidemiology. Occupational cohort studies can be carried out from different approaches, including (1) prospective cohort morbidity and mortality studies and (2) retrospective cohort morbidity and mortality studies. For the prospective cohort study design, rates of disease can be calculated in both the exposed and unexposed groups for a direct measure of the absolute and relative risk. For the retrospective cohort study design, a long time is not required to complete the study because all events (both the exposure and the disease) have already taken place. Occupational cohort studies are usually mortality studies, because records of cause of death are generally more accessible and less biased than the cause of disease records. The central and unique element in occupational cohort studies is the individual work history with detailed exposure information. However, the cohort study design has some limitations: (1) it is inefficient in the evaluation of rare diseases, unless the attributable-risk percent is high; (2) it is expensive and time-consuming (long follow-up of subjects); (3) large numbers of subjects required; (4) the possibility exists of changes in criteria and methods over time; (5) subjects can be lost over time; and (6) administrative problems such as loss of staff and loss of funding occur.

Example 1. Prospective Cohort Mortality Study. Mortality from lung cancer was studied among a large industrial cohort of 26,501 workers who were exposed to formaldehyde.[4] The workers were first employed in 10 plants before January 1, 1966, and were traced to January 1, 1980, to determine vital status. The plant produced a variety of products, including formaldehyde, formaldehyde resins and molding compounds, molded plastic products, decorative laminates, and plywood. Historical exposures to formaldehyde by job, work area, plant, and calendar time were estimated using available monitoring data, and current walk-through surveys were conducted for exposure estimation. The relative risk for lung cancer 20 or more years after first exposure did not rise with increasing exposure to formaldehyde. The lack of a clear exposure-response relationship between lung cancer and formaldehyde exposure in this study is consistent with other reports.[5,33] Mortality from lung cancer was more strongly associated with exposure to other substances, including phenol, melamine, urea, and wood dust than with exposure to formaldehyde. Workers exposed to formaldehyde but not the other substances did not experience an excess mortality from lung cancer. The authors suggested that exposure to phenol, melamine, urea, wood dust, or other exposures may play a more primary role in the development of lung cancer and this association should be further studied in workers involved with resin and molding compound operations.

Example 2. Prospective Cohort Morbidity Study. A four-year longitudinal study conducted in 1972–1976 was designed to evaluate respiratory effects associated with exposure to toluene diisocyanate.[40] The study began with 111 shift workers who were exposed at a polyurethane foam manufacturing plant; 48 of the subjects were still working at the plant on the first Monday of November 1976. Pulmonary function tests including the first second of expiration (FEV_1) were administered to all workers. The workers were divided into three exposure groups; low (< 0.002 ppm), medium (0.002–0.0034 ppm), and high (> 0.0035 ppm). The cumulative exposure of each worker was calculated from the sum of the products of the time spent at the usual job. The cumulative exposure was then divided by the sum of the months spent in the usual job to establish a usual exposure level (in ppm) for each worker during the study period. The decline in FEV_1 (60 ml/year) observed in the high-exposure group exceeded the annual decrement observed in longitudinal studies of normal populations that have demonstrated expected annual declines of 32–47 ml FEV_1. This finding indicates that chronic exposure to levels of toluene diisocyanate greater than 0.0035 ppm results in greater pulmonary function loss than expected.

Case-Control Studies

Case-control studies, also known as retrospective studies, follow a paradigm that proceeds from effect to cause.[30] In a case-control study, individuals with disease (the cases) are selected for comparisons with individuals without the disease (the controls). Cases and controls are compared with respect to exposures associated with the disease under study.

Case-control studies may be preferred if either of the following scenarios exists: (1) the disease of interest is relatively rare and would require a large cohort for follow-up or (2) several occupations or substances may be associated with the disease of interest.

Case-control studies require the exposure to be reasonably common for the study design to be effective. However, some case-control studies might involve few exposed individuals and would not otherwise provide informative data on the epidemiologic problem. Specific individual exposures can be relatively rare from the viewpoint of the general population, but this problem can be overcome by optimizing the particular population for the study.

The application of the case-control approach to studying occupational factors associated with disease is limited primarily by the difficulty in determining the precise nature and extent of past exposures on the basis of an interview. This tends to lead to the use of broadly defined job or industry categories (e.g., usual employment in the leather industry), which dilutes the true risk by including individuals with widely disparate histories of occupational exposures to specific chemicals. Other limitations of case-control study include (1) inefficiency in evaluating rare exposures unless the study is very large or the exposure is common among those with the disease, (2) inability to directly compute incidence rates of disease in exposed and nonexposed individuals, (3) difficulty in establishing the temporal relationship between exposure and disease, and (4) selection and recall bias.

The various sources of systematic error in case-control studies can be referred to as the validity issues. Axelson[3] discussed the various aspects of validity with reference to (1) the possible role of exposure status in the selection of cases and controls, (2) difficulties in obtaining adequate information on exposure among cases and controls, (3) the possible relation of the control entities to one-another (when using persons with diagnoses other than the disease in question) to the exposure, and (4) the effects of confounding factors.

Example 1.   A bladder cancer study was conducted to estimate the risk of bladder cancer associated with occupational exposures in Boston.[8] All new cases of bladder cancer were identified in the defined geographic area during an 18-month period. Control groups were selected from local residents ages 20 to 89. Interviews were conducted to obtain information on occupational history and other factors. For each job held longer than 6 months, demographic variables, nature of the employer's industry, job title, time interval on the job, and specific duties performed were obtained. Relative risks were computed and controlled for age and smoking. The relative risk of bladder cancer among men employed in the leather product industry was 2.25 (95% CI = 1.46–3.46). Among men, excess risk of lower urinary tract cancer also was found in several occupational categories where they had been suspected as a priori: rubber-foreman, leather-foreman, painter, and dyestuffs-laborer.

Example 2.   A study on the association between pancreatic cancer and occupational exposures was conducted in Finland to identify occupational risk factors.[16] Pancreatic cancer is a highly fatal malignancy without a known cause. The Finnish Cancer Register was used to identify 1,419 patients with primary exocrinic pancreatic cancer diagnosed between 1984–1987, at the age of 40–74, and who died by April 1, 1990. The primary controls were 2,510 deceased subjects who were not known to have significant occupational risk factors. For the final study groups, the occupational exposure histories for 595 incident cases of primary exocrinic cancer of the pancreas and 1,622 controls were constructed. The study found elevated odds ratios for ionizing radiation exposure (OR = 4.3, 95% CI = 1.6–11.4) and inorganic dust containing crystalline silica exposure (OR = 2.0, 95% CI = 1.2–3.5).

Example 3.   A case-control study of cancer of the larynx was conducted within a cohort of automobile workers exposed to metal working fluids.[9] Study subjects consisted of 108 cases of laryngeal cancer and 538 controls. Cases were defined as all cohort members with laryngeal cancer detected prior to January 1, 1990, in the metropolitan Detroit and Michigan state cancer registries. Controls were selected from the cohort by incidence density sampling. A risk set was defined for each case and consisted of all subjects at risk of laryngeal cancer at the age of the death (or diagnosis) of the case. Within each risk set, five controls were randomly selected and matched by year of birth, plant, race, and gender. Based on a retrospective exposure assessment, lifetime exposures to straight and soluble metal working fluids, grinding particulate, biocides, selected metals, sulfur, and chlorine were examined. Results suggest that straight mineral oils are associated with almost a twofold excess in laryngeal cancer risk. This finding is consistent with several previous reports in the literature. When categorized exposure variables were examined, the odds ratio increased with increasing exposure, showing evidence of a dose-response relationship: in the highest category of straight metal fluid exposure, > 0.5 mg/m³ years, the odds ratio was 2.23 (95% CI = 1.25–3.98).

Cross-Sectional Studies

Cross-sectional studies examine the relationships between disease and other variables of interest as they exist in a defined population at one particular point in time.[18] This study design is often called a survey or prevalence study. The cross-sectional designs are usually descriptive prevalence studies, using random or probability sampling procedures to select subjects. Cross-sectional studies are especially suited for inquiring into subtle, perhaps even subclinical health effects for which records are unlikely to exist. Cross-sectional studies are essentially prevalence studies, and the relationship between the health effects and time cannot be readily explored. The prevalence of the health effect is compared among subgroups with various occupational exposures, ages, smoking or other medical histories.

Cross-sectional studies are useful for hypothesis generation and health services planning if done by random sampling. If the information was not collected by a random sampling, the estimates of the prevalence of a disease or of an association between a factor and a disease are of little value, since they are not representative of a study base or source population and are subject to many biases. Prevalence studies are considerably less expensive than cohort studies, because it is possible to evaluate the disease prevalence at only one point in time rather than continually searching for incident cases over an extended period. However, in a prevalence survey, it is difficult to ascertain at what age disease first occurred, and it is therefore difficult to determine which exposures preceded the development of disease.

Although cross-sectional designs can sometimes provide etiologic information, the prevalence rate is not ideal for measuring morbidity because of the composite nature of the prevalence.[13] An etiologic cross-sectional study is meaningful only if a close time-relation exists between exposure and morbidity. Diseases of short duration are not good candidates for cross-sectional designs because they, on average, are likely to be missed; conversely, long-duration diseases are usually overrepresented in cross-sectional studies. In occupational settings, cross-sectional studies are likely to include information only on currently employed individuals, thereby missing retired employees and persons who quit due to illness that may be related to an exposure under study.[7]

Example 1.   The National Health Interview Survey, a major data collection program administered by the National Center for Health Statistics, was mandated by the National Health Survey Act of 1956 to provide for a continuing survey to collect information on illness and disability in the United States. In 1988, the survey contained a special section called the Occupational Health Supplement,[37] whose goal was to obtain detailed information on respondent work-related health problems, workplace injuries, and smoking status. Of 42,487 respondents, 1,785 white men indicated that they had work experience in the construction industry. The prevalence rate of asthma per 1,000 construction workers was 19.6.[34]

Example 2.   A cross-sectional survey of farmers found evidence of significant associations between self-reported asthma and the use of carbamate insecticides, according to a respiratory health survey on 1,939 male farmers in 17 municipalities in

Saskatchewan, Canada.[29] Farmers were defined as including every male farmland taxpayer or farm worker in each of the 17 rural municipalities studied. Of 2,375 farmers visited, 1,939 participated in the study, and 83 of the participants (4.3%) were reported to be asthmatics. Interestingly, a significant association with asthma was observed in the use of carbamate insecticides. Of the 83 asthmatics, 32 (38.6%) reported having used carbamate insecticides versus 464 (25.1%) of the 1,856 nonasthmatics. The prevalence odds ratio was 1.9 (95% CI = 1.2–3.0). These findings raised the possibility that exposure to agriculture chemicals could be related to lung dysfunction in exposed farmers.

Ecologic Studies

Ecologic studies provide a crude way of exploring associations between occupation or environment and disease. These studies are considered to be hypothesis-generating rather than hypothesis-testing. Disease rates in various groups defined by specific geographic areas are compared. Several major reservations exist regarding the use of ecologic studies in occupational epidemiology. In some instances, they may provide a reasonable and inexpensive way of generating hypotheses. Alternatively, ecologic studies are limited by the use of proxy data for exposure and disease and by the unavailability of data necessary to control confounding factors.[27] The general problem of inappropriate inferences from ecologic data has been referred to as the ecologic fallacy.[24] Other problems with ecologic studies are related to difficulty in selecting groups of proper size. Groups that are too small will have few cases and unstable rates for the disease in question, or they will be affected by migration.

Example. The National Institute for Occupational Safety and Health published the Work-Related Lung Disease Surveillance Report in 1994.[36] One section of the report presented maps showing the mortality rate for asbestos in the United States for 1989–1990. The maps showed the highest mortality rates for asbestosis in the Northeast, Southeast, and West coasts, locations where the shipbuilding industry was located. A case-control study of lung cancer in coastal Georgia[6] revealed a logical and confirmed association between shipbuilding and lung cancer, possibly as a result of asbestos exposure.

Meta-Analysis

Meta-analysis, an analytic method that has been developed recently, is the process of pooling data from multiple studies that can be used to draw conclusions about therapeutic effectiveness or to plan new studies.[17] The final product has both quantitative and qualitative elements; it takes into account the numerical results and sample sizes of individual studies as well as quality of the data, extent of bias, and strength of the study design. Meta-analysis is a systematic review strategy for addressing research questions that are especially useful when results from several studies disagree with regard to the magnitude or direction of effect. Meta-analysis can be applied to occupational studies with divergent findings.

Example. Meta-analysis of studies on lung cancer among silicotics is reported.[32] In the literature, the association between silicosis and lung cancer has been controversial. The studies among silicotics tend to demonstrate an excess risk of lung cancer, but these studies have been criticized because of possible selection and confounding biases. Data from 29 studies were abstracted. Several of the studies suffered from biases due to competing risks of different cause of death. After adjusting for competing risks, all 29 studies demonstrated lung cancer relative risk estimates to be greater than one. The polled relative risk for the studies combined was 2.2 (95% CI = 2.1–2.4). The results of this meta-analysis demonstrate that increased risks of lung cancer exist for persons diagnosed with silicosis. The authors conclude that the association between silicosis and lung cancer is causal, either due to silicosis itself or due to a direct effect of the underlying exposure to silica.

Epidemiologic Surveillance for Occupational Disease

Occupational surveillance is the collection of relevant data, analysis, and dissemination for the purpose of preventing disease and injury in the workplace. Occupational surveillance data are critical for guiding public policy, planning program objectives, and setting research priorities. Surveillance data also can contribute to more efficient targeting of prevention programs for specific populations and subsequent evaluation of program effectiveness. Dissemination of surveillance data can increase public health awareness among occupational health professionals.

Surveillance for occupational disease should be conducted routinely through the linkage of large data systems containing occupational history and health outcomes. Epidemiologic evaluation of employee health status is becoming an increasingly important component of occupational health objectives, such as estimating baseline rates of morbidity and mortality, providing assistance in the design and interpretation of special studies, and affording prompt response to health-related injuries and participation in health-related programs.[21] NIOSH has undertaken new major initiatives in occupational health surveillance and has developed various epidemiologic occupational surveillance programs. State and local health departments have expanded their capacity to perform surveillance activity and have demonstrated the utility of new surveillance methods. The most universal database for the purpose of occupational surveillance is death certificates that contain the decedent's usual occupation and allow the calculation of proportionate mortality ratios for specific occupational or industrial groups.

Example 1. The National Center for Health Statistics has coded all conditions listed on death certificates since 1968, and the usual occupation and industry of each decedent is available for 25 states since 1985. NIOSH's 1994 Work-Related Lung Disease Surveillance Report,[36] based on mortality data from the National Center for Health Statistics and morbidity data from various sources, showed that the proportionate mortality ratio for coal workers' pneumoconiosis was 100:9 for mining machine operators during 1985–1990. For work-related injury surveillance, NIOSH collected and automated death certificates from 52 vital statistics reporting units in the 50 states, New York City, and the District of Columbia for workers at least 16 years old who died as a result of a work-related injury. This surveillance system is called the National Traumatic Occupational Fatalities surveillance.[35] From 1980–1989, 63,589 workers died from injuries sustained while working. The average annual fatality rate per 100,000 civilian workers decreased from 8.9 in 1980 to 5.6 in 1989.

Example 2. Database in the United Kingdom and Canada. In the United Kingdom, decennial reports and periodic supplements have examined mortality in various occupational groupings.[25] The use of census data on occupation allows estimation of a population at risk and therefore calculation of standardized mortality ratios (SMR). A disadvantage of this approach is that a person who is included in the numerator as a death may not appear in the denominator, since death and census records are not truly linked for individuals. In Canada, a monitoring system has been established by linking a 10% random sample of the workforce to the national mortality register.[14] The occupation of each member of this cohort was reported annually to the Unemployment Insurance Commission as a part of a large study. The value of this monitoring system increases through time, as the cohort matures and latency periods before the onset of disease elapse. The system provides a powerful tool for both generating and testing hypotheses, and this power will increase as further mortality experience is accumulated by the cohort. SMRs were calculated based on this data. The SMRs for the lung cancer in plumbers and pipe fitters were found to be significantly elevated (SMR = 1.68, $p < 0.05$).

Other data bases, such as cancer registries, hospital records, workers' compensation records, and physicians' reports also may be used for surveillance. The major limitations to these sources of data are lack of comparability in occupational data, lack of coding, and underreporting.

Molecular Epidemiologic Studies

The term molecular epidemiology has been used in the literature since 1979.[20] The rapid developments in molecular biology are an integral component of occupational epidemiology because biomarkers of exposure have provided useful information to identify susceptible persons and specify disease entities.[2] Interest has been particularly devoted to the identification of chemical adducts to deoxyribonucleic acid in various working groups. The adducts to DNA can be thought of as markers of exposure or as markers of early adverse health effects.[1] Major advances in molecular epidemiology have helped to identify genes and enzymes that play an important role in many diseases.[12] Thus, molecular epidemiology will probably play an increasing role in occupational epidemiology.

Example. Specific mutations in the p53 gene in liver tumors have been studied.[15] Human hepatocellular carcinoma from patients in Qidong, China, in which both hepatitis B virus and aflatoxin B1 are risk factors, were analyzed for mutations in the p53, a putative tumor-suppressor gene. Eight of 16 patients had a point mutation at the third base position of codon 249. The authors suggest that the mutant p53 may be responsible for a selective clonal expansion of hepatocytes during carcinogenesis. In addition, a comparison of p53 mutations in hepatocellular carcinoma from North America, Europe, Africa, and Asia will be of interest to link etiologic agents with genetic changes occurring during human hepatocellular carcinogenesis.

CONCLUSION

The development of occupational epidemiology has been steadily accelerating, both with regard to methodology and the numbers of various studies being conducted. What future developments are to be expected in occupational epidemiology? Exposure assessments in the work environment will be developed. The traditional types of descriptive and analytic occupational epidemiology also will continue. Psychosocial risk factors in the workplace and their health implications is another field that has been attracting interest.[1] Accidents and injuries in the workplace may gain more attention and will be investigated to determine their association with ergonomic factors. The associations of different occupations with risk factors and lifestyles that cause adverse effects on health deserve much additional epidemiologic research. Another development will be the extensive use of computer technology in epidemiologic studies. The explosion of epidemiologic studies since 1950 is directly related to the development of the computer. Yesterday's epidemiologists usually were directly involved in the design of the studies and collection of data. Today's epidemiologists may have access to the data collected by others that are stored on a computer and ready for analysis. For this reason, today's occupational surveillance records and data are very important for epidemiologists, and they should be maintained for the future. In addition, statistical software for data analysis will be developed. However, the need for careful data analysis and cautious data interpretation is necessary.

The ultimate goals in occupational epidemiology remain the identification or confirmation of new occupational disease and the study of dose-response characteristics in order to prevent occupational diseases and injuries.[22] If occupational epidemiologic studies are well designed and conducted, and if the data are properly analyzed and interpreted, they can provide strong and reliable information on which to base policy and ultimately decision-making affecting the health of workers. There is a growing need for epidemiologic follow-up on the preventive efforts of work-related risks that have been discovered over the years. In the future, many causes of occupational diseases may be practically eliminated or decreased by appropriate technology and control. Continual improvement in occupational health and hazard surveillance will be an essential component of future efforts to prevent and control occupational diseases and injuries in the workplace.

REFERENCES

 1. Axelson O: Some recent developments in occupational epidemiology. Scand J Work Environ Health 20:9–18, 1994.
 2. Axelson O, Soderkvist P: Characteristics of disease and some exposure considerations. Appl Occup Environ Hyg 6:428–435, 1991.
 3. Axelson O: Case-control studies with a note on proportional mortality evaluation. In Karvonen K, Mikheev MI (eds): Epidemiology of Occupational Health. Copenhagen, WHO, 1986, pp 181–199.
 4. Blair A: Mortality from lung cancer among workers employed in formaldehyde industries. Am J Ind Med 17:683–699, 1990.
 5. Bertazzi PA, Pesatori AC, Radice L, et al: Exposure to formaldehyde and cancer mortality in a cohort of workers producing resins. Scand J Work Environ Health 12:461–468, 1986.
 6. Blot WM, Fraumeni JF Jr: Geographical patterns of lung cancer: Industrial correlations. Am J Epidemiol 103:539, 1976.
 7. Checkoway H, Pearce N, Crawford-Brown DJ: Research Methods in Occupational Epidemiology. New York, Oxford University Press, 1989.
 8. Cole P, Hoover R, Friedell GH: Occupation and cancer of the lower urinary tract. Cancer 29:1250, 1972.
 9. Eisen EA, Tolbert PE, Hallock MF, et al: Mortality studies of machining fluid exposure in the automobile industry III: A case-control study of larynx cancer. Am J Ind Med 26:185–202, 1994.
10. Fischman MC, Cadman EC, Desmond S: Occupational cancer. In LaDou J (ed): Occupational Medicine. Norwalk, CT, Appleton & Lange, 1990, pp 182–208.
11. Harting FH, Hesse W: Der Lungenkrebs, die Bergkrankheit in den Schneeberger Gruben. Vierteljahrsschr Gerichtl Med Offentl Gesunheitswesen 30:296–307, 1879.
12. Hemminki K: Use of molecular biology techniques in cancer epidemiology. Scand J Work Environ Health 18(suppl 1):38–45, 1992.
13. Hernberg S: Use of epidemiology in occupational health. In Karvonen M, Mikheev MI (eds): Epidemiology of Occupational Health. Geneva, WHO, 1986, pp 317–340.
14. Howe GR, Lindsay JP: A follow-up study of a ten percent sample of the Canadian labor force. 1. Cancer mortality in males, 1965–1973. J Natl Cancer Inst 70:37–44, 1983.
15. Hsu IC, Metcalf RA, Sun T, et al: Mutational hotspot in the p53 gene in human hepatocellular carcinomas. Nature 350:427–428, 1991.
16. Kauppinen T, Partanen T, Degerth R, Ojajarvi A: Pancreatic cancer and occupational exposures. Epidemiology 6:498–502, 1995.
17. Labbe KA, Detsky AS, Orourke K: Meta-analysis in clinical research. Ann Intern Med 107:224–233, 1987.
18. Last JM: A Dictionary of Epidemiology. 3rd ed. Oxford, Oxford University Press, 1995.
19. Leigh JP, Markowitz S, Fahs M, et al: Costs of occupational injuries and illnesses in 1992. Final NIOSH Report for Cooperative Agreement with E.R.C., Inc. U60/CCU902886, Palo Alto, CA, 1996.

20. Lower GM Jr, Nelson T, Nelson CE, et al: N-Acetyltransferase phenotype and risk in urinary bladder cancer: Approaches in molecular epidemiology. Environ Health Perspect 29:71–79, 1979.

21. Marsh GM: Epidemiology of occupational diseases. In Rom WN (ed): Environmental and Occupational Medicine. Boston, Little, Brown & Co., 1992, pp 35–50.

22. Mausner JS, Kramer S: Epidemiology: An Introductory Text. Philadelphia, WB Saunders, 1985.

23. McLaughlin JK, Brookmeyer R: Epidemiology and biostatistics. In McCunney RJ, Brandt-Rauf PW (eds): A Practical Approach to Occupational and Environmental Medicine. Boston, Little, Brown & Co., 1994, pp 346–357.

24. Morgenstern H: Uses of ecologic analysis in epidemiologic research. Am J Public Health 72:1336–1344, 1982.

25. Registrar General's Decennial Supplements, England and Wales, For 1951, 1961, and 1970–72. Occupational Mortality Tables. London, Her Majesty's Stationery Office, 1993.

26. Rehn L: Blasenkrankungen bei Anilinarbeitern. Verh Dtgch Ges Chir 35:313–318, 1906.

27. Rothman KJ: Modern Epidemiology. Boston, Little, Brown & Co., 1986.

28. Sacks ST, Schenker MB: Biostatistics and epidemiology. In LaDou J (ed): Occupational Medicine, Norwalk, CT, Appleton and Lange, 1990, pp 534–554.

29. Senthilselvan A, McDuffie HH, Dosman JA: Association of asthma with use of pesticides: Results of a cross-sectional survey of farmers. Am Rev Respir Dis 146:884–887, 1992.

30. Schlesselman JJ: Case-Control Studies: Design, Conduct, Analysis. New York, Oxford University Press, 1982.

31. Silvestri GT: Occupational employment: Wide variations in growth in the American work force, 1992–2005. Washington, DC, U.S. Dept. of Labor, Bureau of Labor Statistics, 1994, bulletin 2453.

32. Smith AH, Lopipero PA, Barroga VR: Meta-analysis of studies of lung cancer among silicotics. Epidemiology 6:617–624, 1995.

33. Stayner LT, Elliott L, Blade L, et al: A retrospective cohort mortality study of workers exposed to formaldehyde in the garment industry. Am J Ind Med 13:667–681, 1988.

34. Sullivan P, Bang KM, Hearl FJ, Wagner GR: Respiratory disease risks in the construction industry. Occup Med State Art Rev 10:313–334, 1995.

35. U.S. Department of Health and Human Services, National Institute for Occupational Safety and Health: Fatal injuries to workers in the United States, 1980–1989: A decade of surveillance. Cincinnati, NIOSH, 1992, publication 93-108S.

36. U.S. Department of Health and Human Services, National Institute for Occupational Safety and Health: Work-related lung disease surveillance report 1994. Cincinnati, NIOSH, 1994, publication 94-120.

37. U.S. Department of Health and Human Services, National Center for Health Statistics: Questionnaires from the National Health Interview Survey, 1985–1989. Washington, DC, National Center for Health Statistics, 1993, publication 93-1307.

38. U.S. Department of Labor, Bureau of Labor Statistics: Workplace injuries and illnesses in 1993. Washington, DC, Bureau of Labor Statistics, 1994, USDL-94-600.

39. Waxweiler KJ, Stringer W, Wagoner JK, Jane J: Neoplastic risk among workers exposed to vinyl chloride. Ann N Y Acad Sci 271:40, 1976.

40. Wegman DH: Accelerated loss of FEV1 in polyurethane production workers: A four year prospective study. Am J Ind Med 3:209–215, 1982.

41. Whorton D, Krauss RM, Marshall S, Milby TH: Infertility in male pesticide workers. Lancet 2:1259, 1977.

PAUL K. HENNEBERGER, MPH, ScD

COLLECTION OF OCCUPATIONAL EPIDEMIOLOGIC DATA:

The Use of Surrogate Respondents to Provide Occupational Histories

From the Epidemiological
    Investigations Branch
Division of Respiratory Disease
    Studies
National Institute for Occupational
    Safety and Health
Morgantown, West Virginia

Reprint requests to:
Paul K. Henneberger, MPH, ScD
NIOSH/EPIB
1095 Willowdale Road
Morgantown, WV 26505

Valid measurements of occupational exposures are essential in epidemiologic studies that investigate the relationship between work and disease. Occupational exposures are often characterized by some combination of lifetime work history and quantitative measurements of exposure. Ideally, the work histories are either abstracted from employee records or solicited from the subjects by trained interviewers using a standardized questionnaire. Industrial hygiene measurements should be available for the appropriate substances/conditions and from the relevant locations and times. In practice, occupational exposure data often fall short of the ideal. Issues such as cost, subject confidentiality, and the passage of time frequently conspire to limit the quality and quantity of exposure data.

Sometimes records of employment are unavailable, and some of the subjects are unable to report their own work history. They may be unavailable because they have died, are incompetent due to a neurologic or psychiatric disorder, or simply because they cannot be contacted.[18] The exclusion of subjects with incomplete data can be detrimental for a number of reasons. If most of the subjects are excluded, further investigation is impossible. Even if enough subjects remain, reducing the number of subjects diminishes the power of the study to detect an effect. Also, the exclusion of even a small percentage of the subjects can be devastating if the exclusions are differential by both exposure and outcome. This selection bias can distort the estimate of relative risk either toward or away from the null.[13]

In several studies where the index subjects themselves have been unavailable for interview, surrogate respondents such as family members have provided information about the subject's diet, smoking habits, alcohol use, and work history. Nelson and colleagues provide a comprehensive review of how information from surrogates can affect the estimate of the exposure-disease relationship.[18] The authors discuss issues such as selection of surrogates, sample size requirements, questionnaire design, and statistical analyses.

This chapter focuses on the quality of occupational histories provided by surrogate respondents. The following questions are addressed:

1. How often do surrogates have no knowledge of the index subject's work history, or how often are they unavailable to be interviewed?

2. How often does the information from surrogate respondents match the information from the subjects themselves or from company employee records?

3. What impact does the exposure misclassification that results from using surrogate data have on the estimate of relative risk?

NONRESPONSE OF THE SURROGATE

The primary motivation for using surrogate respondents is the absence of data from any other source. However, the surrogate might not have the desired knowledge about the index subject or might not be available to be interviewed. The nonresponse of surrogates can result in bias or other problems already noted for nonresponse of the subjects themselves.

Several studies have quantified nonresponse of surrogate respondents. For example, surrogates were used in studies of leukemia and nonHodgkin's lymphoma in rural populations.[1,5,6] When asked about the index subject's use of pesticides in farming, the surrogates were more likely than the subjects themselves to give an answer of "don't know." When asked about the use of 38 herbicides, 65% of the surrogates but 35% of the index subjects replied "don't know" to one or more items on the list.[1] The spouse surrogates were less likely to report "don't know" than the other surrogates, who included children, siblings, friends, and neighbors.[6] In a study of reproductive outcomes, the availability of male surrogate respondents appeared to be related to income level.[12] Interviews were completed with 79.8% of the male partners for private patients but with only 48.6% of the male partners for public clinic patients.

The failure of the surrogate to provide any answer to a question about the index subject was investigated by Pickle et al. in case-control studies of respiratory cancer in three communities in the United States.[20] Trained interviewers used a standardized questionnaire that sought information on smoking, occupation, medical history, and demographics. If a subject was deceased, a surrogate was sought in the following order of priority: spouse, offspring, sibling, and other (parents, nieces and nephews, in-laws, friends). Surrogates provided data for about 83% of the 2,606 subjects. A surrogate's failure to provide information in response to a question was considered a nonresponse. The overall nonresponse percentages were low for several questions (lung disease, 1%; education, 3%; county of birth, 4%; ever worked in shipbuilding, 4%) and higher for several other items (ever handled asbestos, 12%; smoking category, 12%; years smoked, 15%; detailed smoking history, 44%; parents' cancer, 26%; grandparents' cancer, 69%). The percentage of nonresponse for the occupational questions varied by type of respondent (Table 1). The "other" surrogates were the least able to provide information about occupation. Also, the

TABLE 1. Nonresponse Rates (%) by Type of Respondent When Asked about the Subject's Work (Sample Size = 2,606)

Questions	Self	Spouse	Sibling	Child	Other	Overall Nonresponse Percentage
Has the subject ever handled asbestos?	1	13	14	12	22	12
Has the subject worked in the ship building industry for 6 months or more?	1	4	1	2	14	4

Adapted from Pickle LW, Brown LM, Blot WJ: Information available from surrogate respondents in case-control interview studies. Am J Epidemiol 118:99–108, 1983.

nonresponse percentage for the asbestos question varied by gender, with female respondents doing worse (15% nonresponse) than the male respondents (3%). The contrast by gender in nonresponse was less evident for the shipbuilding question (4% female, 1% male).

Pickle et al. reach several general conclusions about surrogate respondents.[20] Surrogate respondents other than spouse, sibling, or offspring should be avoided. Nonresponse increases as more detail is requested and as time elapses since the events occurred. The nonresponse among surrogates is positively associated with the probability that the subject had been exposed. For example, men were more likely than women to have handled asbestos or worked in shipbuilding, and nonresponse to the occupational questions was greater when the index subject was male rather than female. At least for smoking and family history of cancer, surrogates should be sought who shared the subject's household during the time that the relevant events took place. Thus, siblings do better with questions related to the subject's early life, and spouses and offspring do better with issues of adult life. However, for the occupational questions, which relate to the subject's adult life, the percentage of nonresponse of siblings was about equal to that of spouse and offspring (see Table 1).

SURROGATE-SUBJECT AND SURROGATE-RECORD AGREEMENT

Measurement validity has been defined as "an expression of the degree to which a measurement measures what it purports to measure."[15] Completely valid data are free from bias. Interviews with surrogate (or proxy) respondents are usually conducted in lieu of interviews with subjects. The level of agreement between the two sources of information addresses the validity of the surrogate data, assuming that the data gathered from the subjects themselves can be considered the "gold standard." However, if one considers the subject's data as possibly flawed, the surrogate-subject comparison is more appropriately viewed as an indicator of reliability. Reliability is concerned with "the degree to which the results obtained by a measurement procedure can be replicated."[15] In this context, the surrogate-subject reliability should best be judged against the standard of the subject-subject reliability, and yet such a comparison is rarely made.[18]

The usual method for evaluating surrogate data is to compare them to information provided by the subject or abstracted from company employee records. The most common measurement of concordance is the overall percentage agreement between the two sources of data. The kappa statistic is also used to evaluate agreement.[10] Other studies use sensitivity, specificity, and positive predictive value, with the subject-reported data or employee records as the gold standard.[13] In at least one study, the investigators examined specific agreement for positive response.[28]

A report about the quality of work histories provided by surrogates was published by Rogot and Reid in 1975.[23] From a study of cancer among British and Norwegian migrants to the United States, the investigators found a 77% agreement for usual occupation between next-of-kin and self reports. Subsequent studies that evaluate occupational histories from surrogate respondents address a variety of outcomes including different types of cancer,[1–4,6,8,11,14,16,19,20] neurologic disorders,[7,22,25,28] reproductive outcomes,[12,24] and chronic lung disease.[26] The most common finding is that the surrogate-subject or surrogate-record agreement declines when there is more detail to recall (Table 2). For example, the percentage agreement is greater for reports of (1) usual or last job rather than for the entire job history;[3,16,22] (2) jobs rather than specific exposures;[3,4,6,7,14,16,19,25,26,28] (3) industry or occupation category rather than the specific industry or occupation.[8] Also, the surrogate is less likely to provide

TABLE 2. Examples of Decline in Quality of Surrogate Occupational Data When Answer Involves Greater Detail*

Reference	General Information	Specific Information
Bond et al., 1988[3]†	70.8% agreement for usual assignment	48.4% agreement for all assignments; 2.6% agreement for specific agents
Boyle & Brann, 1992[4]	General question like "ever lived/worked on a farm/ranch": sensitivity = 73%, specificity = 88%, and positive predictive value = 83%	Specific occupational exposures: usually sensitivity < 40% and specificity > 90%, and positive predictive value 0–78%
Brown et al., 1991[6]	83–100% agreement for yes/no questions re agricultural pesticide use	30.4–66.7% agreement for frequency of using specific pesticides
Chong et al., 1989[7]	Agreement for job description (75–94%)	Agreement lower for job titles (36–64%), number of jobs (24–50%), and number of departments (20–46%); slight to fair agreement for specific substances (most kappas < 0.40)
Coggon et al., 1985[8]	Agreement for industry category (66%) and occupation category (60%)	Agreement for industry (59%) and occupation (43%)
Johnson et al., 1993[14]	87–93% agreement for general farming questions	70–73% for overall pesticide use; 68–74% for specific pesticides
Lerchen & Samet, 1986[16]	Agreement for usual job (industry 84%, occupation 78%) and last job (industry 74%, occupation 70%)	Lower % agreement for lifetime jobs (industry 51%, occupation 48%) and low agreement for most specific exposures
Pershagen & Axelson, 1982[19]†	99% agreement for ever worked in copper smelter	For subset of smelter workers, 68% agreement for high arsenic exposure
Rocca et al., 1986[22]	86% agreement for last job	63% agreement for lifetime jobs
Semchuk & Love, 1995[25]	Sensitivities for rural work ranged from 46–67%	Sensitivities for use of agricultural chemicals ranged from 17–60%
Shalat et al., 1987[26]	81% agreement for solvent exposure by occupation-exposure linkage system	58% agreement by questionnaire alone for solvent exposure
Wang et al., 1994[28]	Concordance on positive history: 73.9% for crop farming, 71.4% for agricultural work	Concordance on positive history: 64.0% for pesticide use, 52.2% for fertilizer use

* Occupational histories from surrogate respondents compared to data from the subjects themselves or from company employee records.
† Interview data compared to company employment records.

all the information correctly if the subject has a complex job history. For example, in a study in which interview data were compared to company employee records, the percentage of subjects and surrogates who correctly reported the subject's longest work assignment was 80.4% when the subject's lifetime number of assignments was one, declined to 66.8% with two lifetime assignments, and declined to 59.1% with three lifetime assignments.[3] In a study of reproductive outcomes by Schnitzer et al., both the mother and father were questioned about the father's occupation during a 7-month period around conception.[24] In 3,602 cases, the mother's report matched the father's report less often if the father had more jobs. The percentage agreement went from 65.4% with one job to 16.5% with two jobs and 2.7% with three jobs. The same pattern was observed for the controls.

Another common trend is for surrogates to report fewer jobs and exposures than the subjects report[1,2,4,6,8,16,22,25] or employee records indicate.[19] However, there are instances in which the surrogates more often overreport than underreport the subject's exposure.[14]

There are several examples in the medical literature where the surrogate more easily recalled jobs that the subject held for a longer time. Shalat et al. interviewed 26 spouse pairs about the husband's occupation and exposure to solvents.[26] The job histories reported by surrogates were used with an occupation-exposure linkage system to determine the husband's solvent exposure status. The percentage agreement between spouse pairs was 81% (kappa = 0.71, sensitivity = 71%, specificity = 92%) but increased to 88% (kappa = 0.78, sensitivity = 77%, specificity = 100%) for greater than 5 years of solvent exposure. In a case-control study by Boyle and Brann, 270 male cancer patients and their surrogates were interviewed.[4] The sensitivity of the surrogate responses for eight categories of jobs improved an average of 17% when the subject had held the job for at least five years. In a study of lung cancer by Bond et al., information for 591 of 734 subjects (80.5%) was provided by surrogates.[3] With data combined from both self and surrogate respondents, the percentage agreement with company employee records for usual work area improved with the number of years the subjects had the assignment: 44.7% for < 1 year, 70.9% for 1–4.9 years, and 73.2% for > 5 years. In another study of lung cancer, spouse surrogates underreported short-term jobs (i.e., less than 1 year) more often than jobs of longer duration.[16]

Several factors associated with a higher percentage agreement for surrogate data have been reported less frequently, as follows: a shorter time elapsed between the subject's job and the surrogate interview;[3] spouse surrogates rather than other types of surrogates;[4] higher levels of income for the subjects and surrogates;[12,24] and higher levels of education for the subjects and surrogates.[24]

THE IMPACT OF MISCLASSIFICATION ON ESTIMATES OF RELATIVE RISK

The opportunity for biased estimates of relative risk is limited if the occupational data from surrogates are nearly identical to the gold standard (i.e., self-reported data or employee records). However, the agreement of surrogate data with the gold standard is often in the 60–90% range for general occupational information and is lower for more specific information (Table 2). The possibility of bias exists with these levels of agreement. Information bias results from "systematic differences in the way data on exposure or outcome are obtained from the various study groups."[13] In other words, the data for the study groups are not comparable and can lead to an underestimation or overestimation of the true exposure-disease relationship. This can arise from the study participants (recall bias) or the researchers (observation or interviewer bias). Recall bias occurs in case-control studies when the subjects report their exposure differentially based on disease status. Those who have had a disease might be more inclined to report past exposures than the disease-free control subjects. In cohort studies, those who have had certain exposures might be particularly interested in reporting certain outcomes. The other type of information bias, observation or interviewer bias, occurs when the interviewer or investigator evaluates exposure differentially based on the subject's outcome status or evaluates the outcome differentially based on the subject's exposure status. For example, an interviewer might differentially probe for data based on the subject's study group status.

With recall bias and observation/interviewer bias, the misclassification of exposure is differential by study group, and the estimate of relative risk can be biased in either direction. When the misclassification of exposure is random or nondifferential, it occurs in equal proportions in both outcome groups. This type of misclassification of dichotomous exposure variables biases true non-null results toward the null.[13] Nondifferential misclassification of a polychotomous exposure measurement can bias relative risk estimates either toward or away from the null.[9] Dosemeci et al. used hypothetical data to demonstrate that "an estimate of trend in an ordered polychotomous exposure can change direction in the presence of nondifferential misclassification."[9] In another example of nondifferential misclassification with three levels of exposure, there was no change in the odds ratios.[27] Thus, when surrogates are used and exposure variables have more than two levels, there is no way to predict if nondifferential misclassification will result in bias, and if bias occurs there is no way to predict the direction.

Given the unpredictable impact of differential and (sometimes) nondifferential misclassification, there is a need to evaluate the direction and magnitude of these potential biases whenever surrogate respondents are used. Knowing the agreement percentage for all surrogate respondents, or even separately for cases and controls, is not sufficient to understand how the relative risk estimate might be biased. It is necessary to know the direction and extent of the misclassification separately for cases and controls. This need is demonstrated by Johnson et al. in a study of cancers and agricultural chemicals.[14] The odds ratios based on data from surrogates were compared with the ORs computed with self-reported data. For general farming experience and overall pesticide use, the surrogate ORs tended to be less. For specific pesticide use, the surrogate ORs were split between those greater than and those less than the ORs based on self-reported data. The findings for the pesticides atrazine and trifluralin are presented in Table 3. The percentage agreements for leukemia cases and controls were similar for the two pesticides. However, the biases introduced by the proxy data went in opposite directions for these two compounds. The proxy OR for atrazine was 4.7 times the self OR, and the proxy OR for trifluralin was 0.7 times the self OR. The investigators noted that when the surrogate OR was greater (e.g., atrazine), the surrogates for controls usually underreported exposure and the surrogates for cases usually overreported exposure. When the surrogate OR was less than the self OR (e.g., trifluralin), the surrogates for controls overreported exposure more than the surrogates for cases. The researchers conclude that both nondifferential and differential misclassification of pesticide exposure can occur when using data provided by surrogate respondents.[14] These findings highlight the need to evaluate surrogate data for both cases and controls in order to measure adequately the effect of misclassification on estimates of relative risk.

TABLE 3.   Exposure to the Pesticides Atrazine and Trifluralin

	Atrazine				Trifluralin			
Agreement between self and proxy respondents (%)	*Controls* 74		*Cases* 70		*Controls* 76		*Cases* 74	
Reported subject was exposed (%)	*Controls*		*Cases*		*Controls*		*Cases*	
	Self 12	*Proxy* 5	*Self* 13	*Proxy* 22	*Self* 8	*Proxy* 12	*Self* 11	*Proxy* 12
Difference (Proxy–Self)	-7		+9		+4		+1	
Odds ratio (OR)	*Self* 1.1		*Proxy* 5.2		*Self* 1.5		*Proxy* 1.0	
Ratio of proxy OR to self OR			4.7				0.7	

The cases were incident cases of leukemia.
Adapted from Johnson RA, Mandel JS, Gibson RW, et al: Data on prior pesticide use collected from self- and proxy respondents. Epidemiology 4:157–164, 1993.

Other researchers also have investigated bias that results from surrogate misclassification of occupational exposure. An example of recall bias among surrogate respondents was revealed by Greenberg et al. in a reanalysis of an earlier study.[11] Two different mortality studies of the same nuclear shipyard had conflicting results. A 1978 proportional mortality study used next of kin to provide information about radiation exposure and reported an excess of all cancers (56 observed, 31.5 expected) among nuclear workers.[17] A 1981 cohort study used the shipyard files to determine radiation exposure and reported a slightly reduced standardized mortality ratio for all cancers among nuclear workers (SMR = 92).[21] In a reanalysis of the data from the 1978 study, the files from the shipyard were used to validate the information on nuclear work provided by the next-of-kin surrogates.[11] It was discovered that the next of kin tended to report the subjects who had died of noncancer causes as never having done nuclear work when in fact they had. The relatives of cancer decedents did not demonstrate the same tendency. The differential misclassification of exposure biased the estimate of the nuclear work-cancer association away from the null.

In a study by Blot et al. with 458 cases of lung cancer and 553 controls, 76% of the interviews were conducted with surrogate respondents.[2] The ORs for shipbuilding were nearly the same for self-respondents (OR = 1.5) and next-of-kin surrogates (OR = 1.6). Simultaneous self and surrogate interviews were conducted with only 24 subjects, and the respective ORs for the two groups were not reported.

For 30% of the cases and controls in a study by Semchuk and Love of Parkinson's disease, surrogate respondents (83% spouse, 17% offspring) also were interviewed.[25] Controlling for other risk factors with conditional logistic regression, the adjusted ORs for herbicide use were 3.09 (95% CI = 1.27–7.56) with self data alone and 2.60 (95% CI = 1.11–6.09) when 30% of the data were replaced with surrogate data. Similar reductions in ORs were observed for other risk factors. The investigators conclude that the pooling of data from self and proxy respondents might lead to biased estimates of relative risk.[25]

A study of leukemia and nonHodgkin's lymphoma by Brown et al. was initiated to investigate possible associations with agricultural exposures.[6] The surrogates more often underestimated than overestimated exposure. The effect of underreporting was explored with hypothetical distributions of exposure to selected pesticides. There were three levels of exposure based on the number of days per year worked with the pesticides. The misclassifications resulted in changes in the estimates of relative risk, but the researchers concluded that the misclassified data did not substantially distort the trends in risk.

CONCLUSIONS

Surrogate respondents should not be the first choice for information on occupation. Company employee records or interviews of the subjects themselves are usually better sources.

When surrogates are used, interviewing them requires the same care that is needed when interviewing the subjects themselves. That is, the instrument must be developed, tested, and administered carefully to prevent information bias. Using a structured questionnaire with explicit instructions about administering it can minimize the chances of bias introduced by the interviewer and the subject. Blinding the researchers to the study group status of the subjects helps to prevent observation bias. Blinding the subjects to their own study group status or keeping them unaware of the study hypothesis helps to prevent recall bias. However, many studies of occupational groups are reported by the mass media, and the suspected exposure-disease links are made public. Both surrogates and subjects often have a vested interest in the outcome of the study and might consciously or unconsciously try to influence the findings with their answers to the questionnaire.

It is evident from the studies reviewed that a number of features are potentially associated with the ability of the surrogate to provide complete and valid occupational data. The surrogate nonresponse is reduced if a spouse or close relative is the surrogate; as the subject's and surrogate's incomes increase; as less detail is requested; if the events in question are more recent; and if there is little chance that the subject ever worked in the industry or occupation in question. Several researchers have reported that the quality of surrogate data improves when the usual or last job is requested rather than the entire work history; jobs rather than specific exposure compounds are requested; the subject's work history is relatively simple; and the subject had the job for a relatively long time. It has been reported less frequently that the following factors also contribute to higher quality surrogate data: the time between job and interview is short; the subject's spouse is the surrogate; the subject and surrogate had higher levels of income; and the subject and surrogate had higher levels of education.

Misclassification of exposure is likely to occur even when great care is taken to select and interview the surrogate respondents. The unpredictable impact of exposure misclassification on relative risk estimates needs to be addressed. When a study includes a mixture of surrogate and self respondents, nondifferential misclassification can be explored by stratifying the analyses on respondent status.[27] Since differential misclassification also might occur, a study that uses surrogate respondents should include an evaluation component. The occupational information provided by at least a subset of the surrogates should be compared to a gold standard of employee records or self-reported information. If surrogate data is used for both cases and controls, both groups should be evaluated to understand the impact of misclassification on odds ratios. The measurements of bias can then be used to either formally or informally adjust estimates of relative risk that are based on surrogate data.[18]

REFERENCES

1. Blair A, Zahm SH: Patterns of pesticide use among farmers: Implications for epidemiologic research. Epidemiology 4:55–62, 1993.
2. Blot WJ, Harrington JM, Toledo A, et al: Lung cancer after employment in shipyards during World War II. N Engl J Med 299:620–624, 1978.

3. Bond GG, Bodner KM, Sobel W, et al: Validation of work histories obtained from interviews. Am J Epidemiol 128:343–351, 1988.
4. Boyle CA, Brann EA: Proxy respondents and the validity of occupational and other exposure data. Am J Epidemiol 136:712–721, 1992.
5. Brown LM, Blair A, Gibson R, et al: Pesticide exposures and other agricultural risk factors for leukemia among men in Iowa and Minnesota. Cancer Res 50:6585–6591, 1990.
6. Brown LM, Dosemeci M, Blair A, Burmeister L: Comparability of data obtained from farmers and surrogate respondents on use of agricultural pesticides. Am J Epidemiol 134:348–355, 1991.
7. Chong JP, Turpie I, Haines T, et al: Concordance of occupational and environmental exposure information elicited from patients with Alzheimer's disease and surrogate respondents. Am J Ind Med 15:73–89, 1989.
8. Coggon D, Pippard EC, Acheson ED: Accuracy of occupational histories obtained from wives. Br J Ind Med 42:563–564, 1985.
9. Dosemeci M, Wacholder S, Lubin JH: Does nondifferential misclassification of exposure always bias a true effect toward the null value? Am J Epidemiol 132:746–748, 1990.
10. Fleiss JL: Statistical Methods for Rates and Proportions. 2nd ed. New York, Wiley & Sons, 1981.
11. Greenberg ER, Rosner B, Hennekens C, et al: An investigation of bias in a study of nuclear shipyard workers. Am J Epidemiol 121:301–308, 1985.
12. Hatch MC, Misra D, Kabat GC, Kartzmer S: Proxy respondents in reproductive research: A comparison of self- and partner-reported data. Am J Epidemiol 133;826–831, 1991.
13. Hennekens CH, Buring JE: Epidemiology in Medicine. Boston, Little, Brown & Co, 1987.
14. Johnson RA, Mandel JS, Gibson RW, et al: Data on prior pesticide use collected from self- and proxy respondents. Epidemiology 4:157–164, 1993.
15. Last JM: A Dictionary of Epidemiology. 3rd ed. New York, Oxford University Press, 1995.
16. Lerchen ML, Samet JM: An assessment of the validity of questionnaire responses provided by a surviving spouse. Am J Epidemiol 123:481–489, 1986.
17. Najarian T, Colton T: Mortality from leukemia and cancer in shipyard nuclear workers. Lancet 1:1018–1020, 1978.
18. Nelson LM, Longstreth WT Jr, Koepsell TD, van Belle G: Proxy respondents in epidemiologic research. Epidemiol Rev 12:71–86, 1990.
19. Pershagen G, Axelson O: A validation of questionnaire information on occupational exposure and smoking. Scand J Work Environ Health 8:24–28, 1982.
20. Pickle LW, Brown LM, Blot WJ: Information available from surrogate respondents in case-control interview studies. Am J Epidemiol 118:99–108, 1983.
21. Rinsky RA, Zumwalde RD, Waxweiler RJ, et al: Cancer mortality at a naval nuclear shipyard. Lancet 1:231–235, 1981.
22. Rocca WA, Fratiglioni L, Bracco L, et al: The use of surrogate respondents to obtain questionnaire data in case-control studies of neurologic diseases. J Chronic Dis 39:907–912, 1986.
23. Rogot E, Reid DD: The validity of data from next-of-kin in studies of mortality among migrants. Int J Epidemiol 4:51–54, 1975.
24. Schnitzer PG, Olshan AF, Savitz DA, Erickson JD: Validity of mother's report of father's occupation in a study of paternal occupation and congenital malformations. Am J Epidemiol 141:872–877, 1995.
25. Semchuk KM, Love EJ: Effects of agricultural work and other proxy-derived case-control data on Parkinson's disease risk estimates. Am J Epidemiol 141:747–754, 1995.
26. Shalat SL, Christiani DC, Baker EL Jr: Accuracy of work history obtained from a spouse. Scand J Work Environ Health 13:67–69, 1987.
27. Walker AM, Velema JP, Robins JM: Analysis of case-control data derived in part from proxy respondents. Am J Epidemiol 127:905–914, 1988.
28. Wang F-L, Semchuk KM, Love EJ: Reliability of environmental and occupational exposure data provided by surrogate respondents in a case-control study of Parkinson's disease. J Clin Epidemiol 47:797–807, 1994.

AARON BLAIR, PhD
RICHARD B. HAYES, DDS, PhD
PATRICIA A. STEWART, PhD
SHELIA HOAR ZAHM, ScD

OCCUPATIONAL EPIDEMIOLOGIC STUDY DESIGN AND APPLICATION

From the Occupational
  Epidemiology Branch
Division of Cancer Epidemiology
  and Genetics
National Cancer Institute
Bethesda, Maryland

Reprint requests to:
Aaron Blair, PhD
Occupational Epidemiology Branch
Division of Cancer Epidemiology
  and Genetics
National Cancer Institute
Executive Plaza North
Room 418
Bethesda, MD 20892-7364

Epidemiologic studies of occupational groups have been undertaken to ensure a safe and healthy work environment and to use the "occupational laboratory" to identify hazards that may be of significance for the population at large.[5] Occupational studies have a long and productive history and have been especially important in identification of carcinogenic agents. Most exposures classified by the International Agency for Research on Cancer as human carcinogens occur primarily in the occupational setting.[98] Recently, objectives of epidemiologic investigations have been expanded to characterize exposure-response gradients, to understand mechanisms of action, to identify susceptible individuals, and to provide information for disease prevention. These additional objectives have imposed new and sometimes difficult demands upon study design.

The optimal study design to evaluate potential occupational hazards varies according to research objectives, disease of interest, understanding of etiology, and location of the study populations. Basic designs have been well described in texts on occupational epidemiology.[26,67] This chapter provides a brief description of the application of the most frequently used epidemiologic designs for occupational studies and focuses on issues especially important in hypothesis-testing investigations of chronic diseases such as cancer.

BASIC OCCUPATIONAL EPIDEMIOLOGIC DESIGNS

A variety of study designs are available for the generation and testing of hypotheses about occupationally associated risks of disease. The quality of studies forms a continuum from those with limited information on important epidemiologic considerations to highly analytic investigations that obtain information necessary to address most important methodologic issues. This continuum is often dichotomized into hypothesis-generating and hypothesis-testing investigations. Hypothesis-generating studies usually include ecologic correlation, proportionate mortality or morbidity, cross-sectional, and case series designs, while hypothesis-testing investigations typically employ cohort or case-control approaches. However, the hypothesis-testing/hypothesis-generating dichotomy depends upon the detail and quality of the information gathered rather than the overall study design. In general, however, data assembled in case series, proportionate mortality, and ecologic correlation studies are usually limited and can address only a few of the criteria required for the determination of causality in hypothesis-testing studies. On the other hand, cohort and case-control investigations can often address most of the issues crucial to determine causality, such as avoiding confounding and bias and evaluating exposure-response relationships.[44] In addition, the distinction between hypothesis-generating and hypothesis-testing analyses can even be blurred within a single study. An investigation may be hypothesis-testing for some factors and hypothesis-generating for others. For example, quantitative exposure assessment may be performed for some exposures in a cohort study but not for others, and interviews in case-control studies may be detailed and comprehensive for some areas of interest but brief and simplistic for others.

Although hypothesis-generating studies may be unable to resolve etiologic questions, they have played an important role in occupational health. Several of the classic advances in our understanding of occupational disease have begun with a report on a case series, including the observations of soot-related occupational scrotal cancer, aromatic amine-related bladder cancer, and vinyl chloride-related angiosarcoma of the liver.[5]

Cross-sectional studies relate cause to effect at one point in time. Because this design lacks a time dimension, it is most appropriate for assessment of relatively immediate biologic responses, e.g., acute toxicity. With certain assumptions, however, cross-sectional designs can be used to evaluate exposure-effect relationships involving chronic diseases. The chief assumptions are that current exposures are good surrogates for longer-term exposures and that the duration of disease is independent of exposure status. A considerable body of epidemiologic evidence on occupational diseases has been developed from cross-sectional surveys.

Hypothesis-generating studies often use data collected for administrative purposes. The availability of vital statistics records on mortality and occupation/industry in England and Wales[35] and the United States;[22] record linkage efforts developed in Sweden,[61] Canada,[104] and Denmark;[70] and tumor registries in United States[21,109] are just a few examples of use of such resources. These resources provide opportunities to evaluate new ideas and sharpen hypotheses quickly and inexpensively.

COHORT AND CASE-CONTROL DESIGNS

Although hypothesis-generating designs have provided important information regarding occupational health and should be encouraged, this chapter focuses on hypothesis-testing studies. Cohort and case-control designs are the two main approaches used for hypothesis-testing in occupational epidemiology. Increasingly, nested case-control approaches are used that incorporate elements of both designs. The quality of an investigation is determined by the details of the study methods, i.e., avoidance of bias, control for confounding, validity and level of detail in the assessment of exposure, the accuracy of diagnosis, power, and appropriate analysis and interpretation. These factors should be considered when evaluating the advantages and disadvantages of these two designs.

Population Base

Occupational cohorts and subjects of nested case-control designs are often assembled from the workforce of one or a few companies. Unions and professional associations are sometimes used, but their record systems usually lack detailed work histories and other information required for quantitative exposure assessment. Consequently, company-based studies with personnel records providing fairly detailed work histories are preferred. Because of practical problems associated with conducting a study at many locations, cohort investigations have, by and large, been restricted to larger companies. This exclusion of workers from small companies could have unintended consequences on our understanding of occupational hazards. Large companies typically have more resources and greater expertise to control exposures,[68] and patterns of exposure may differ between large and small companies. Thus, evaluations of disease risk from occupational exposure based on cohort studies of large companies may have focused on the lower end of the exposure spectrum, and hazards may have been missed or underestimated. Reliance upon large companies for cohorts may also partially account for the poor record of including women and minorities in occupational studies[110] because many small workplaces employ proportionally more minorities and women than larger establishments. A large fraction of the U.S. workforce is employed in small establishments,[32] and it is unfortunate that this population has been largely excluded from study by the cohort design.

In contrast, this underrepresentation of small businesses is atypical in case-control studies. Subjects in case-control studies are usually a sample of the general population, and subject participation is not restricted by company size. It appears, therefore, that results from cohort and case-control investigations are based on quite different segments of the working population, and this could account for the differences sometimes observed between results from these two designs. A disadvantage of case-control studies is that the proportion of subjects exposed to specific occupational hazards may be quite small. This difficulty can sometimes be partially overcome by locating case-control studies in geographic areas that enhance the probability of enrolling of subjects in certain occupations or with specific exposures. For example, location of studies of lymphatic and hematopoietic cancers in midwestern states with small urban populations increased the proportion of farmers in the studies and provided better power to evaluate pesticide exposures.[19,23,45,111]

Breadth of Evaluation

Cohort and case-control designs typically differ in the scope of exposure-disease evaluations possible. Cohort mortality studies offer the opportunity to evaluate associations between many different causes of death and a limited number of exposures, while case-control studies offer the reverse, i.e., evaluation of the relationship between one or a few diseases and many exposures. Each can be designed to overcome its limitation. For example, cohort studies focusing on complex industries, such as steel[55] and rubber,[65] or studies that include many workplaces with a particular exposure, such as formaldehyde,[12,13,15] may allow the evaluation of health effects from many exposures. Multiple diseases could be included in case-control designs, such as the approach used by Siemiatycki in Montreal.[80]

The choice of whether to use a case-control or cohort design may depend on whether the overall purpose of the study is to evaluate disease risk from a specific exposure or to investigate the etiology of a specific disease. Case-control investigations are usually better for assessing a wide range of possible risk factors. The availability of appropriate data resources also affects the choice of design. Lack of company personnel records on workers with specific exposures may make a cohort study impossible, while inability to perform quantitative exposure assessment may discourage the case-control approach.

Accurate Disease Determination

Accurate determination of disease is important in all epidemiologic investigations because misclassification of disease affects the estimates of relative risk.[52] If misclassification of disease is nondifferential, i.e., the level of misclassification is similar among the exposed and unexposed, relative risks are biased toward the null for dichotomous outcomes (as is the usual situation for disease). Effects of nondifferential misclassification are more complicated in polychotomous situations. If differential, i.e., the degree of disease misclassification is associated with exposure status, the bias can be toward or away from the null, depending upon the pattern of misclassification.

The likelihood of disease misclassification varies by type of disease and how disease is ascertained. For example, on death certificates, cancer is typically determined more accurately as an underlying cause of death than nonmalignant respiratory disease, although the accuracy of cancer diagnosis differs by site. Percy, in comparing diagnostic information on death certificates with that from hospital records, found that concordance between diagnoses from death certificates and hospital records was high for cancers of the lung, colon, breast, and bladder (more than 90%) but poor for soft tissue sarcoma, liver, pharynx, and pancreas (less than 60%).[72] Because of these diagnostic differences, the accuracy of disease determination may differ between cohort and case-control studies. In cohort studies, outcomes are often based on death certificates, but in case-control designs they are more likely to be based on hospital or other medical records. Thus, case-control studies are likely to have less disease misclassification than cohort mortality studies. This difference could contribute to contradictory findings that sometimes occur between studies with these designs.

For diseases that are poorly determined from death certificates, investigators sometimes seek hospital records to validate the death certificate diagnosis. This is useful and appropriate as long as the correction procedure is applied to both the exposed and unexposed populations. Many cohort studies, however, use the general population as the unexposed, and it is usually impractical to make adjustments in the diagnoses of the general population because of the effort required. In these situations, it is inappropriate to remove inaccurate diagnoses from the exposed cohort and not from the referent (i.e., the general population) because this action artificially biases relative risk estimates toward the null.

Exposure Assessment

Establishment of a dose-response relationship is an important criterion for establishing causality.[67] Because measurements of dose (internal concentrations of an agent) are rarely available for studies of diseases with long latencies, occupational investigators usually rely on measurements of external exposures. Even these are seldom available for any but the most recent years. Crude classifications such as ever/never exposed or duration of exposure have been widely used, but these have a potential for substantially misclassifying subjects.[86] Misclassification of exposure has similar effects on estimates of relative risks as misclassification of diseases, i.e., nondifferential misclassification biases risk estimates toward the null for dichotomous exposures, and differential misclassification can bias the estimates toward or away from the null.

Nondifferential misclassification of polychotomous exposure categories is more complicated since errors occur between levels of exposure as well as between exposed and unexposed individuals. In some situations nondifferential misclassification may move the relative risk estimate away from the null.[31] This never occurs, however, in the highest exposure category. Here nondifferential misclassification only diminishes the estimates of relative risk. These different effects by level of exposure occur because if high-exposure (and therefore high-risk) individuals are misclassified into a lower exposure category, the relative risk of that category will be increased. At the highest exposure level, however, only lower exposed individuals may be misclassified into this category because no higher exposed subjects exist. Transfer of individuals with lower exposure (and therefore lower risk) into the high category can only diminish the estimate of the relative risk.

In theory, exposure assessments need not vary by study design, but in practice they do. When the study population is assembled from one or a small number of companies, as in most cohort studies, considerable information can be assembled on each company from historical records, plant visits, industrial hygiene measurements, and interviews. In contrast, lifetime work histories in case-control studies identify a large number of employers. Because contact with each workplace is not practical, exposure assessment in case-control studies has historically been restricted to qualitative or semiquantitative evaluations.

Hypothesis-testing studies require high-quality, quantitative exposure assessments. This is difficult, however, because exposure misclassification can arise from many sources. Most retrospective exposure assessments are made on administrative designations (e.g., jobs that are held by individuals rather than the individuals themselves because the latter is so impractical). The goal of such an approach is to obtain maximum homogeneity of exposure within the group and maximum heterogeneity of exposure between the groups. However, if job descriptions are unclear, production processes vague, or monitoring data limited, subjects may be grouped inappropriately, which causes exposure misclassification. Construction of homogeneous exposure grouping may be more error-prone in case-control studies than in cohort studies because of the larger number of occupations and industries included and the more limited information on job tasks and workplace practices.

The techniques used to develop quantitative estimates of exposure are another source of misclassification. A number of estimation techniques have been used. In cohort studies, these approaches can be classified as arithmetic calculations, statistical prediction models, and professional judgment.[87] Calculation of means from monitoring data is the most desirable approach because it is simple, reproducible, and requires few assumptions. This approach, however, requires monitoring data for all exposure groups over the entire study period, a situation that rarely occurs for diseases with long latencies.

When monitoring data are available for some exposure/calendar year job combinations but missing for others, statistical models can sometimes be used to predict the missing exposures.[28,47] Statistical modeling has the advantage of developing unbiased estimates in a fairly reproducible manner and is generally applicable when there are a small number of exposure groups relative to the number of measurement data. Predictive models are limited, however, in that they require some measurement data for all workplace conditions and situations being predicted. For example, measurements are required before and after workplace changes that influence exposures, such as changes in production techniques, installation of ventilation equipment, and reduction of leaks.

When neither the arithmetic mean nor statistical predictive models can be used, investigators have often relied on "professional judgment" approaches to develop quantitative estimates. In this approach qualitative information, such as descriptions of job tasks, is combined with the limited measurement data to develop exposure estimates for unmonitored work assignment/time periods. Currently, there are no standardized methods for this approach. Historically, descriptions of how estimates based on professional judgment were developed have typically been brief and vague, and poor documentation makes evaluation of these estimates difficult, reduces reproducibility of the estimates, and invites criticism of the study. Descriptions of the information available and the procedures used to estimate exposures, therefore, need to be more comprehensive and describe the assessment process in more detail. In some more recent studies, detailed descriptions of the assessment process are provided.[6,28,30,47,74,85,108] One approach to improve documentation involves the creation of two complementary computerized systems: one for storing information available on each job (e.g., process description, tasks, location)[88] and the other for recording how each exposure estimate was developed.[94]

Calculation of arithematic means or statistical modeling has generally not been possible in community-based, case-control studies of chronic disease because of the lack of measurements. Information about the job and workplace has traditionally been obtained from interviews with the study subject or proxy respondent, and epidemiologic analyses were based on job titles or simple job-exposure matrices (a cross tabulation of jobs and exposure).[46]

Siemiatycki and colleagues developed the first major improvement in procedures to assess occupational exposures for case-control studies.[80] They used chemists to obtain detailed information from subjects on job tasks, work procedures, and materials to provide a clearer picture of possible exposures.[37] Concentration, frequency, and duration of exposure were estimated. These procedures have recently been modified for use in a computer-assisted system.[90,91] Computerized questionnaires matched to the reported job title seek information on specific jobs on tasks, procedures, and materials, which supplements the traditional, generic work history.[92,93] The interview data are promptly reviewed by an industrial hygienist to determine whether subjects need to be asked additional questions to clarify ambiguous or contradictory exposure information. Explicit evaluation criteria to assess this type of information has been suggested.[91] The procedures of Siemiatycki and Gerin[37,91] and Stewart[92,93] obtain information to address the inherent variability of exposures within a job title and should allow a more accurate assessment of exposure. Because these efforts improve the quality of exposure assessment, they increase the statistical power to detect a disease risk.[29]

Misclassification of exposure occurs in all exposure evaluation procedures. Efforts to evaluate the accuracy and reliability of the exposure estimates should be included, wherever possible, to provide information on the likely degree of misclassification and to appraise its effect on estimates of relative risk. With such information, one can predict the direction and magnitude exposure that misclassification may have on estimates of relative risk.[75] Reliability and validity approaches include using multiple types of estimation techniques,[47] withholding a subset of measurement data,[95] and reconstructing exposures.[30]

Incorporation of Biologic Markers

There are increasing opportunities to incorporate biologic monitoring of exposures, markers of effect, and disease susceptibility into occupational studies. To be useful to determine dose in studies of chronic diseases, biologic exposure markers must persist in tissue, such as organohalides and metals. Investigators have explored the association with serum organohalide levels and cancers of the breast[33,53,107] and lung[8] and blood leads,[73] where tissue levels have been used as biologic dosimeters. Biologic tissues are easier to obtain in case-control studies; their use in cohort studies entails long-term storage of a large number of samples and, therefore, requires a significant commitment of resources. In some circumstances, materials collected for other purposes may be successfully used in epidemiology.[8,49,53] The key issue for incorporating biologic markers of exposure in case-control and cohort studies is the determination of the added benefit provided over exposure assessment based on job and work practices.

In contrast to its limited role in exposure specification, biologic specification of disease has made important contributions to occupational epidemiology. Early use for biologic specification of disease is illustrated by histologic classification of disease in the angiosarcoma of the liver-vinyl chloride and nasal adenocarcinoma-wood dust relationships.[5] Molecular markers recently have also been used to characterize the disease. Aflatoxin exposure, common to agricultural occupations in many countries,[3] has been associated with a specific mutation of the p53 tumor suppressor gene.[39] In another study, *ras* oncogene activation has been associated with solvent exposure in cases of acute myeloid leukemia.[96] Molecular disease classification offers considerable promise, although further research is required to determine to what extent disease-related molecular alterations are indeed exposure-specific and related to development of disease.

A third use of biologic markers in occupational epidemiology is the evaluation of genetic susceptibility. Experimental investigations have demonstrated the importance of metabolic transformation in the carcinogenicity of many occupational carcinogens.[103] Applying these procedures to human investigations promises to improve our efforts to identify carcinogens by focusing on individuals where relative risks may be high because of their metabolic characteristics. This in turn should enhance our understanding of human cancer by relating cancer risk in populations to the underlying biology.[77]

The relationship between activation of chemicals and deactivation of them or their metabolites is important in determining cancer risk. Many genotoxic occupational chemicals are not direct-acting carcinogens and require metabolic activation.[40] Aromatic amines, polycyclic aromatic hydrocarbons, and benzene are examples in the occupational environment. Some chemicals, such as the alkylating agent melphalan and bis-chloromethyl ether, are direct-acting carcinogens. Although these chemicals react directly with cellular macromolecules, including genomic deoxyribonucleic acid (DNA), enzymes involved in deactivation could play a protective role. Wide interindividual variation in activation and deactivation activity is characteristic for many of these enzymes and, in some cases, this variability is due to inherited polymorphisms. Genetic polymorphisms have been associated with cancer of the lung, bladder, colon, and other sites in population studies.[24]

The use of biologic markers and monitoring is growing in epidemiologic studies.[41] Because of the relatively specific nature of occupational exposures, opportunities to include biologic markers, especially for genetic susceptibility, in
epidemiologic investigations offer unique promise. Biologic markers can strengthen
occupational investigations, and opportunities for inclusion of such techniques
should be carefully considered in all high-quality, hypothesis-testing occupational
investigations.

Confounding and Bias

Consideration of confounding and bias is important in all epidemiologic investigations, and cohort and case-control designs have offered different capabilities
with regard to these issues. Because case-control studies typically include interviews with study subjects, it is relatively easy to obtain information on many important confounding factors and to control for them in the analysis. On the other hand,
information on confounders is usually sparse, if not absent, in cohort mortality studies. This is because study data in cohort designs are usually obtained from personnel
records, which lack information on lifestyle confounders and because interviewing
subjects who worked at a company many years in the past is impractical. Lack of information on other risk factors, however, does not necessarily mean that relative risk
estimates from cohort studies are confounded. Very specific conditions are required
before confounding can occur,[18] and the likelihood that these conditions occur can
be assessed to evaluate the probability and magnitude of confounding.[14] Axelson has
shown that even a strong risk factor such as cigarette smoking is unlikely to explain
relative risks for lung cancer from occupational exposures of greater than 1.6.[9] This
lack of strong confounding of occupational risks by tobacco use also has been
shown empirically.[10,81]

Cohort studies offer advantages with regard to selection and information bias.
Case-response bias (a form of differential information bias) is a concern in case-
control studies, but it cannot occur in cohort designs, where information on exposure is obtained prior to diagnosis of disease. The frequency of occurrence of
case-response bias in case-control studies is unclear,[27] but questions should be built
into any interview to obtain an appraisal of its potential occurrence.[16]

Collection of information on lifestyle and other disease risk factors in occupational investigations offers opportunities to evaluate interaction and effect modification in addition to the ability to control for confounding. Occupational studies have
rarely obtained information on nonoccupational factors, perhaps because of the reliance on the cohort design. When data on other actual or potential risk factors are
collected, however, they often have been used to identify subgroups of workers at
especially high risk or to provide explanations for complicated risk patterns.
Examples include lung cancer, smoking, and asbestos exposure;[78] nonHodgkin's
lymphoma, family history of cancer, and agricultural exposures;[112] nonHodgkin's
lymphoma, nitrates, and diet;[102] and lung cancer, formaldehyde, and other occupational exposures.[12]

Power

Cohort and case-control studies offer contrasting advantages with regard to statistical power. Statistical power, defined as the ability of a study to detect a significant
difference in the outcome measure, is a function of the sample size, the level of statistical significance desired, the prevalence of the outcome in the referent population,
and the magnitude of the expected effect. Cohort studies, by including selected work

populations, increase the number and the proportion of the study subjects exposed to the substance of interest. This effectively increases study power for moderately frequent to common diseases. The weakness of the cohort design is that extraordinarily large cohorts are required to provide reasonable numbers of cases of rare diseases. Case-control studies are typically based on the general population, and the proportion of subjects exposed to any particular substance often can be quite small. On the other hand, since case-control studies are based on the general population, which is quite large, it is usually quite easy to assemble large numbers of cases of rare diseases.

A key element in assessing power is usually the number of **exposed** cases, although in some situations power can be limited because of the small number of unexposed cases. The number of exposed cases provides a useful gauge for comparing power of studies of different designs. The studies of formaldehyde and cancer are useful to demonstrate power issues in cohort and case-control studies. Both designs have been used to study cancer risks from exposure to this chemical. Cohort investigations have been conducted among facilities producing or using formaldehyde. Some of these studies were quite large and had considerable power to evaluate moderate to common causes of death.[1,13,84] For rare causes such as nasal cancer (the site that was excessive in animal bioassays), however, the power in cohort studies was very low. For example, in the largest cohort study, only two exposed cases of nasal cancer occurred.[13] In contrast, case-control studies[42,71,76,99] of nasal cancer designed to evaluate formaldehyde exposure all had more exposed cases than two and, thus, had more power. Even with only a few percent of the cases expected to be exposed to formaldehyde, these case-control studies had more exposed cases than occurred in the cohort studies.

The traditional methods of calculating power assume a dichotomous exposure variable. If the exposure is continuous and risk increases monotonically with exposure, power calculations that treat the exposure as dichotomous will indicate the need for more subjects than if the continuous nature of the exposure variable is taken into account.[57] Larger sample sizes are needed when causality has already been established, and studies are being conducted to distinguish between proposed exposure-response gradients[58] or when the interest is in possible genetic-environmental interactions.[48]

Power is an important component in planning a study. After a study is completed, however, it takes on a different aspect. A study with low power is informative if an effect is observed, but it is less informative if no effect is observed. The lack of effect in a study of low power is unconvincing and cannot be taken as evidence of safety.[2,17,43]

Comparison Groups

The principles that guide the selection of the optimal referent population are similar in both case-control and cohort occupational studies. The referent population should represent the population that gave rise to the cases or the exposed cohort, have the same quality of information on exposure and outcome variables, minimize confounding, and be practical in terms of resources and time needed for their inclusion.[26,67,100,101]

Case-Control Studies

POPULATION-BASED CONTROLS

In case-control studies where all cases within an identifiable base population are ascertained, the controls should be a random sample of the population that gave rise to the cases. The controls can be identified through use of population rosters or other methods thought to reach all or most of the population, such as random-digit dialing. A distinct advantage of population-based controls is that results can be readily inferred to the entire population.[67] Population-based controls, however, are usually more expensive to identify and interview than hospital and other types of controls, and response rates are generally lower.[69,83]

Population-based controls may be inappropriate if case ascertainment has been incomplete. Other types of controls should be considered, such as hospital controls, neighborhood controls, friends, and relatives.

HOSPITAL CONTROLS

Hospital controls are used when cases are not population-based. It is hoped that the controls will be partially matched on factors that led cases to seek medical care from the same hospital. The problem is that because the hospital's catchment area may not be the same for all diagnoses, the controls may not be drawn from the exact same population as the cases. The choice of which hospital patients to choose for controls is critical. To minimize possible confounding, one should exclude persons admitted for diseases or conditions known to be related to the exposure of interest. It is often useful to include several disease entities in the control series to avoid using a diagnosis that might unknowingly be related to the exposure. While patients should be excluded from the control series if their current admission is for a disease related to the exposure of interest, it is not necessary to exclude patients who merely have a previous history of the disease unless cases with similar histories are also excluded.[58] Generally, hospital controls are more convenient to identify, yield better response rates, and more comparable information to the cases than population controls.[69,83]

NEIGHBORHOOD CONTROLS

When it is not feasible to sample the general population through rosters or other methods, a possible alternative is to use neighborhood controls. These are obtained by selecting households near the case's residence and then identifying controls within those households. To be valid, the selection process must strictly follow the sampling protocol, without substitution for convenience. Use of neighborhood controls may control for factors associated with neighborhood but may result in overmatching. In addition, the method may fail in neighborhoods where it is difficult to enumerate and access some households (e.g., high-rise apartments). Neighborhood controls also may not be appropriate if there has been substantial migration either into or out of the neighborhood since the case was diagnosed.

RELATIVES, FRIENDS, AND OTHER CONTROLS

Relatives and friends of cases also have served as controls. These subjects are convenient and inexpensive to identify but may also result in overmatching.[100] Some researchers have encountered great reluctance among cases to name friends for the investigations.[50,79] Hospital visitors were used as controls in a war-torn country where traditional methods of selecting neighborhood controls were not possible.[7] Because visiting hospitalized friends and relatives was a social obligation in that country, the hospital visitors approximated a cross-section of the country's population.

CANCER CONTROLS

Due to the existence of cancer registries and other special data resources, many studies have used other cancer cases as controls. They are relatively easy and inexpensive to identify compared to other types of controls and may minimize recall and interviewer bias.[54,82] Cancer controls may introduce bias, however, if the exposure is related to several cancers, as some are. They also present an inferential problem because relative risks are not relative to being healthy but to having other cancers.

PROXY RESPONDENTS

In epidemiologic studies in which information must be obtained directly from study subjects (rather than records), proxy respondents are sometimes used when subjects are unavailable to be interviewed due to disease, death, or other reasons. This is quite common for rapidly fatal diseases, including many cancers. In some circumstances, proxies may even be preferred if their information is more accurate than the subject's (e.g., mother's report of a subject's childhood illnesses or a wife's report on food preparation practices for her husband's meals). Proxies have been used extensively and successfully in nonoccupational, epidemiologic research, generally providing reliable though usually less detailed data than the subjects themselves.[11,20,101] In occupational studies, however, proxies generally report fewer jobs, less detailed exposure information, and sometimes inflate the status of the deceased's occupation.[25]

DECEASED CONTROLS

Information bias may be introduced if more proxies are used for cases than for controls or vice versa. The severity and rapidly fatal nature of many diseases often creates situations in which it is difficult to interview cases directly. To minimize information bias, researchers have sometimes matched on vital status[38,62,100,101] (a deceased control is selected for deceased cases). This may ensure comparable information between cases and controls. The major problem is that deceased persons are not representative of the population that gave rise to the cases, because they had more exposure to factors that lead to premature mortality, such as tobacco and alcohol.[38,62] Excluding certain causes of death from the control group can reduce but probably not eliminate this problem.[63] One suggestion is to select living controls to minimize confounding but to interview their proxies to avoid information bias. This procedure, however, is awkward and makes no sense to study participants. Further, it does not necessarily eliminate information bias because information from a proxy for a living subject may not be comparable to information from a proxy for a deceased subject.

Cohort Studies

The optimal referent group for an occupational cohort study would be another working population that resembles the exposed population in all characteristics except the exposure of interest. Major issues in selecting a referent population include the healthy worker effect,[64] socioeconomic differences, and short-term worker biases.[89] Because the optimal group is usually impossible to identify, several alternatives have been used.

NATIONAL POPULATION GROUP

Occupational cohort mortality studies have traditionally used the total population as a referent group to generate expected numbers of deaths after adjusting for gender, race, age, and calendar time. National rates are used because the comparison population is large and national mortality rates are readily available. In the United States, the general population is frequently used and may be the only choice if the study cohort comes from multiple locations across the country. However, national rates are available for few outcomes other than mortality and cancer incidence.

LOCAL POPULATION

The local population (e.g., state, county) may be a more appropriate referent population if the disease rates in the area where the cohort is located vary significantly from the general U.S. population rates. Often both national and local referent populations are used in occupational cohort studies.[36] There are some limitations to using local rates. The occupational cohort under study must constitute a small proportion of the local population or else the study would be tantamount to comparing the cohort with itself. Migration patterns also may affect the appropriateness of use.[36] If the workers come into the area to work or migrate out of the area before disease or death, the local population might not be an appropriate referent population.

OTHER WORKERS

Comparing an employed population with the general or local population, which consists of employed and unemployed persons, often results in the phenomenon known as the healthy worker effect.[34,64] The relatively lower mortality experienced by employed persons is thought to be due to selection of healthy persons into the workforce and early removal of unhealthy persons from the workforce.[53,66,106] Employed persons also may differ from the general population with respect to socioeconomic status, smoking, alcohol consumption, and other factors that affect mortality.[52,66,106] A serious public health consequence of the healthy worker effect is that a real excess risk caused by occupational exposures may go undetected if the risk is not substantially larger than the healthy worker effect.

Occupational cohorts whose members experience a range of exposures can be analyzed using cohort members with little or no exposure to the substance of interest as an internal referent group, and exposure-response gradients can be examined within the cohort. The number of unexposed workers, however, is often small, which can introduce considerable variability in the estimates of relative risks. Unexposed members of the cohort also may differ socioeconomically from the exposed because the unexposed tend to disproportionately hold white-collar jobs. Bias can be introduced if socioeconomic status or lifestyle factors associated with socioeconomic status are associated with disease risk.

Workers from outside the study cohort may serve as a referent population. Studies with a separate cohort (e.g., police for a study of firefighters) typically must expend as much information to identify and trace the referent cohort as the exposed cohort, and this can substantially increase the cost of the study. Studies that use a single referent cohort also run the risk that the exposures experienced by the referent may have unforeseen health effects. This is similar to the bias that can be introduced by the use of a single disease as referent in a case-control study.

Combining several occupational groups to form a working referent population avoids the potential pitfalls of a single occupational referent cohort. Many European countries have national mortality data on all employed persons,[4,59,61,105] but the United States does not. The National Cancer Institute and the National Institute for Occupational Safety and Health, however, have recently developed a Computerized Occupational Referent Population System (CORPS), which combines all occupational cohort studies conducted by the two agencies.[97] The broad range of occupations and industries included in CORPS should minimize bias that might occur with only one referent cohort, while still providing a large, working population for comparison. Subsets of CORPS can be selected to tailor the referent population to the study cohort in terms of geographic location and worker characteristics such as race, gender, blue collar/white collar, employment status, and minimum employment duration.

MULTIPLE REFERENT GROUPS

In case-control or cohort studies, researchers may propose to use multiple referent groups to overcome limitations associated with any one group. If the results across the different reference groups are similar, interpretation is easy. If the results differ, however, one must decide which group is the most appropriate. If one group is inherently preferable, the epidemiologist should probably use if from the beginning rather than risk misinterpretation from chance differences. If multiple referent groups control for potential confounding in different ways or control for different confounders, each group could be viewed as an independent investigation of the hypothesis, i.e., replication, but usually multiple groups introduce confusion.

PROSPECTIVE STUDY DESIGNS

In an epidemiologic cohort study, a group with one or more exposures of interest is identified and observed over time to determine disease occurrence.[26,67] Most occupational cohort studies have been retrospective (both cohort identification and the observation period have occurred in the past). The time frame for completion of retrospective studies depends on the time required for data collection and analysis. In a prospective study, however, the researchers identify a current working population and follow them into the future to observe disease occurrence. A prospective study may take years or decades to complete. Prospective studies are, therefore, typically much more time-consuming and expensive than retrospective studies. If a hypothesis can be adequately investigated through quicker, less expensive retrospective studies, one would not launch a prospective study. The amount of information favorable for the initiation of a prospective cohort study is narrow. There must be sufficient evidence to warrant the sizable effort and expense associated with a prospective investigation but not so much evidence to make the study redundant or obsolete before its completion. Existing evidence must be sufficient to make the hypothesis credible but not so strong that the prospective study is unnecessary.

A decided advantage of prospective studies is the opportunity for improved exposure assessment. If exposure information can be adequately assessed retrospectively, there is usually little reason to launch a prospective study. If, however, information is difficult to assess retrospectively or is subject to case-response bias, a prospective study design may be preferred. For example, retrospective exposure assessment of solvents is extremely difficult in industries in which there has been frequent substitution of individual solvents over time and use has varied among workers in the same job categories. A prospective study would provide the opportunity to regularly assess the workers' current exposures and practices via questionnaire, monitoring, or other techniques. This should improve the quality of the exposure assessment because monitoring and other assessments can be made periodically during the study. In addition, exposure assessment in a prospective study occurs, by definition, prior to the development of disease. Thus, a prospective study design eliminates the possibility of case-response bias, a charge often levied (albeit rarely substantiated) against case-control studies.

If the exposure assessment procedure for a prospective study requires repeated access to a workplace, the continued cooperation of industry management and labor throughout the study is necessary. This is an important consideration in determining the feasibility of a proposed prospective cohort study of occupational exposures.

Because of the large cost and effort required by researchers, a prospective study should be launched only for important, high-priority topics. There will need to be significant scientific opportunities and results over the short term to warrant the expense of such an investigation and to sustain the researchers' enthusiasm while waiting for sufficient time to pass to address the main issues under investigation.

SUMMARY

Occupational epidemiologic investigations have provided, and will continue to provide, important information to understand environmental causes of disease. High-quality investigations designed to test hypotheses have several requirements. They must include valid quantitative assessments of exposure, some information on lifestyle risk factors, and include biologic monitoring and marker components whenever possible. Availability of these data allows a clear evaluation of potential confounders and biases, assessment of interaction among risk factors, and provides the opportunity to identify susceptible subgroups.

REFERENCES

1. Acheson ED, Gardner MJ, Pannett B, et al: Formaldehyde in the British chemical industry. Lancet 1:611–616, 1984.
2. Ahlbom A, Axelson O, Hansen ES, et al: Interpretation of "negative" studies in occupational epidemiology. Scand J Work Environ Health 16:153–157, 1990.
3. Alavanja MCR, Malker H, Hayes RB: Occupational cancer risk associated with the storage and bulk handling of agricultural food stuff. J Toxicol Environ Health 22:247–254, 1987.
4. Alderson M: Occupational studies: The use of national and industrial comparisons or an internal analysis. In Peto R, Schneiderman M (eds): Banbury Report 9. Quantification of Occupational Cancer. Cold Spring Harbor, NY, Cold Spring Laboratory, 1981, pp 599–610.
5. Alderson M: Occupational Cancer. London, Butterworth & Co., 1986.
6. Amandus HE, Wheeler R, Jankovic J, Tucker J: The morbidity and mortality of vermiculite miners and millers exposed to tremolite-actinolite: Part I. Exposure estimates. Am J Ind Med 11:1–14, 1987.
7. Armenian HK, Lakkis NG, Sibai AM, Halabi SS: Hospital visitors as controls. Am J Epidemiol 127:404–406, 1988.
8. Austin H, Keil JE, Cole P: A prospective follow-up study of cancer mortality in relation to serum DDT. Am J Public Health 79:43–46, 1989.
9. Axelson O, Steenland K: Indirect methods of assessing the effects of tobacco use in occupational studies. Am J Ind Med 13:105–118, 1988.
10. Blair A, Hoar S, Walrath J: Comparison of crude and smoking-adjusted standardized mortality rates. J Occup Med 27:881–884, 1985.
11. Blair A, Kross B, Stewart PA: Comparability of information on pesticide use obtained from farmers and their proxy respondents. J Agr Safety Health 1:165–176, 1995.
12. Blair A, Stewart PA, Hoover RN: Mortality from lung cancer among workers employed in formaldehyde industries. Am J Ind Med 17:683–699, 1990.
13. Blair A, Stewart P, O'Berg M, et al: Mortality among industrial workers exposed to formaldehyde. J Natl Cancer Inst 76:1071–1084, 1986.
14. Blair A, Stewart WF, Sandler DP, et al: A philosophy for dealing with hypothesized uncontrolled confounding in epidemiologic studies. Med Lav 86:108–112, 1995.
15. Blair A, Stewart PA, Hoover RN, et al: Cancers of the nasopharynx and oropharynx and exposure to formaldehyde. J Natl Cancer Inst 78:191–193, 1987.
16. Blair A, Zahm SH: Patterns of pesticide use among farmers: Implications for epidemiologic research. Epidemiology 4:55–62, 1993.
17. Blair A, Zahm SH: Over interpretation of small numbers in the Dow 2,4-D cohort study. J Occup Environ Med 37:363–365, 1995.
18. Breslow NE, Day NE: Statistical methods in cancer research. Vol. 1—The analysis of case-control studies. Lyon, France, International Agency for Research on Cancer, 1980, IARC scientific publication 32.
19. Brown LM, Blair A, Gibson R, et al: Pesticide exposures and other agricultural risk factors for leukemia among men in Iowa and Minnesota. Cancer Res 50:6585–6591, 1990.
20. Brown LM, Dosemeci M, Blair A, Burmeister L, et al: Comparability of data obtained from farmers and surrogate respondents on use of agricultural pesticides. Am J Epidemiol 134:348–355, 1991.

21. Brownson RC, Zahm SH, Chang JC, Blair A: Occupational risk of colon cancer: An analysis by anatomic subsite. Am J Epidemiol 130:674–675, 1989.
22. Burnett CA, Dosemeci M: Using occupational mortality data for surveillance of work-related diseases of women. J Occup Med 36:1199–1203, 1994.
23. Cantor KP, Blair A, Everett G, et al: Pesticides and other agricultural risk factors for non-Hodgkin's lymphoma among men in Iowa and Minnesota. Cancer Res 52:2447–2455, 1992.
24. Caporaso N: Genetic susceptibility in the occupational setting: Introduction to the workshop. Med Lav 86:199–206, 1995.
25. Checkoway H, Demers PA: Occupational case-control studies. Epidemiol Rev 16:151–162, 1994.
26. Checkoway H, Pearce N, Crawford-Brown DJ: Research Methods in Occupational Epidemiology, Monographs in Epidemiology and Biostatistics. Vol 13. New York, Oxford University Press, 1989.
27. Coughlin SS: Recall bias in epidemiologic studies. J Clin Epidemiol 43:87–91, 1990.
28. Dement JM, Harris RL, Symons MJ: Exposures and mortality among chrysotile asbestos workers. Part I: Exposure estimates. Am J Ind Med 4:399–419, 1983.
29. Dewar R, Siemiatycki J, Gerin M, et al: Loss of statistical power associated with the use of a job-exposure matrix in occupational case-control studies. Appl Occup Environ Hyg 6:508–515, 1991.
30. Dodgson J, Cherrie J, Groat S: Estimates of past exposure to respirable man-made mineral fibers in the European insulation wool industry. Ann Occup Hyg 31:567–582, 1987.
31. Dosemeci M, Wacholder S, Lubin JH: Does nondifferential misclassification of exposure always bias a true effect toward the null value? Am J Epidemiol 132:746–748, 1987.
32. Dun and Bradstreet: Dun's Yellow Pages. Dialog Information Service, Inc., Mountain Lakes, NJ, 1988.
33. Falck F, Ricci A, Wolff MS, Godbold J, et al: Pesticides and polychlorinated biphenyl residues in human breast lipids and their relation to breast cancer. Arch Environ Health 47:143–146, 1992.
34. Fox AJ, Collier PF: Low mortality rates in industrial cohort studies due to selection for work and survival in the industry. Br J Prev Soc Med 30:225–230, 1976.
35. Fox AJ, Goldblatt PO: Longitudinal study of sociodemographic mortality differential, 1971–1975, Office of Population Censuses and Surveys. London, Her Majesty's Stationery Office, 1980, series LS, no 1.
36. Gardner MJ: Considerations in the choice of expected numbers for appropriate comparisons in occupational cohort studies. Med Lav 77:23–47, 1986.
37. Gerin M, Siemiatycki J, Kemper H, Begin D: Obtaining occupational exposure histories in epidemiologic case-control studies. J Occup Med 27:420–426, 1985.
38. Gordis L: Should dead cases be matched to dead controls? Am J Epidemiol 115:1–5, 1982.
39. Greenblatt MS, Bennett WP, Hollstein M, et al: Mutations in the p53 tumor suppressor gene: Clues to cancer etiology and pathogenesis. Cancer Res 54:4855–4878, 1994.
40. Guengrich FP: Metabolic activation of carcinogens. Pharmacol Ther 54:17–61, 1992.
41. Hayes RB: Genetic susceptibility and occupational cancer. Med Lav 86:206–213, 1995.
42. Hayes RB, Raatgever JW, De Bruyn A, et al: Cancer of the nasal cavity and paranasal sinuses and formaldehyde exposure. Int J Cancer 37:487–492, 1986.
43. Hernberg S: Negative results in cohort studies—how to recognize fallacies. Scand J Work Environ Health 7(suppl 4):121–126, 1981.
44. Hill AB: The environment and disease: Association or causation? Proc R Soc Med 58:295–300, 1965.
45. Hoar SK, Blair A, Holmes FF, Boysen CD, et al: Agricultural herbicide use and risk of lymphoma and soft-tissue sarcoma. JAMA 256:1141–1147, 1986.
46. Hoar SK, Morrison AS, Cole P: An occupation and exposure linkage system for the study of occupational carcinogenesis. J Occup Med 22:722–726, 1980.
47. Hornung RW, Greife AL, Stayner LT: Statistical model for prediction of retrospective exposure to ethylene oxide in an occupational mortality study. Am J Ind Med 25:825–836, 1994.
48. Hwang S-J, Beaty TH, Liang K-Y: Minimum sample size estimation to detect gene-environment interaction in case-control designs. Am J Epidemiol 140:1029–1037, 1994.
49. Jellum E, Andersen A, Lund-Larsen P: The JANUS serum bank. Sci Total Environ 1993 (Nov 1):139–140, 527–535, 1993.
50. Jones S, Silman AJ: Re: Problems ascertaining friend controls in a case-control study of lung cancer. Am J Epidemiol 134:673–674, 1991.
51. Kleinbaum DG, Kupper LL, Morgenstern H: Epidemiologic Research—Principles and Quantitative Methods. Belmont, CA, Lifetime Learning Publications, 1982.
52. Koskela RS: Occupational mortality and morbidity in relation to selective turnover. Scand J Work Environ Health 8(suppl 1):34–49, 1982.

53. Krieger N, Wolff MS, Hiatt RA, et al: Breast cancer and serum organochlorines: A prospective study among white, black, and Asian women. J Natl Cancer Inst 86:589–599, 1994.
54. Linet MS, Brookmeyer R: Use of cancer controls in case-control cancer studies. Am J Epidemiol 125:1–11, 1987.
55. Lloyd JW, Ciocco A: Long-term mortality study of steelworkers: I. Methodology. J Occup Med 11:299–310, 1969.
56. Lubin JH, Gail MH: On power and sample size for studying features of the relative odds of disease. Am J Epidemiol 131:552–566, 1990.
57. Lubin JH, Gail MH, Ershow AG: Sample size and power for case-control studies when exposures are continuous. Stat Med 7:363–376, 1988.
58. Lubin JH, Hartge P: Excluding controls: Misapplication in case-control studies. Am J Epidemiol 120:791–793, 1984.
59. Lynge E, Thygesen L: Use of surveillance systems for occupational cancer: Data from the Danish national system. Int J Epidemiol 17:493–500, 1988.
60. MacMahon B, Pugh T: Epidemiology: Principles and Methods. Boston, Little, Brown & Co., 1970.
61. Malker HSR: Register-epidemiology in the identification of cancer risks. Arbete Och Halsa 21:7–50, 1988.
62. McLaughlin JK, Blot WJ, Mehl ES, Mandel JS: Problems in the use of dead controls in case-control studies. I. General results. Am J Epidemiol 121:131–139, 1985.
63. McLaughlin JK, Blot WJ, Mehl ES, Mandel JS: Problems in the use of dead controls in case-control studies. II. Effect of excluding certain causes of death. Am J Epidemiol 122:485–494, 1985.
64. McMichael AJ: Standardized mortality ratios and the "healthy worker effect": Scratching beneath the surface. J Occup Med 18:165–168, 1976.
65. McMichael AJ, Spirtas R, Kupper LL: An epidemiologic study of mortality within a cohort of rubber workers. 1964–72. J Occup Med 16:458–464, 1974.
66. Monson RR: Observations on the healthy worker effect. J Occup Med 28:425–433, 1986.
67. Monson RR: Occupational Epidemiology. 2nd ed. Boca Raton, FL, CRC Press, 1990.
68. National Institute for Occupational Safety and Health: National occupational hazard survey. Vol III. Survey analysis and supplemental tables. Cincinnati, NIOSH, 1977.
69. Norell S, Ahlbom A: Hospital or population controls? Presented at The International Occupational Epidemiology Meeting, Como, Italy, 9/85.
70. Olsen JH, Jensen OM: Occupation and risk of cancer in Denmark. Scand J Work Environ Health 13(suppl 1):1–91, 1987.
71. Olsen JH, Jensen SP, Hink M, et al: Occupational formaldehyde exposure and increased nasal cancer risk in man. Int J Cancer 34:639–644, 1984.
72. Percy C, Stanek E, Gloeckler L: Accuracy of cancer death certificates and its effect on cancer mortality statistics. Am J Public Health 71:242–250, 1981.
73. Rappaport SM: Biological monitoring and standard setting in the USA: A critical appraisal. Toxicol Lett 77:171–182, 1995.
74. Rice C, Harris RL, Lumsden JC, et al: Reconstruction of silica exposure in the North Carolina dusty trades. Am Ind Hyg Assoc J 45:689–696, 1984.
75. Rosner B, Willett WC, Spiegelman D: Correction of logistic regression relative risk estimates and confidence intervals for systematic within-person measurement error. Stat Med 8:1051–1069, 1989.
76. Roush GG, Walrath J, Stayner LT, et al: Nasopharyngeal cancer, sinonasal cancer, and occupations related to formaldehyde: A case-control study. J Natl Cancer Inst 79:1221–1224, 1988.
77. Schulte PA, Perera FP (eds): Molecular Epidemiology: Principles and Practices. San Diego, Academic Press, 1993.
78. Selikoff IJ, Seidman H, Hammond EC: Mortality effects of cigarette smoking among amosite asbestos factory workers. J Natl Cancer Inst 65:507–513, 1980.
79. Shaw GL, Tucker MA, Kase RG, Hoover RN: Problems ascertaining friend controls in a case-control study of lung cancer. Am J Epidemiol 133:63–66, 1991.
80. Siemiatycki J, Day N, Fabry J, et al: Discovering carcinogens in the occupational environment: A novel epidemiologic approach. J Natl Cancer Inst 66:217–225, 1981.
81. Simonato L, Vineis P, Fletcher AC: Estimates of the proportion of lung cancer attributable to occupational exposure. Carcinogenesis 9:1159–1165, 1988.
82. Smith AH, Pearce NE, Callas PW: Cancer case-control studies with other cancers as controls. Int J Epidemiol 17:298–306, 1988.
83. Stavraky KM, Clarke EA: Hospital or population controls? An unanswered question. J Chronic Disord 36:301–307, 1983.
84. Stayner LT, Elliott L, Blade L: A retrospective cohort mortality study of workers exposed to formaldehyde in the garment industry. Am J Ind Med 13:667–681, 1988.

85. Stewart PA, Blair A, Cubit DA, et al: Estimating historical exposures to formaldehyde in a retrospective mortality study. Appl Ind Hyg 1:34–41, 1986.
86. Stewart PA, Herrick RF: Issues in performing retrospective exposure assessment. Appl Occup Environ Hyg 6:421–427, 1991.
87. Stewart PA, Lees PSJ, Francis M: Quantification of historical exposures in occupational cohort studies. (manuscript).
88. Stewart PA, Lemanski D, White D, et al: Exposure assessment for a study of workers exposed to acrylonitrile. I. Job Exposure profiles: A computerized data management system. Appl Occup Environ Hyg 7:820–825, 1992.
89. Stewart PA, Schairer C, Blair A: Comparison of jobs, exposures, and mortality risks for short-term and long-term workers. J Occup Med 32:703–708, 1990.
90. Stewart WF, Stewart PA: Occupational case-control studies: I. Collecting information on work histories and work-related exposures. Am J Ind Med 26:297–312, 1994.
91. Stewart PA, Stewart WF: Occupational case-control studies: II. Recommendations for exposure assessment. Am J Ind Med 26:313–326, 1994.
92. Stewart PA, Stewart WF, Heineman EF, et al: A novel approach to data collection in a case-control study of cancer and occupational exposures. Int J Epidemiol (in press).
93. Stewart PA, Stewart WF, Siemiatycki J, et al: Questionnaires for collecting detailed occupational information for community-based case-control studies. Appl Occup Environ Hyg (in press).
94. Stewart PA, Triolo H, Zey J, et al: Exposure assessment for a study of workers exposed to acrylonitrile. II. A computerized exposure assessment program. Appl Occup Environ Hyg 10:698–706, 1995.
95. Stewart PA, Zey JN, Hornung R, et al: Exposure assessment for a study of workers exposed to acrylonitrile. III. Evaluation of exposure assessment methods (manuscript).
96. Taylor JA, Sandler DP, Bloomfield CD, et al: Ras oncogene activation and occupational exposure in acute myeloid leukemia. J Natl Cancer Inst 84:1626–1632, 1992.
97. Thomas TL, Mason TJ, Ramsbottom RI, et al: Development of a computerized occupational referent population system (CORPS) for epidemiologic studies. Am J Epidemiol 123:918–919, 1986.
98. Vainio H, Hemminki K, Wilbourn J: Data on the carcinogenicity of chemicals in the IARC Monographs programme. Carcinogenesis 6:1653–1665, 1985.
99. Vaughan TL, Strader C, Davis S, et al: Formaldehyde and cancers of the pharynx, sinus and nasal cavity: I. Occupational exposures. Int J Cancer 38:677–688, 1986.
100. Wacholder S, McLaughlin JK, Silverman DT, et al: Selection of controls in case-control studies: I. Principles. Am J Epidemiol 135:1019–1028, 1992.
101. Wacholder S, McLaughlin JK, Silverman DT, et al: Selection of controls in case-control studies: II. Types of controls. Am J Epidemiol 135:1029–1041, 1992.
102. Ward MH, Zahm SH, Weisenburger DD, et al: Diet and drinking water source: Association with non-Hodgkin's lymphoma in eastern Nebraska. In McDuffie HH, Dosman JA, Semchuk KM, et al (eds): Agricultural Health and Safety. Boca Raton, FL, Lewis Publishers, 1995, pp 143–150.
103. Williams GM, Weisburger J: Chemical carcinogens. In Klaasen CD, Amdur MO, Doull J (eds): Casarett and Doull's Toxicology. The Basic Science of Poisons. New York, Macmillan, 1987.
104. Wigle DT, Semenciw RM, Wilkins K, et al: Mortality study of Canadian male farm operators: Non-Hodgkin's lymphoma mortality and agricultural practices in Saskatchewan. J Natl Cancer Inst 82:575–582, 1990.
105. Wiklund K, Einhorn J, Wennstrom G, Rapaport E: A Swedish cancer-environment registry available for research. Scand J Work Environ Health 7:64–67, 1981.
106. Wilcosky T, Wing S: The healthy worker effect: Selection of workers and work forces. Scand J Work Environ Health 13:70–72, 1987.
107. Wolff MS, Toniolo PG, Lee EW, et al: Blood levels of organochlorine residues and risk of breast cancer. J Natl Cancer Inst 85:648–652, 1993.
108. Yu RC, Tan W-Y, Mathew RM, et al: A deterministic mathematical model for quantitative estimation of historical exposure. Am Ind Hyg Assoc J 51:194–201, 1990.
109. Zahm SH, Brownson RC, Chang JC, et al: Study of lung cancer histologic types, occupation, and smoking in Missouri. Am J Ind Med 15:565–578, 1989.
110. Zahm SH, Pottern LM, Lewis DR, et al: Inclusion of women and minorities in occupational cancer epidemiologic research. J Occup Med 36:842–847, 1994.
111. Zahm SH, Weisenburger DD, Babbitt PA, et al: A case-control study of non-Hodgkin's lymphoma and the herbicide 2,4-dichlorophenoxyacetic acid (2,4-D) in eastern Nebraska. Epidemiology 1:349–356, 1990.
112. Zahm SH, Weisenburger DD, Saal RC, Babbitt PA, Blair A: The role of agricultural pesticide use in the development of non-Hodgkin's lymphoma in women. Arch Environ Health 48:353–358, 1993.

GARY M. MARSH, PhD

BASIC OCCUPATIONAL EPIDEMIOLOGIC MEASURES

From the Department of
Biostatistics
Graduate School of Public Health
University of Pittsburgh
Pittsburgh, Pennsylvania

Reprint requests to:
Gary M. Marsh, PhD
Department of Biostatistics
Graduate School of Public Health
University of Pittsburgh
130 DeSoto Street
Pittsburgh, PA 15261

Occupational epidemiology has evolved during the past several decades as a distinct sub-discipline within the broader fields of epidemiology and occupational medicine. It applies the concepts and methods of these fields to the health determinants of working populations. A major objective of occupational epidemiology is to determine the health consequences of workplace exposures and to make or recommend remedial efforts when indicated. Other objectives are to provide data useful for setting standards for the protection of workers exposed to toxic substances and to make projections of risk to members of the population at large, who typically experience lower-intensity exposures than occur in the workplace. Problems of a more basic scientific nature, such as elucidating mechanisms of toxicity and exposure-response relationships, can also be addressed in occupational epidemiology.

The estimability of exposure-response relationships depends largely on the quantity and quality of available historical exposure data. In practice, complete and accurate historical exposure data are often nonexistent or unavailable and therefore must be approximated. In addition to an accurate workplace exposure characterization, the estimation of meaningful exposure-response relationships requires an accurate quantification of the presence or occurrence of disease.

This chapter focuses on the "response" side of the exposure-response relationship and summarizes some of the measures of disease frequency and measures of effect that are commonly used in occupational epidemiologic research. An appendix illustrates measures of disease occurrence and effect. The chapter also covers some basic statistical standardization procedures that are used to help compare these measures among groups that differ with respect to age or other factors. The statistical measures and standardization procedures are presented in the context of the classical occupational epidemiologic study designs. A complete discussion of these designs is found in the next chapter.

MEASURES OF DISEASE OCCURRENCE
The occurrence of disease among working populations is measured using rates and proportions. The choice of a particular measure depends on the study design, the health endpoint of interest, and whether occurrence is to be measured at a specific point in time or during a specific time interval. The following measures of disease occurrence have specific meanings.

Rate Measures
One approach to quantifying the population disease frequency during a specific time interval is to compute the number of newly occurring, or *incident cases*, during the time interval of study per number of *person-years of observation*. This quantity is a disease *incidence rate*. The denominator of the incidence rate, person-years, is a quantity used to combine the number of persons with their *follow-up time*. For example, one person followed one year and two persons each followed one-half year both yield one person-year of observation. Other terms for incidence rate are *incidence density, instantaneous risk, force of morbidity* and *hazard rate*. In general, the term *rate* is used to denote the number of newly occurring cases per person-time units.

The *mortality rate* is a special form of incidence rate that expresses the incidence of death. For example, if 1,000 workers are followed for one year and each of 10 new lung cancer deaths occur at mid year, the mortality rate for lung cancer is $10/(1000 - .5(10)) = 0.01005$. For large-scale studies, several computer programs are available for performing person-year and rate calculations.[20,22,23,26,32]

Probability and Risk Measures
A second approach to measuring disease occurrence over a specified time interval is to compute the number of incident cases per number of persons at risk at the beginning of the time interval. This quantity is a disease *risk* and represents the *probability* of developing or dying from a particular disease during the time interval of study. Thus, in the above example, the one-year probability or risk of mortality from lung cancer is $10/1000 = 0.01$, which is slightly less than the one-year mortality rate.

Rates are generally more informative than risks because they take into account the person-time of observation, which in many settings is likely to vary among study members when deaths (or cases) occur at variable points in time. Rates are the central measures of disease occurrence in cohort studies.

Prevalence Measures
Prevalence measures denote the number of cases of disease that exist in the population. *Point prevalence* refers to the prevalence at one point in time and is usually expressed as a *proportion* or *percentage*. Unlike incidence measures, which focus on events, point prevalence focuses on disease status. For example, if a group of 500 workers are surveyed, and 75 report symptoms of respiratory disease and 125 have symptoms of skin disease, the prevalence of respiratory disease is 75/500

(15%), and the prevalence of skin disease is 125/500 (25%). Point prevalence, like risk, does not indicate the rate at which persons develop disease. *Period prevalence* denotes the number of cases that existed during a period of time. Period prevalence is more difficult to interpret because it combines initial point prevalence with subsequent incidence rates.

Prevalence measures are seldom used in etiologic applications of occupational epidemiologic research because differences in prevalence across time or among groups may be the result of differences in the incidence or duration of disease, or both. This occurs because prevalence (P) is approximately equal to the incidence rate (I) times average disease duration $\bar{D}$ when P is small and I is constant over time:

$$P \cong I\bar{D}$$

Prevalence measures arise primarily in cross-sectional studies and are particularly useful for studying classes of diseases with unmeasurable or uncertain moments of onset such as congenital malformations and nonlethal degenerative diseases.[30]

MEASURES OF EFFECT

In occupational epidemiologic research, the term *effect* refers to the difference in disease occurrence between two groups of workers who differ with respect to a causal exposure characteristic.[30] Two types of measures of effect are used in occupational epidemiology, *absolute effects* and *relative effects*. The choice of effect measure is guided by the health endpoint under study and the nature of the inferences to be drawn from the results of the study.

Absolute effect is expressed as the differences in risks, rates, or prevalence between an exposed group and an unexposed but otherwise comparable baseline or reference group. *Relative effect* is based on the ratio of the absolute effect to a baseline rate. For example, if I_1 and I_0 are the incidence rates among exposed and unexposed workers, respectively, the absolute effect is $(I_1 - I_0)$ and the relative effect is $(I_1 - I_0)/I_0 = (I_1/I_0) - 1$. Occupational epidemiologists usually refer only to the ratio component (I_1/I_0), which is known as the *relative risk, relative rate* or simply *rate ratio*.

The absolute effect measure is often more useful for estimating the magnitude of the occupational health problem presented by the exposure. Also, the absolute effect, unlike the relative effect, is not affected by changes in the baseline incidence rate of disease. On the other hand, the relative effect measure is the preferred measure for etiologic research because it is often a clearer indicator of the strength of an association or, under appropriate circumstances, causal role.[9]

SUMMARY MEASURES OF DISEASE OCCURRENCE AND EFFECT

The measures of disease occurrence and effect described above can be expressed as overall summary measures for a group (e.g., *crude rates*) and as measures for homogeneous subgroups defined by age, race, sex or other variables. *Crude summary rates* have limited usefulness in occupational studies because they are not mutually comparable across groups that differ with respect to variables associated with the event under study (e.g., age, race and sex). If this occurs, the relationship between exposure and the study event is said to be confounded by the variable. For example, if two groups (e.g., exposed and unexposed) have different age distributions, age is a *confounding variable* if disease rates are associated with age. However, while subgroup-specific measures generally provide a more complete and accurate

TABLE 1. Layout of Crude Data for a Cohort Study Using Rates and Person-Years

	Study (Exposed) Group	Reference (Unexposed) Group	Total
Events (cases or deaths)	a	b	M
Person-Years	N_1	N_0	T
Rate	$R_1 = a/N_1$	$R_0 = b/N_0$	$R_T = M/T$

characterization of disease occurrence than do crude summary measures, their utility is limited in studies that contain sparse subgroup-specific data or that involve comparisons of populations that are finely stratified (i.e., subdivided) according to several variables. Two approaches that can be taken to summarize measures such as rates across subgroups of a confounding variable, while maintaining the unique information contained in subgroup-specific rates, are to compute either *standardized* or *pooled rates.*

Cohort Studies

Table 1 summarizes measures of risk most frequently encountered in occupational cohort studies that use rates and person-years. A *standardized rate* (SR) is simply a weighted average of the subgroup-specific rates. This can be expressed as

$$SR = \sum_i W_i R_i / \sum_i W_i$$

where i represents the subgroups and W_i and R_i are are the subgroup-specific weights and incidence (or mortality) rates, respectively. Weights can be derived either internally from the distribution of the confounder variable (e.g., age) in the study (exposed) group or externally from the confounder distribution of a comparison, or reference (assumed unexposed), group. The latter approach is known as the *direct method of standardization.*

The comparison of a study group with a reference group is usually made by taking the ratio of their respective standardized rates. This rate ratio (RR_s) is expressed as

$$RR_s = \sum_i W_i R_{1i} / \sum_i W_i R_{0i}$$

If the W_i are taken from the confounder distribution of the study group (i.e., $W_i = N_{1i}$), the RR_s reduces to the commonly used *standardized mortality ratio* (SMR):

$$SMR = \sum_i a_i / \sum_i N_{1i} R_{0i}$$

The SMR represents the ratio of the sum of the observed number of events in the study group to the sum of the expected numbers in the study group, where the expected numbers are based on the rates in the reference group.

The SMR is a type of *indirectly standardized measure* because its weights are derived internally. The product of the SMR and the crude summary rate in the study group is known as the *indirectly standardized rate* (ISR):

$$ISR = SMR \cdot R_1$$

If for RR_s the W_i are taken externally from the confounder distribution of the reference group (i.e., $W_i = N_{0i}$), then RR_s reduces to the *standardized rate ratio* (SRR) described by Miettinen:[25]

$$SRR = \sum_i N_{0i} R_{1i} / \sum_i b_i$$

The SRR represents the ratio of the number of expected events in the reference group, based on rates in the study group, to the number of observed events in the reference group. The SRR is also referred to as the *comparative mortality figure* (CMF).[3,11]

Note that analogous to the expression for ISR, the *directly standardized rate* (DSR) from above can be expressed as the product of the SRR and the crude summary rate in the reference group:

$$DSR = SRR \cdot R_0$$

Pooling is an alternate approach to summary rate ratio estimation that involves computing a weighted average of the subgroup-specific rate ratios rather than the ratio of weighted averages of subgroup-specific rates as in the RR_s. Here the summary rate ratio is expressed as

$$RR'_s = \sum_i W_i (R_{1i}/R_{0i}) / \sum_i W_i$$

The *Mantel-Haenszel method*[18] provides the usual choice of weights for RR'_s where $W_i = b_i N_{1i}/T_i$. With these weights RR'_s becomes

$$RR_{M-H} = \sum_i a_i (N_{0i}/T_i) / \sum_i b_i (N_{1i}/T_i)$$

Proportional Mortality Studies

In some occupational studies it is not possible to enumerate a population at risk, but it is possible to measure the number of events (usually deaths) of interest. In this case, the proportion of deaths from a specific cause (relative to total deaths) can be used in place of death rates to derive summary measures of disease occurrence that resemble and approximate those based on rates.

Table 2 summarizes measures of proportional mortality.

If, in Table 1, the total person-years of observation in the ith subgroup of the study and reference groups, N_{1i} and N_{0i}, respectively, are replaced by the corresponding total number of observed deaths, D_{1i} and D_{0i}, and the rates in the study and reference groups, R_{1i} and R_{0i}, are replaced by the corresponding proportional mortalities, a/D_{1i} and b/D_{0i}, the expression for SMR above becomes the *standard proportional mortality ratio*:

$$SPMR = \sum_i a_i / \sum_i D_{1i} (b_i/D_{0i})$$

and the expression for SRR above becomes

$$SePMR = \sum_i D_{0i} (a_i/D_{1i}) / \sum_i b_i$$

TABLE 2. Layout of Crude Data for Proportional Mortality Studies

	Study (Exposed) Group	Reference (Unexposed) Group	Total
Cause-Specific Deaths	a	b	M
Total Deaths	D_1	D_0	D
Proportional Mortality	a/D_1	b/D_0	M/D

the *externally standardized proportional mortality ratio* described by Zeighami and Morris[34] and Marsh et al.[24] The SPMR and SePMR also can be computed within specific disease categories. For example, site-specific cancer mortality can be expressed as a proportion of all cancer mortality in a *proportional cancer mortality ratio* (PCMR). The appendix provides a numerical example that illustrates the computation of the summary measures of effect described above.

Several authors have discussed methodologic issues related to the use of these summary measures of effect.[4,6,7,10,12–15,17,21,24,27,28,33] Some of the major points are summarized below.

1. All ratio estimates express disease frequency on a multiplicative scale. Some absolute estimates of effect, expressed on an additive scale, are discussed by Monson.[27]

2. When the rate ratio is constant across all subgroups of the confounder, the SMR, SRR, and RR_{M-H} are equal. Also, for a specific subgroup of the confounder, all three measures provide the same unbiased estimate of the rate ratio.

3. The directly standardized measures (DSR, SRR and SePMR) are generally more valid than their indirectly standardized counterparts (ISR, SMR and SPMR) for comparing two or more study groups with different confounder distributions. This follows from the fact that the former measures derive their weights externally from a common reference group; however, the weights of indirect standardization are derived internally from each of the compared study groups.

4. The utility of the directly standardized measures is often limited by the inability to construct stable subgroup-specific rates or proportions within the study groups. This explains the relative popularity of the less valid but more reliable indirect measures, such as the SMR, which are usually based on very stable reference population rates. Thus, the choice between the SMR and SRR as a summary measure of effect involves a trade-off between validity (bias) and reliability (precision).

5. While the proportional mortality based measures (SPMR and SePMR) are quickly and easily computed, their interpretation relative to the rate-based measures is limited, because the number of deaths available for study may not be representative of all deaths occurring in the population and the constraint that proportional mortalities across all causes of death must sum to one.

Breslow and Day[3] and Checkoway et al.[6] provide a more complete discussion of these measures along with related statistical inferential procedures. Computer programs, such as the Occupational Cohort Mortality Analysis Program (OCMAP) developed at the University of Pittsburgh,[5,19,20,22] are also available for the analysis of occupational studies that use these standard measures.[26,32] A new version of the program, OCMAP-PLUS, enables the comprehensive analysis of cohort data that include complex, multifactor work history and exposure data.[23]

Case-Control Studies

In contrast to the cohort study, the case-control study, often termed a *case-referent* or *retrospective study*, involves the comparison of the exposure profiles of workers who developed the disease of interest (cases) with other workers who were presumably free of the disease at the times when the cases were identified (controls). Ideally, cases and controls should be comparable with respect to the a priori probability of exposure, the method of ascertainment, the method of collection, and the reliability and validity of data on exposure status and potentially confounding variables and all characteristics (other than exposure) that relate both to the health outcomes and exposure variables under study (i.e., confounding variables). Because it

TABLE 3. Layout of Crude Data for a Case-Control Study

	Exposed	Unexposed	Total
Cases (Events)	a	b	M_1
Controls (Nonevents)	c	d	M_0
Total	N_1	N_0	T

is usually not possible at the outset of a study to ascertain the comparability of cases and controls with respect to potential confounders, efforts are generally made to control for confounding bias either through design (matching cases to one or more controls on the basis of one or more confounders) or through analysis (stratification by levels of one or more confounders).

Case-control studies can be used to estimate the measures of effect derivable only in cohort studies while reducing the cost and problems of following a cohort (and obtaining data on exposures and confounders on all subjects). Case-control studies do not provide direct measures of disease incidence, but they do yield odds ratios that estimate relative risks. Table 3 shows crude data layout for a case-control study.

The *crude odds ratio* (OR) is defined as the ratio of the odds of exposure among the cases to the odds of exposure among the controls:

$$OR = (a/b) / (c/d) = ad / bc$$

The case-control study analysis may be stratified by levels of one or more possible confounding variables (e.g., age or smoking status). If this is done, a *pooled summary odds ratio* is given by Mantel and Haenszel[18] as

$$OR_{M-H} = \sum_i a_i (d_i/T_i) / \sum_i b_i (c_i/T_i)$$

where summation is taken across all subgroups of the cases and controls. That the odds ratio estimates the relative risk is apparent upon comparing OR and OR_{M-H} to the expressions for RR_s and RR_{M-H} presented previously.

Two basic types of case-control studies are used in occupational epidemiologic research. A cohort-based study, often called a *nested case-control study*, is conducted within the framework of an existing occupational cohort, which provides both a basis for complete case ascertainment and a sampling frame for the selection of controls. Nested case-control studies are usually indicated when it is not feasible to obtain data on exposures or potential confounders for all cohort members.

In nested case-control studies, controls are usually selected from the cohort using a procedure called *incidence density sampling*. This involves considering each case in turn and randomly selecting one or more controls from the risk set of persons who were at risk at the age the individual was identified as a case. In some cases, the selection of controls is restricted by certain matching variables (i.e., controls are further matched to cases on one or more factors), which may include living or dead status (i.e., to avoid differential recall bias) or by diseases (or deaths) that are believed to be unrelated to the exposure under study. The cumulative exposures of the case and the controls and the status of any confounding variables are then evaluated as of this age. The relative risk is estimated by forming the ratio of the average exposure of the cases to the average exposure of the controls while adjusting for the confounding variables.

Another strategy for selecting controls in nested case-control studies is referred to as the *case-cohort design*.[29] In this approach, controls are selected at the beginning of the cohort study as a stratified random sample of the entire cohort. This approach eliminates the need to identify cases prior to control selection and can provide controls for several simultaneous case-control studies of various diseases.[16] The utility of the case-cohort design is limited by its analytic complexity and the paucity of available statistical methods that allow control for multiple confounders.

Beaumont et al. have developed a useful computer program for incidence density sampling.[1] OCMAP-PLUS also contains an incidence density sampling algorithm that creates risk sets for use in *relative risk regression analysis*.[23] A thorough review of analytic methods for case-control studies is provided by Breslow and Day.[2] Other aspects of case-control studies are discussed by Cole[8] and Schlesselman.[31]

REFERENCES

1. Beaumont JJ, Steenland K, Minton A, Meyer S: A computer program for incidence density sampling of controls in case-control studies nested within occupational cohort studies. Am J Epidemiol 129:212–219, 1989.
2. Breslow NE, Day NE: Statistical Methods in Cancer Research. Vol 1: The Analysis of Case-Control Studies. Lyon, France, International Agency for Research on Cancer, 1980.
3. Breslow NE, Day NE: Statistical Methods in Cancer Research. Vol 2: The Design and Analysis of Cohort Studies. Lyon, France, International Agency for Research on Cancer, 1987.
4. Breslow NE, Lubin JH, Marek P, Langholz B: Multiplicative models and cohort analysis. J Am Stat Assoc 78:1–12, 1983.
5. Caplan RJ, Marsh GM, Enterline PE: A generalized effective exposure modeling program for assessing dose-response in epidemiologic investigations. Comp Biomed Res 16:587–596, 1983.
6. Checkoway H, Pearce NV, Crawford-Brown DJ: Research Methods in Occupational Epidemiology. New York, Oxford University Press, 1989.
7. Chiazze L: Problems of study design and interpretation of industrial mortality experience. J Occup Med 18:169–170, 1976.
8. Cole P: The evolving case-control study. J Chron Dis 32:15–27, 1979.
9. Cornfield J, Haenszel W: Some aspects of retrospective studies. J Chron Dis 11:523–534, 1960.
10. Decoufle P, Thomas TL, Pickle LW: Comparison of the proportionate and cause-specific mortality among workers at an energy research laboratory. Br J Ind Med 42:525–533, 1980.
11. Fleiss J: Statistical Methods for Rates and Proportions. 2nd ed. New York, John Wiley & Sons, 1981.
12. Gaffey WR: A critique of the standardized mortality ratio. J Occup Med 18:157–160, 1976.
13. Gilbert ES: Some confounding factors in the study of mortality and occupational exposure. Am J Epidemiol 116:177–188, 1982.
14. Greenland S: Interpretation and estimation of summary ratios under heterogeneity. Stat Med 1:217–227, 1982.
15. John LR, Marsh GM, Enterline PE: Evaluating occupational hazards using only information known to employers: A comparative study. Br J Ind Med 40:346–352, 1983.
16. Kupper LL, McMichael AJ, Spirtas R: A hybrid epidemiologic study design useful in estimating relative risk. J Am Stat Assoc 70:524–528, 1975.
17. Kupper LL, McMichael AJ, Symons MJ, Most BM: On the utility of proportional mortality analysis. J Chron Dis 31:15–22, 1978.
18. Mantel N, Haenszel W: Statistical aspects of the analysis of data from retrospective studies of disease. J Natl Cancer Inst 22:719–748, 1959.
19. Marsh GM, Co-Chien H, Rao BR, Ehland J: OCMAP: Module 6—a new computing algorithm for proportional mortality analysis. Am Stat 43:127–128, 1989.
20. Marsh GM, Ehland J, Paik M, et al: OCMAP/PC: A user oriented cohort mortality analysis program for the IBM PC. Am Stat 40:308–309, 1986.
21. Marsh GM, Ehland J, Sefcik S: Mortality and Population Data System [technical report]. Pittsburgh, University of Pittsburgh, Department of Biostatistics, 1987.
22. Marsh GM, Preininger ME: OCMAP: A user-oriented occupational cohort mortality analysis program. Am Stat 34:245–246, 1980.
23. Marsh GM, Sefcik S, Alcorn C, Youk A: A new occupational cohort mortality analysis program for multifactor work history and exposure-based analysis. Occup Hyg 3:xiv, 1996.
24. Marsh GM, Winwood J, Rao BR: Prediction of the standardized risk ratio via proportional mortality analysis. Biometrical J 29:355–368, 1987.
25. Miettinen OS: Standardization of risk ratios. Am J Epidemiol 96:383–388, 1972.
26. Monson RR: Analysis of relative survival and proportional mortality. Comp Biomed Res 7:325–332, 1974.

27. Monson RR: Occupational Epidemiology. 2nd ed. Boca Raton, FL, CRC Press, 1990.
28. Pott P: Chirurgical Observations. London, Hawes, Clarke and Collins, 1775.
29. Prentice RL: A case-cohort design for epidemiologic cohort studies and disease prevention trials. Biometrika 73:1–11, 1986.
30. Rothman KJ: Modern Epidemiology. Boston, Little, Brown & Co., 1986.
31. Schlesselman JJ: Case-Control Studies: Design, Conduct, Analysis. New York, Oxford University Press, 1982.
32. Waxweiler RJ, Beaumont JJ, Henry JA, et al: A modified life-table analysis program system for cohort studies. J Occup Med 25:115–124, 1983.
33. Wong O, Decoufle P: Methodologic issues involving SMR and PMR in occupational studies. J Occup Med 24:299–304, 1982.
34. Zeighami E, Morris M: The measurement and interpretation of proportionate mortality. Am J Epidemiol 117:90–97, 1983.

APPENDIX

Measures of Disease Occurrence and Effect: An Illustration

Appendix Table 1 presents data from a hypothetical cohort study in which total death rates and death rates from lung cancer are compared between a low-exposure study group and a high-exposure study group with an external population serving as the common reference group (Appendix Table 2). The data layout is presented in Tables 1 and 2 in the text.

Appendix Table 1 shows that the low- and high-exposure groups have virtually identical crude death rates for lung cancer (0.0084 and 0.0086, respectively). However, the age-specific rates are uniformly larger in the high-exposure group, suggesting that lung cancer mortality may be associated with level of exposure. In this example, age, which is related both to exposure group and to lung cancer

APPENDIX TABLE 1. Data from a Hypothetical Cohort Study

		Study Group 1 (High Exposure)			Study Group 2 (Low Exposure)			
		Deaths				Deaths		
		All Causes	Lung Cancer			All Causes	Lung Cancer	
Age Subgroup i	Person-Years N_{1i}	Number D_{1i}	Number a_i	Rate R_{1i}	Person-Years N_{1i}	Number D_{1i}	Number a_i	Rate R_{1i}
20–44	2500	8	3	.0012	1000	4	1	.0010
45–64	1000	14	4	.0040	1500	18	3	.0020
65+	1500	130	36	.0240	2500	202	38	.0152
Total	5000	152	43	.0086	5000	224	42	.0084

APPENDIX TABLE 2. Reference Group for Hypothetical Study Described in Appendix Table 1

| | | Deaths | | |
| | | All Causes | Lung Cancer | |
Age Subgroup i	Person-Years N_{0i}	Number D_{0i}	Number b_i	Rate R_{0i}
20–44	50,000	100	5	.0001
45–64	35,000	400	49	.0014
65+	15,000	1000	66	.0044
Total	100,000	1500	120	.0012

rates, is confounding the association between exposure and lung cancer as measured by the crude rates. To control for confounding by age, the techniques of standardization and pooling can be used to compute various summary measures of effect. For example, the lung cancer SMR for the high exposure group would be computed as

$$\text{SMR}_{\text{High}} = \frac{(3+4+36)}{2500(.0001) + 1000(.0014) + 1500(.0044)} = \frac{43}{8.25} = 5.21$$

Summary measures expressed as rate ratios (RR_s) are usually multiplied by 100 so that deviations from 100 represent percent excesses or deficits in mortality. Thus, $\text{SMR}_{\text{High}} = 5.21 * (100) = 521$, indicating that the high-exposure group had a 421% excess in lung cancer mortality relative to the reference population. Similarly, the SMR for the low-exposure group is found as

$$\text{SMR}_{\text{Low}} = \frac{(1+3+38)}{1000(.0001) + 1500(.0014) + 2500(.0044)} * 100 = 318$$

indicating a 218% excess in lung cancer mortality. Therefore, because $\text{SMR}_{\text{Low}} < \text{SMR}_{\text{High}}$, the standardized data suggest an association between exposure and lung cancer.

The directly standardized lung cancer SRR can also be computed for both study groups as

$$\text{SRR}_{\text{High}} = \frac{(50,000)(.0012) + (35,000)(.0040) + (15,000)(.0240)}{(5+49+66)} * (100) = 467$$

$$\text{SRR}_{\text{Low}} = \frac{(50,000)(.0010) + (35,000)(.0020) + (15,000)(.0152)}{(5+49+66)} * (100) = 290$$

While the SRR values differ somewhat from the SMR values, the relationship $\text{SRR}_{\text{Low}} < \text{SRR}_{\text{High}}$ holds, again suggesting an association between exposure and lung cancer mortality. Because the age distributions differ in study groups 1 and 2, and age is also related to exposure, the directly standardized SRR is the preferred summary measure.

Using the summary measures computed above the indirectly standardized rates (ISR) for the two study groups are

$$\text{ISR}_{\text{High}} = (5.21)(.0086) = .0448$$
$$\text{ISR}_{\text{Low}} = (3.18)(.0084) = .0267$$

and the directly standardized rates (DSR) are

$$\text{DSR}_{\text{High}} = (4.67)(.0012) = .0056$$
$$\text{DSR}_{\text{Low}} = (2.90)(.0012) = .0035$$

While the absolute values of ISR and DSR are arbitrary, depending solely on the choice of the reference population, both summary measures again indicate a pattern of greater mortality in the high versus low exposure group.

Pooling can also be used to compute RR_{M-H} in both groups as

$$RR_{\text{M-H,High}} = \frac{3(50,000/52,500) + 4(35,000/36,000) + 36(15,000/16,500)}{5(2500/52,500) + 49(1000/36,000) + 66(1500/16,500)} * (100) = 519$$

$$RR_{\text{M-H,Low}} = \frac{1(50,000/51,000) + 3(35,000/36,500) + 38(15,000/17,500)}{5(1000/51,000) + 49(1500/36,500) + 66(2500/17,500)} * (100) = 316$$

The RR_{M-H} values are close to the SMR values and reflect the same association between exposure and lung cancer.

Proportional mortality measures could also be computed from Appendix Tables 1 and 2 in the situation where the person-years at risk values, N_{1i} and N_{0i}, were unknown. These would be

$$SPMR_{High} = \frac{(3 + 4 + 36)}{8(5/100) + 14(49/400) + 130(66/1000)} * (100) = 402$$

$$SPMR_{Low} = \frac{(1 + 3 + 38)}{4(5/100) + 18(49/400) + 202(66/1000)} * (100) = 267$$

Also, the directly standardized SePMRs would be computed as

$$SePMR_{High} = \frac{100(3/8) + 400(4/14) + 1000(36/130)}{(5 + 49 + 66)} * (100) = 357$$

$$SePMR_{Low} = \frac{100(1/4) + 400(3/18) + 1000(38/202)}{(5 + 49 + 66)} * (100) = 233$$

Although the absolute values of the proportional mortality measures differ from their rate-based counterparts, the pattern of both SPMRs and SePMRs again reveals the association between exposure and lung cancer mortality.

The above results are summarized in Appendix Table 3, which shows that all of the standardized or pooled summary measures of effect reflect the true underlying pattern in age-specific lung cancer rates (i.e., larger in higher exposure group). This pattern was obscured in the comparison or crude rates between groups 1 and 2, due to confounding by age.

APPENDIX TABLE 3.   Results of a Hypothetical Cohort Study

Summary Measure	Study Group 1 (High Exposure)	Study Group 2 (Low Exposure)
Crude Rate (R)	0.0086	0.0084
SMR	521	318
SRR	467	290
RR_{M-H}	519	316
ISR	0.0448	0.0267
DSR	0.0056	0.0035
SPMR	402	267
SePMR	357	233

DAVID F. GOLDSMITH, MSPH, PhD

IMPORTANCE OF CAUSATION FOR INTERPRETING OCCUPATIONAL EPIDEMIOLOGY RESEARCH:

A Case Study of Quartz and Cancer

From the California Public Health
Foundation
Berkeley, California

Reprint requests to:
David F. Goldsmith, MSPH, PhD
California Public Health Foundation
2001 Addison Street, Suite 210
Berkeley, CA 94704-1103

A crucial role for the discipline of epidemiology is providing a guide for the derivation of a causal link between exposure and disease. Interpretation of epidemiologic research and placement within biologic knowledge are essential for advances in public health as well as occupational medicine. Much of epidemiologists' contribution to causal thinking in the 20th century has focused on environmental and consumer health protection in areas such as provision of safe drinking water and sewage services, control of air pollution, childhood vaccines, wearing of seat belts, and safe handling of food. The approach to causal processes for chronic disease prevention and derivation of effective policies in the workplace have illustrated the interplay between epidemiology and other occupational health disciplines such as industrial hygiene, medical surveillance, statistics, and worker and management collaboration. This chapter discusses the criteria for causation considered by the U.S. Surgeon General, the International Agency for Research on Cancer, and others to place the evidence in historical context. As a case study, the criteria for judging the evidence for potential carcinogenicity of silica dust are examined. Lastly, the importance of effective communication with workers and corporate management about causal concerns from workplace exposures is discussed.

CAUSATION DEFINED

The need for criteria related to causation of chronic diseases evolved from the classic logic of

Henle-Koch's postulates for demonstrating infectious disease causation. These postulates, modified by Lilienfeld and Stolley in 1994, are as follows:

1. The organism must be found in all cases of the disease.
2. It must be possible to isolate the organism from patients with the disease and grow it in culture.
3. When pure culture is inoculated into susceptible animals or humans, it must reproduce the disease.[42]

Thus, a causal microorganism is a bacteria or virus meeting these criteria for the occurrence of disease in humans; it must meet the necessary condition for producing disease but need not be sufficient. In other words, exposure to an infectious agent produces illness, but it probably needs susceptible hosts to manifest the disease and to be detected.

In 1976, Evans proposed a synthesis of Henle-Koch postulates with more current concepts that are applicable to both chronic (noninfectious) and infectious diseases.[15]

1. The incidence or prevalence of disease needs to be significantly greater in subjects exposed to the proposed causal factors than among unexposed controls.
2. Exposure to the hypothesized cause should be more frequent among subjects with the disease than among disease-free controls after controlling for all risk factors.
3. The disease should follow exposure to the hypothesized cause.
4. Various host responses should follow exposure to the putative agent along a biologic gradient from mild to severe.
5. A measurable host response after exposure to the cause should appear in subjects unaffected before exposure (i.e., biomarkers) or should increase if present before exposure and should not be observed among unexposed controls.
6. Reproduction or production of disease should occur more frequently among exposed than among unexposed subjects (this experiment could be observed in laboratory animals or volunteers or demonstrated after workplace exposure).
7. Elimination or control of causal exposures or vectors should decrease or eliminate the disease (e.g., near elimination of byssinosis with technologic control of cotton bract exposures).
8. Modification of host response to the hypothesized cause should reduce or eliminate risk (e.g., immunization).
9. All of the observed relationships should be rational biologically and epidemiologically.

The accumulation of powerful epidemiologic evidence of the role of smoking in the causation of lung cancer throughout the developed world after World War II led to the need to measure the evidence for judging the sufficiency of data in order to provide rational public health policies. The proposed criteria were built on Henle-Koch's logic but placed much more emphasis on epidemiologic findings, whereas Henle-Koch's principles tended to rely on bacteriology and transmissibility of agent to uninfected hosts (such as exposure of hospital staff to patients with tuberculosis), which may not apply to long-latent chronic illnesses. A confluence of causal thinking emerged in the middle 1960s with the release of the U.S. Surgeon General's first report on smoking and health in 1964[68] and Sir Austin Bradford Hill's paper on the criteria for causation in environmental health in 1965.[34]

At this juncture, it is worth defining the difference between association and causation. Two variables such as high concentration of automobile dealers and AIDS cases in the United States may show some association compared with locations in which concentrations of car dealers are low. However, *no known* evidence indicates that employment in automobile sales is part of any causal linkage between exposure and disease variables, despite their statistical correlation. Thus, one could say that there is an *association* between the concentration of car dealers and AIDS, but *no biologic or clinical causal link exists.* On the other hand, workplace exposure to asbestos dust and the risk of asbestosis are known to be associated; more importantly, chronic inhalation of respirable asbestos fibers is causally related to contracting the occupational pulmonary disease called asbestosis.

From the work of Hill (1965), the U.S. Surgeon General, (1964 and 1982), and Lilienfeld and Stolley (1994), the criteria for judging causation for chronic diseases, particularly for cancer, may be stated as follows[34,42,67,68]:

- Strength of the correlation or high relative risk
- Dose-response relationship
- Consistency of findings
- Biologic plausibility, including experimental evidence
- Temporal cogency
- Control of confounding and bias
- Specificity
- Overall coherence.

These criteria are applied to determine whether there is sufficient evidence to conclude or to have a strong suspicion that the putative exposure(s) or risk factors and disease are causally linked. Causation can be inferred *even if all the criteria are not fully met,* thus reenforcing the requirement for careful and cautious application of professional judgment to causality assessment. Caution is necessary because etiologic determinations have implicit social, legal, and public health effects. Thus, a causal "web" exists when sufficient evidence indicates that exposures or defined factors increase the probability of disease and that management of or intervention in one or more of these exposures or risk factors lowers or prevents the occurrence of disease. The etiologic factor or exposure does not need to be the sole cause of the disease, and it may modify other diseases.

High Relative Risk or Strength of the Correlation

Many epidemiologists consider a relative risk or odds ratio to be strong if it exceeds 2.0; that is, if the disease risk among exposed subjects is more than doubled compared with a control group. A relative risk > 2.0 produces an attributable risk or attributable fraction[42] of over 50% and thus can be defined as more likely than not to be linked with a defined risk factor or exposure. Given a relative risk of 1.3–1.8 (i.e., a weak association), a causal link must be determined on the basis of other research findings. However, a modest association repeatedly reported from high-quality epidemiology studies can still be relevant for effective occupational health policy. An example might be an ergonomic factor that reduces back injuries by 50%, which may be of major concern for both industrial and public health officials. The strength of the correlation is the first clue leading to serious concern of biologic effect for workplace exposures and supports the development of causality in conjunction with other evidence.

Dose-Response Relationship

If an occupational exposure is causally related to disease, the risk should be related to the extent of exposure to the agent. In other words, the data should show a dose-response gradient; the most clear-cut demonstration is the powerful trend for increasing chronic disease risks and amount of lifetime cigarette smoking. Despite instances in which disease risk does not follow an exposure-response pattern or quantification of exposure is difficult, dose-response findings add weight to a presumed etiologic pattern. Gradients may be seen for both cumulative dose and exposure duration. Many retrospective occupational studies rely on proxy measures of exposure, such as time employed in a work area, although new methods of biomonitoring (of blood, hair, urine) will increase the precision of dose estimation. There are also studies of radon film badges or silica dust levels in which historical reconstruction of doses may be considered of high quality and results (with and without dose-responses) should be accorded greater weight than studies with poor or missing exposure information. There also may be concerns about possible censoring of exposure-response findings because of loss of more sensitive subjects or long survival of nonsusceptibles.

Consistency of Findings

Different studies in which various investigators apply different study methods and find the same or similar results add strength to the causal exposure-disease link. Epidemiologic consistency is the logical equivalent of laboratory scientists who produce the same results under differing experimental or field conditions. An example is the consistent finding of leukemia among benzene-exposed workers throughout the world.

Biological Plausibility Including Experimental Evidence

Epidemiologists seek to label causal effects that are biologically relevant, because to do otherwise means that our discipline would not be bounded by cumulative knowledge in chemistry, toxicology, and clinical medicine. Thus, observations in epidemiology must be biologically plausible. For example, it makes powerful biologic sense that toxic substances that produce sterility and angiosarcoma of the liver in laboratory animals (such as dibromochloropropane [DBCP] and vinyl chloride) are likely to do so among workers. By way of contrast, scientists would not expect eye color to be related to workplace accidents because of biologic implausibility, even if there were a statistical association between the two factors. Thus, for this type of evidence, epidemiologists must consider exposure pathways to specific tissues or organs, including metabolism of compounds, and be willing to change views when new biochemical or experimental findings provide support for linkages previously considered nonexistent.

Temporal Cogency

For chronic diseases such as cancer, temporal cogency has two components: the disease must follow exposure in time (rather than being coincident with or preceding first exposure) and must occur after sufficient duration of exposure. Duration is likely to be a minimum of 10–15 years after initiation of exposure, and thus some relevant latent time becomes part of the causal picture. As an example, pleural or peritoneal mesothelioma from asbestos exposure has latent periods ranging from 20–40 years from first exposure. Another component of this causal criterion is reduction in risk after cessation of exposure. The best example is the well-documented decline in lung cancer risk among people who remain exsmokers for 10 years or more compared with people who continue to smoke.[67]

Control of Confounding and Bias

Because of the observational nature of occupational epidemiology, randomized clinical trials have no role in industrial health studies. Thus causal linkages must stand on research that has controlled for possible confounding and bias. An example is the extensive debate about possible bias of subjects' prior knowledge of use of defoliants and herbicides when the Scandinavian findings of soft-tissue sarcomas and exposure to phenoxyacetic acid herbicides were reported.[29] When other cancers known not to be related to herbicides were assessed in case-control studies, they were not found to have elevated risks, thus confirming that subjects' overclassification was not the reason for the high risk levels for soft-tissue sarcomas.

Specificity

To avoid fuzzy thinking about matters of causation, it is relevant to specify the exposure or industrial process and the concomitant disease(s). This includes pathognomonic findings of unique exposures producing single types of pathology such as hepatic angiosarcoma among vinyl chloride monomer-exposed workers or mesotheliomas in workers with past exposure to asbestos. In 1994, Lilienfeld and Stolley include "specificity of the association" as part of the criteria of causation, although they admitted that single exposure producing only one disease is contrary to what epidemiologists have learned about carefully researched causal exposures such as tobacco smoking and asbestos, both of which produce many diseases.[42] In the same way, health scientists have come to learn that a disease can have many potential causal factors, each independent and all necessary (or none sufficient) for producing etiologic links. An example is combined exposure to aflatoxin and hepatitis, which may produce liver cancer. Specific thinking tries to narrow the focus of epidemiologists so that association of rubber and tire manufacture with risks of lymphatic cancer is focused on a causal link between leukemia and exposure to benzene in tire building or pliofilm production.

Overall Coherence

Because of the social and commercial effects of the judgments used in assessing causation, one must ask whether all of the evidence together is coherent. The review process should not indict innocent exposures or industries. A false-positive determination also threatens the credibility of occupational epidemiologists when new exposure and disease associations reach critical stages of evaluation that require policy changes. Thus, assessment of coherence becomes useful in looking backward at overall strength of the causal evidence and forward to the effectiveness of risk assessment and risk management policies that are derived from them. An example of coherence may be the validity of concluding that exposure to respirable asbestos fibers is the cause of many diseases—asbestosis, mesothelioma, and lung and other cancers. However, an extension of causal thinking leading to policies of removal of sealed (nonfriable) asbestos from every public school building in the U.S. overlooks both the excessive cost and the understanding that the risk applies to workers and has not been linked with building users because of absence of exposure.

In 1965 Hill proposed that analogy was part of the criteria for causation. That is, if chemicals with similar structures (Hill's example was thalidomide) produce chronic diseases, analogous chemicals also should be considered etiologically linked. Epidemiologists must use analogy as a means to develop or test hypotheses, but since other criteria address questions of causation, this point of evidence should not be considered part of the etiologic criteria.

IARC CLASSIFICATION OF CARCINOGENICITY

The International Agency for Research on Cancer (IARC) has developed through its monograph series a process to evaluate exposures and industries for carcinogenicity. The IARC classification process goes beyond the causal assessment criteria to classify materials by the degree of carcinogenicity. Furthermore, IARC considers evidence from experimental tumor biology in its evaluation process and emphasizes the point by stating: "in the absence of adequate data on humans, it is biologically plausible and prudent to regard agents and mixtures for which there is sufficient evidence of carcinogenicity in experimental animals as if they presented a carcinogenic risk to humans."[38] The purpose of the IARC carcinogen classification is to weigh and summarize results from the evaluation of data about many chemicals and occupational processes in order to identify and communicate conclusions concerning likely risk from human exposure to these chemicals and industrial processes.

From the preamble of every IARC monograph the classification criteria used by each working group of expert scientists are spelled out. For humans, there are four categories of carcinogenesis: sufficient, limited, inadequate, and lack of evidence. The **sufficient** category is similar to the causal criteria defined above. **Limited** means that "a positive association has been observed between exposure to the agent, mixture or exposure circumstance and cancer for which a causal interpretation is considered to be credible, but chance, bias or confounding could not be ruled out with reasonable confidence. **Inadequate** classification is made when "the available studies are of insufficient quality, consistency or statistical power to permit a conclusion regarding the presence or absence of a causal association, or no data on cancer in humans are available." **Lack of carcinogenicity** is defined by the following:

> There are several adequate studies covering the full range of levels of exposure that human beings are known to encounter, which are mutually consistent in not showing a positive association between exposure to the agent, mixture, or exposure circumstance and any studied cancer or at any observed level of exposure. A conclusion of "evidence suggesting lack of carcinogenicity" is inevitably limited to the cancer sites, conditions and levels of exposure and length of observation covered by the available studies. In addition, the possibility of a very small risk at the levels of exposure studied can never be excluded.[38]

Carcinogenicity in experimental animals studies is classified into four categories: sufficient, limited, inadequate, and evidence suggesting lack of carcinogenicity. **Sufficient** evidence is determined by "a causal relationship has been established between the agent or mixture and an increased incidence of malignant neoplasms or an appropriate combination of benign and malignant neoplasms in (a) two or more species of animals or (b) in two or more independent studies in one species carried out at different times or in different laboratories or under different protocols." **Limited** evidence includes "data (that) suggest a carcinogenic effect but are limited for making a definitive evaluation because, e.g., (a) the evidence of carcinogenicity is restricted to a single experiment; or (b) there are unresolved questions regarding the adequacy of the dosing, conduct or interpretation of the study; or (c) the agent or mixture increases the incidence only of benign neoplasms or lesions of uncertain neoplastic potential, or of certain neoplasms which may occur spontaneously in high incidences in certain strains." **Inadequate** evidence includes "studies (that) cannot be interpreted as showing either the presence or absence of a carcinogenic effect because of major qualitative or quantitative limitations, or no data on cancer in experimental animals are available." **Lack of carcinogenicity** is defined as "adequate studies involving at least two species are available which show that, within the limits of the tests used, the agent or mixture is not carcinogenic. A conclusion of evidence suggesting lack of carcinogenicity is inevitably limited to the species, tumor sites and levels of exposure studied."

IARC reviewers also consider other relevant genotoxicity and tumor pathology types, pharmacokinetics, structure activity findings, and mechanistic studies if interpretation of either human or animal findings is uncertain.

An overall evaluation is conducted to place the agent or industrial process into a grid (Table 1) reflecting the strength of the evidence. **Group 1** is characterized by sufficient evidence of carcinogenicity in humans, regardless of the degree of animal evidence. **Group 2** includes agents and industrial processes for which the degree of carcinogenicity in humans is almost sufficient, as well as those for which no human data exist, but there is sufficient evidence for carcinogenicity in animals. **Group 2A** chemicals or industrial processes are classified as probably carcinogenic to humans when there is sufficient evidence in animals with limited evidence in humans, sufficient animal evidence plus strong supporting/relevant genotoxicity evidence, or limited human evidence and supporting evidence. **Group 2B** exposures are judged to be possibly carcinogenic to humans with limited human evidence or sufficient animal evidence or limited animal evidence plus supporting genotoxic evidence. **Group 3** includes chemicals that are not classifiable as to their carcinogenicity to humans; this classification includes chemicals with studies that are inadequate in humans and inadequate or limited in animals (unless there is some supporting evidence). **Group 4** are agents or occupational exposures for which cancer risk is significantly less than expected.

From 1971–1994 the IARC assessment program has reviewed 775 agents or industrial processes. In 1995, McDonald and Saracci provided a compilation of IARC reviews and found 63 chemicals or industrial processes labeled as group 1; 50 labeled as group 2A; 209 labeled group 2B; 452 labeled group 3; and 1 chemical (caprolactan) labeled as group 4.[44] There are so few group 4 chemicals because IARC generally reviews chemicals for which there are some suspicious findings among either humans or animals.

EXAMPLE OF SILICA DUST EXPOSURE

Issues of Silica Causation

The carcinogenicity of crystalline silica (also known as free silica, quartz, alpha quartz or SiO_2) has been debated in the scientific community since the 1930s.[21,27] Silica dust exposures that occur during mining and smelting of metal ores have been known almost since biblical times to produce many types of respiratory disease that coalesce around the diagnosis of miners' phthisis, or potters' rot or asthma, or consumption. Today we know these conditions as silicosis, silicotuberculosis, and other

TABLE 1. IARC Classification Scheme for Human and Animal Evidence

Human Evidence	Animal Evidence			
	Sufficient	Limited	Inadequate	(-) Carcinogenicity
Sufficient	Group 1	Group 1	Group 1	Group 1
Limited	Group 2A	Group 2B	Group 2B	Group 2B
Inadequate	Group 2B	Group 3	Group 3	Group 3
(-) Carcinogenicity	Group 2B	Group 4	Group 4	Group 4

less specific fibrotic respiratory ailments. The debate about the carcinogenicity of silica has been thoroughly evaluated only in the last decade.

In the 1930s, J. Henry Dible, a Liverpool pathologist, published a review of 14 autopsied cases of silicosis in which four patients were found to have cancers, including one woman with leukemia, two men with lung tumors (one also having a colon cancer), and a third man with liver cancer. On the basis of this uncontrolled evidence, he suggested a link between silica exposure and cancer.[14] From the mid-1930s until the 1980s there were periodic exchanges in the medical literature about the chronic disease risks among "dusty trades" workers, but there was more published information about the risk of silicosis,[11,76] its clinical sequelae, and its medicolegal implications than concern about possible carcinogenicity from the inhalation of quartz dust.

It is interesting to note the positions of leading scientists in earlier assessments of silica's carcinogenicity. In 1963 Wagoner and colleagues reported a follow-up study of a group of metal ore miners. The authors reported a significant standardized mortality rate (SMR) of 292 (47 observed and 16.1 expected deaths; $p < 0.01$) for respiratory system cancers and an SMR of 149 (51 observed and 34.2 expected deaths; $p < 0.01$) for digestive system neoplasms. The authors examined several factors, including age, smoking, immigration, urbanization, social class, autopsy and diagnostic rates for tumors, and radon levels and rejected each as a possible explanation. The authors considered silica and silicosis as possible reasons for the excessive cancer but rejected them based on studies from South Africa, England, and the U.S.[70] There was no mention of studies supportive of a role for silica and silicosis, including Dible (1934), Collis and Yule (1933), and Klotz (1939).[10,14,39] In their seminal review of silicosis in 1976, Ziskind et al. stated the following:

> there is no indication that silicosis is associated with increased risk for the development of cancer of the respiratory or other systems. When there is combined exposure to silica and other substances such as arsenic, nickel, or chromate, the increased susceptibility to cancer appears to be related to the other material. There is no indication of a synergistic increase of susceptibility to cancer after exposure to such other dusts and silica.

However, there were no citations to support their statements.[76] Despite Selikoff's own data related to silica-exposed New York City tunnel workers, which showed an apparent dose-response for lung cancer risk (based on attained years from first employment and number of years worked after minimum 20 years latency), he concluded "with reasonable confidence" that "silica does not lead to cancer, merely because of its elemental nature, nor because of its potential for fibrosis."[61] Although Selikoff cited two case reports from 1935 supporting initial links between asbestos and lung cancer, he did not cite similar reports from 1934–1939 supporting an association between silica and lung cancer.

In the past decade, the link between silica exposure and cancer risk has undergone a transformation. This renewed focus began with a 1982 article in which evidence for lung cancer risks among silica-exposed workers and laboratory animals was evaluated.[25] The general consensus among pulmonary specialists was that silica exposure and silicosis were not risk factors for lung (or any) cancer.[11,31,37,45,53,61,76] Since Goldsmith et al. raised the issue in 1982, researchers and agencies have given consideration to the alternative view that silica is a probable or likely human carcinogen.[38,54,62] The foundation for this position is based on findings in rats[50,58,59] and excessive pulmonary cancer risks among silica-exposed workers, particularly among silicotics.[2,3,18,21,23,25,26,28,34,38,39,43,49,58,62]

For the past 10 years IARC has judged the animal evidence to be sufficient and the human evidence to be limited. Thus silica is a probable human carcinogen with a classification of 2A. IARC will reexamine its classification of silica as a probable human carcinogen in the fall of 1996. Tumor sites other than the lung, including lymphatic and gastrointestinal malignancies, have been reported in the literature and will be assessed by IARC.

This review focuses on research that addresses the causal evaluation related to silica, including a separate assessment for workers with silicosis. Relevant points concerning interpretation of studies include the following: the quality of and correlation with industrial hygiene data or any surrogate estimate of dust exposure or "dose" (such as length of employment); the means by which smoking is adjusted; and the presence of confounding from other sources such as radon, arsenic, or diesel emissions. These factors are addressed as possible explanations for observed cancer risk.

Does Silica Exposure or Silicosis Cause Cancer?

Determining whether silica causes cancer involves comparison of the evidence with standard criteria for determining causation. This assessment was undertaken in 1987 by IARC and in 1988 by the State of California.[38,54] Other agencies such as the National Institute of Occupational Safety and Health and the National Toxicology Program adopted IARC's evaluation although the U.S. Environmental Protection Agency has not done so. In both cases, one must ask whether the current data comply with the following criteria: strong relative risk; dose-response (including reliable exposure data); consistency; biologic plausibility (including experimental animal findings); temporal cogency; control for confounding and bias; specificity; and overall coherence.

STRONG RELATIVE RISK

For silica-exposed workers, levels of lung cancer risk seem to be consistently elevated, with a range of 1.3–3.7. Especially noteworthy are the relatively modest risks for granite workers, tunnelers, and sandblasters, who generally do not have mixed exposures. Gold miners throughout the world seem to have elevated lung cancer risks, with the exception of Homestake miners in South Dakota, who show a slightly elevated relative risk (RR) of 1.13 for lung cancer and 2.54 for other pulmonary cancers.[65] By contrast, the work of Hnizdo and Sluis-Cremer showed a smoking-adjusted RR among miners that increased with silica dose.[36] Some iron and tin ore miners show elevated lung cancer risks, although evidence suggests that lung cancer may be related to radon exposure, perhaps in combination with silica exposure.[22] Foundry workers also have some elevated lung cancer risks, but with the exception of the study by Fletcher, linkage with silica exposure remains elusive.[19] Several cohorts have elevated rates of digestive and lymphatic cancer, particularly gold miners.[41,65]

For silicotics, there is a strong set of relative risks. With the exception of autopsy studies that show risks less than the null value (relative risk of 1.0), 27 of 29 epidemiologic studies of silicotics throughout the world (reviewed recently by Goldsmith and by Smith et al.[21,63]) show strikingly significant risks that range from 1.4 in Austria to 6.5 in Japan.[9,51] Only Hessel and coworkers from South Africa have shown no association between silicosis and lung cancer,[32,33] and their study has been challenged by Hnizdo and Sluis-Cremer, who found a relative risk of 3.9 among those with silicosis of hilar lymph glands.[36] Also noteworthy are the recent elevated risks for lung cancer among silicotics in North Carolina, reported by Amandus et al.; among a national sample of metal ore miners, reported by Amandus and Costello; among California silicotics, reported by Goldsmith et al.; in Ontario, reported by Finkelstein; and in Italy, reported by Merlo et al.[2,3,17,23,47]

DOSE-RESPONSE GRADIENTS

For a material to be biologically active, increasing the dose must increase the risk. Among silica-exposed workers, there are several examples of dose-related gradients, but some tended to be indirect measures of exposures, such as length of time employed (e.g., Selikoff[61]) or increased risk for dustier jobs (e.g., Fletcher[19]). However, the work of Winter et al., Hnizdo and Sluis-Cremer, and Checkoway et al. demonstrated a dose-response for cumulative industrial hygiene/respirable particle exposure[7,36,73] and confirms the previous indirect associations, thus strengthening the link between silica dust and lung cancer. Fu and colleagues and McLaughlin et al. found significant dose-responses between lung cancer and total dust and silica among Chinese tin miners, a gradient that remained after adjustment for smoking.[20,46] Among silicotics, only indirect data link workplace silica concentrations to lung cancer risk. However, four positive studies show a gradient for the degree of silicosis disability as a risk factor for lung cancer.[8,36,48,52] Goldsmith et al. showed a gradient for lung cancer (but not for malignancies of the large intestine) by level of compensation awarded—a surrogate for degree of silicosis.[23] To the extent that severity of silicosis reflects silica exposure, then silicotics share the dose-related gradients demonstrated in studies of silica exposure.

All of the occupational and industrial groups considered have a history of high dust exposure to crystalline silica. The best exposure data exist for quartz-exposed workers rather than for silicotics, because obtaining individual dust concentrations is or was not practical. The exception is sampling data from the North Carolina Dusty Trades monitoring,[56] but Amandus et al. did not present these data in their paper.[3] Some studies presented indirect exposure measures such as years employed[61] or duration underground. However, the most powerful exposure data are presented for respirable quartz in the tin mines of China by McLaughlin et al. and Fu et al. (1992); for California diatomaceous earth workers by Checkoway et al.; among U.K. ceramic workers by Winter et al.; and in South African gold mines by Wyndham et al. and Hnizdo and Sluis-Cremer.[7,20,36,46,73,74] All studies found measurable lung cancer risks correlated with cumulative silica exposures after adjustment for smoking.

Absence of silica exposure data in cancer epidemiology studies is a function of either a lack of quartz measurements or an inability to recreate exposure or dust levels (for silicotics). In studies in which quality silica dust exposures have been developed or reported from other sources, dose-response lung cancer gradients have been found.[7,20,36,46,74] The exceptions reported by Steenland and Brown for gold mining[65] and McLaughlin et al. for tungsten and iron-copper mining[46] do not diminish the strength of the positive exposure-response gradients in the published literature.

CONSISTENT FINDINGS

The relative risks for silica-exposed workers and for silicotics have been consistent among investigators and dusty industries and across national boundaries and study designs. The consistency for the findings among epidemiologic studies of silicotics is impressive, and the associations hold true in Europe, Asia, and North America.

BIOLOGIC PLAUSIBILITY (INCLUDING ANIMAL FINDINGS)

Respirable silica interacting with pulmonary tissue to produce lung cancer is the pathway outlined by Goldsmith et al. in 1982 when the issue of biologic plausibility arose over a decade ago.[25] Silica exposure is multipathologic, causing silicosis, cor pulmonale, autoimmune diseases, silicotuberculosis, and probably nephritis.[4,22] Understanding one precise mechanism by which quartz produces cancer does not mean that it cannot induce cancer through different pathways. In 1982 Goldsmith et al. suggested that quartz could act directly or via a fibrotic mechanism (similar to foreign body tumorigenesis), and there is no agreement as to which is more likely.[25] In 1986 Saffiotti suggested that release of cell mediators during the fibrotic process, which are especially reactive when exposed to freshly fractured quartz, could stimulate cell proliferation in adjacent tissue and ultimately neoplasia.[57] Saffiotti's most recent thinking, based on experimental work in his laboratory at the U.S. National Cancer Institute, suggests that the complex biologic and neoplastic capability of silica requires host susceptibility via the production of or access to reactive oxygen species,[58] including the ability of silica to bind with DNA.[12]

Ample animal evidence supports the carcinogenicity of silica, as recognized in 1987 by IARC, which judged the findings to be sufficient. Since 1987, biologists studying rodent cancer have demonstrated that lifetime exposure to DQ12 quartz is carcinogenic via inhalation at doses as low as 1 mg/m³.[50,64] It is also clear that quartz produces fibrosis in the lung and that it either precedes or appears to show some species specificity, because rats (along with humans) demonstrate that silica produces fibrotic and neoplastic diseases, whereas other rodents (such as hamsters and guinea pigs) do not. Saffiotti[57,60] has developed several lines of research to explain this paradox and the mechanisms for carcinogenesis.[12,72]

TEMPORAL COGENCY

In both silica-exposed workers and among silicotics, data support appropriate time-related events. That is, cancer risk is not elevated until at least 20 years employment, which is consistent with what has been learned about other workplace carcinogens such as asbestos and arsenic. The lung cancer excesses among silicotics have emerged *after* the diagnosis of silicosis (not coincidentally) and again usually after decades of employment or exposure to silica. No epidemiologic studies of former silica workers with reduced cancer risks were discovered during an online search on this topic.

CONTROLS FOR CONFOUNDING

As pointed out in 1987 by IARC Monograph panel members, lack of adjustment for smoking was the biggest confounder in both types of early cancer studies.[38] However, adjusting for smoking when data are incomplete and when data are present does not alter the risk of lung cancer.[23,47] In studies of foundry workers, other environmental exposures (such as polycyclic aromatic hydrocarbons and metal oxide fumes) may continue to confound a suggestive link with silica dust. IARC panelists also observed that selection bias may play a role in the elevated risk for silicotics, who were more likely to have physicians' attention. Thus lung tumors were more likely to be found because of chronic pulmonary disease.[45] However, given the strong likelihood of histologic confirmation for lung cancers, this argument does not blunt the strong and consistent finding of significantly elevated lung cancer rates among silicotics. There may be unmeasured types of confounding in some of the lymphatic and gastrointestinal cancer excesses.

SPECIFICITY

Specificity of the association is confirmed by the fact that the review assessing causation for cancer among workers with silica exposure or with defined silicosis. For those reasons one should not address cancer risk in industries such as coal, asbestos, and uranium mining because silica is not the primary or specific exposure of concern. Specificity is increased because the assessment focuses on pulmonary effects from exposure to respirable particulates and the target organ (for the most part) is the lung. Almost every study demonstrates clear-cut excessive mortality and morbidity risks for silicosis and for nonmalignant pulmonary diseases, including tuberculosis.

OVERALL COHERENCE

Silica-exposed workers have a moderate relative risk that is consistent across industries, countries, and investigators, and there are excellent dose-response data from the U.S., South Africa, and China for lung cancer. After confounding by age and smoking has been adjusted, the elevated lung cancer risk remains; there are good exposure data, with biologic specificity and a powerful animal model; and no chronologic violations of temporal cogency. On these bases, it is logical to conclude that occupational silica exposure is carcinogenic for humans (Table 2).

Silicotics have strong relative risks for lung cancer that are consistent among countries, investigators, and industries giving rise to fibrotic lung disease. Despite limited information about silica exposure, several studies support an increased risk according to severity of fibrosis—an indirect measure of silica dose. Furthermore, selection, smoking, and radon do not appear to account for the consistently high relative risks. The animal model is less clear-cut, but the findings are consistent with biologic specificity and are temporally correct. Thus, it is rational to argue that silicosis predisposes to an increased lung cancer risk and that risk is due to high silica exposure, fibrotic processes, or both (see Table 2).

Summary of Evidence of Human Cancers Related to Silica Exposure

Many studies have examined the cancer risk in silicotics and nonsilicotics separately.[2,8,23,52,75] The presence of silicosis itself may be an independent risk factor for pulmonary neoplasia, an indicator variable for duration and/or intensity of exposure, or a marker of genetic susceptibility to pulmonary damage by respirable size crystalline silica. The general trend is that silicotics show increased risk of pulmonary neoplasia compared both with those exposed to silica without silicosis and with the general population.

TABLE 2. Criteria for Cancer Causation for Silica Exposure and for Silicosis

Point of Evidence	Silica Exposed Workers	Workers with Silicosis
Strong relative risk	+	+++
Dose-response gradient	++	+
Consistent findings	++	+++
Controlled confounding	+	+
Biologic plausibility	++	±
Temporal cogency	+	+
Specificity	++	++
Overall coherence	Yes	Yes

+ = criteria met; ± = incomplete evidence.

Winter et al. among U.K. ceramic workers, Fu et al. and McLaughlin et al. among Chinese tin miners, Hnizdo and Sluis-Cremer among South African gold miners, and Checkoway et al. among U.S. diatomaceous earth workers demonstrated excessive lung cancer risk associated with occupational exposure to crystalline silica and dose-response relationships.[7,20,36,46,73] These studies also demonstrated greater than additive interaction between crystalline silica and tobacco smoke. Other epidemiologic studies demonstrated dose-response gradients for the association between silicosis and lung cancer,[8,36,48,52] but exposures from polycyclic aromatic hydrocarbons, metal oxide fumes, and radon confound the evidence.[21,24,35]

Besides increases in pulmonary cancer in silicotics and nonsilicotic workers exposed to silica, epidemiologic studies also have demonstrated evidence of increased risk for other tumors. Increases in the risk of lymphatic malignancies were demonstrated by Brown et al. and Steenland and Brown, Kurppa et al., Mirer et al., and Redmond et al.[6,40,49,55,66] Similarly, Wagner et al. demonstrated increases in lymphatic cancers in crystalline silica-exposed animals.[69] Finkelstein et al. showed a consistent excess of gastric cancer among Ontario silicotics,[16,18] and Kusiak et al. reported similar results among Ontario gold miners.[41] In 1995 Goldsmith et al. reported a two-fold excess for cancer of the large intestine among California silicotics.[23]

Taken together with the positive animal findings and the ability of silica to bind with DNA, IARC's assessment[38] that there is sufficient evidence for the carcinogenicity of quartz does not appear to be in doubt. Furthermore, the most current human evidence for the carcinogenicity of silica appears to be sufficient based on the findings from both silica-exposed workers and silicotics.[5,21] Thus, a large body of scientific evidence supports the conclusion that occupational silica dust exposure is carcinogenic to humans.

Communicating the Potential Cancer from Silica

If worker exposure to silica or silicosis is a causal risk for cancer, how can one effectively communicate this potential to workers, management, and communities? Because it appears that the cancer risks are greatest for those with extant silicosis,[5] the existing dust control methods—which are effective in lowering silicosis risks—are also likely to prevent cancer.[27] The Occupational Safety and Health Administration (OSHA) recently initiated a "Special Emphasis Program for Silicosis" to raise the index of concern for all stakeholders in the silica and industrial health community.[13] It is disappointing that OSHA seems to be unaware that current concern about silicosis and the need for special attention arose because minority workers, particularly poorly educated Afro-Americans, Mexican-Americans, and other immigrants, are becoming sick with acute and accelerated silicosis.[71] Employers have a strong role in prevention, and if minority workers are overexposed in the workplace, they and their communities will bear the brunt of the adverse health effects, including premature deaths[11] and cancer.

Several attempts have been made to derive cancer and noncancer risk assessments; however, there appears to be no consensus about methods.[26,30] Furthermore, if the 1996 IARC panel judges the evidence for human silica exposure and carcinogenicity to be sufficient, lowering current occupational standards for silica and other quartz minerals also may be rational. Reducing industrial exposures to quartz is likely to lead to reduced risk for cancer, silicosis, and other related health effects. Current efforts at preventing exposure with effective industrial hygiene sampling, wet methods, and effective exhaust ventilation will probably be effective in managing silica dust in the workplace and general environment. Such efforts must include medical screening and surveillance of workers. When alternatives to silica exist, as in abrasive blasting, less toxic abrasives should replace silica.

CONCLUSION
One of the most important roles for occupational epidemiology is to provide a scientific basis for assessing causation. In general, the process requires critical judgment of the risk evidence, with particular attention to the criteria of strong relative risk, dose-response, consistency, control for confounding, biologic plausibility, temporal cogency, and specificity. If the data are biologically rational and make clinical sense from the view of prevention, the process is most likely coherent. This reassurance is needed to ensure that exposures or industrial processes are not misjudged as false positives. Applying the criteria to the current evaluation of silica dust exposure as a carcinogen strongly suggests that epidemiologic research findings meet the causal criteria for both silica-exposed workers and silicotics. Thus, one can conclude that the evidence for human carcinogenicity for silica dust exposure is sufficient. Prevention policies suggest that controlling silica dust emissions will lower the risk of silicosis, autoimmune diseases, silicotuberculosis, and cancer.

REFERENCES
1. Abraham JL, Wiesenfeld SL: Two cases of fatal PMF in an ongoing epidemic of accelerated silicosis in oilfield sandblasters: Lung pathology and mineralogy. In Inhaled Particles VIII. Cambridge, British Occupational Hygiene Society, 1996.
2. Amandus H, Costello J: Silicosis and lung cancer in U.S. metal miners. Arch Environ Health 46:82–89, 1991.
3. Amandus HE, Shy CM, Wing S, et al: Silicosis and lung cancer in North Carolina dusty trades workers. Am J Ind Med 20:57–70, 1991.
4. Balaan MR, Banks DE: Silicosis. In Rom WN (ed): Environmental and Occupational Medicine. Boston, Little, Brown, 1992, pp 345–358.
5. Berry G: Crystalline silica: Health impacts and possible lung cancer risks. J Occup Health Safe Aust N Z 12:157–167, 1996.
6. Brown DP, Kaplan SD, Zumwalde RD, et al: Retrospective cohort mortality study of underground gold mine workers. In Goldsmith DF, Winn DM, Shy CM (eds): Silica, Silicosis, and Cancer: Controversy in Occupational Medicine. New York, Praeger, 1986, pp 335–350.
7. Checkoway H, Heyer NJ, Demers PA, Breslow NE: Mortality among workers in the diatomaceous earth industry. Br J Ind Med 50:586–597, 1993.
8. Chia SE, Chia KS, Phoon WH, Lee HP: Silicosis and lung cancer among Chinese granite workers. Scand J Work Environ Health 17:170–174, 1991.
9. Chiyotani K, Saito K, Okubo T, Takahashi K: Lung cancer risk among pneumoconiosis patients in Japan, with special reference to silicotics. In Simonato L, Fletcher AC, Saracci R, Thomas TL (eds): Occupational Exposure to Silica and Cancer Risk. Lyon, France, International Agency for Research on Cancer (IARC), 1990, pp 95–104.
10. Collis EL, Yule GU: The mortality experience of an occupational group exposed to silica dust compared with that of the general population and an occupational group exposed to dust not containing silica. J Ind Hyg 15:395–417, 1933.
11. Craighead JE: Silicosis and Silicate Disease Committee of NIOSH: Diseases associated with exposure to silica and nonfibrous silicate materials. Arch Pathol Lab Med 112:673–720, 1988.
12. Daniel LN, Mao Y, Williams AO, Saffiotti U: Direct interaction between crystalline silica and DNA—proposed model for silica carcinogenesis. Scand J Work Environ Health 21(Suppl 2):22–26, 1995.
13. Dear JA: Special Emphasis Program (SEP) for Silicosis. Washington, DC, U.S. Department of Labor, Occupational Safety and Health Administration, 1996.
14. Dible JH: Silicosis and malignant disease. Lancet ii:982–983, 1934.
15. Evans AS: Causation and disease: The Henle-Koch postulates revisited. Yale J Biol Med 49:175–195, 1976.
16. Finkelstein M: Kusiak RS, Suranyi G: Mortality among miners receiving workmen's compensation for silicosis in Ontario: 1940–1975. J Occup Med 24:663–667, 1982.

17. Finkelstein MM: Silicosis, radon, and lung cancer risk in Ontario miners. Health Physics 85:396–399, 1995.
18. Finkelstein MM, Liss GM, Kramer F, Kusiak RA: Mortality among surface-industry workers receiving workers' compensation awards for silicosis in Ontario: 1940–1984. Br J Ind Med 44:588–594, 1987.
19. Fletcher AC: The mortality of foundry workers in the United Kingdom. In Goldsmith DF, Winn DM, Shy CM (eds): Silica, Silicosis, and Cancer: Controversy in Occupational Medicine. New York, Praeger, 1986, pp 385–401.
20. Fu H, Jing X, Yu S, et al: Quantitative risk assessment for lung cancer from exposure to metal ore dust. Biomed Environ Sci 5:221–228, 1992.
21. Goldsmith DF: Silica exposure and pulmonary cancer. In Samet JM (ed): Epidemiology of Lung Cancer. New York, Marcel Dekker, 1994, pp 245–298.
22. Goldsmith DF: Health effects of silica dust exposure. Rev Mineral 29:545–606, 1994.
23. Goldsmith DF, Beaumont JJ, Morrin LA, Schenker MB: Respiratory cancer and other chronic disease mortality among silicotics in California. Am J Ind Med 28:459–467, 1995.
24. Goldsmith DF, Guidotti TL: Combined silica exposure and cigarette smoking: A possible synergistic effect. In Goldsmith DF, Winn DM, Shy CM (eds): Silica, Silicosis, and Cancer: Controversy in Occupational Medicine. New York, Praeger, 1986, pp 451–459.
25. Goldsmith DF, Guidotti TL, Johnston DR: Does occupational exposure to silica cause lung cancer? Am J Ind Med 3:423–440, 1982.
26. Goldsmith DF, Wagner GR, Saffiotti U, et al: Special Issue—Second International Symposium on Silica, Silicosis, and Cancer, San Francisco. Scand J Work Environ Health (Suppl 2):1–117, 1995.
27. Goldsmith DF, Wagner GR, Saffiotti U, et al: Future research needs in the silica, silicosis, and cancer field. Scand J Work Environ Health 21(Suppl 2):115–117, 1995.
28. Goldsmith DF, Winn DM, Shy CM (eds): Silica, Silicosis, and Cancer: Controversy in Occupational Medicine. New York, Praeger, 1986, p 536.
29. Hardell L, Sandstrom A: Case-control study: Soft tissue sarcomas and exposure to phenoxyacetic acids or chlorophenols. Br J Cancer 39:711–717, 1979.
30. Hardy TS, Weill H: Crystalline silica: Risks and policy. Environ Health Perspect 103:152–155, 1995.
31. Heppleston AG: Silica, pneumoconiosis, and carcinoma of the lung. Am J Ind Med 7:285–294, 1985.
32. Hessel PA, Sluis-Cremer GK: Case-control study of lung cancer and silicosis. In Goldsmith DF, Winn DM, Shy CM (eds): Silica, Silicosis, and Cancer: Controversy in Occupational Medicine. New York, Praeger, 1986, pp 351–355.
33. Hessel PA, Sluis-Cremer GK, Hnizdo E: Silica exposure, silicosis, and lung cancer: A necropsy study. Br J Ind Med 47:4–9, 1990.
34. Hill AB: The environment and disease: Association or causation? Proc R Soc Med 58:295–300, 1965.
35. Hnizdo E: Risk of silicosis in relation to fraction of respirable quartz [letter]. Am J Ind Med 25:771–772, 1994.
36. Hnizdo E, Sluis-Cremer GK: Silica exposures, silicosis, and lung cancer: A mortality study of South African gold miners. Br J Ind Med 48:53–60, 1991.
37. Hueper WC: Occupational and environmental cancers of the respiratory system. Rec Results Cancer Res 3:1–159, 1966.
38. International Agency for Research on Cancer: IARC Monographs on the Evaluation of the Carcinogenic Risk of Chemical to Humans. Silica and Some Silicates, monograph no. 42. International Agency for Research on Cancer, Lyon, France, 1987.
39. Klotz MO: Association of silicosis and carcinoma of the lung. Am J Cancer 35:38–49, 1939.
40. Kurppa K, Gudbergsson H, Hannunkari I, et al: Lung cancer in silicotics in Finland. In Goldsmith DF, Winn DM, Shy CM (eds): Silica, Silicosis, and Cancer: Controversy in Occupational Medicine. New York, Praeger, 1986, pp 311–319.
41. Kusiak RA, Ritchie AC, Springer J, Muller J: Mortality from stomach cancer in Ontario miners. Br J Ind Med 50:117–126, 1993.
42. Lilienfeld DE, Stolley PD: Foundations of Epidemiology, 3rd ed. New York, Oxford University Press, 1994.
43. McDonald C: Mineral dusts and fibers. In McDonald JC (ed): Epidemiology of Work Related Diseases. London, BMJ Publishing Group, 1995, pp 87–116.
44. McDonald J, Saracci R: Metals and chemicals. In McDonald JC (ed): Epidemiology of Work Related Diseases. London, BMJ Publishing Group, 1995, pp 7–37.
45. McDonald JC: Silica, silicosis and lung cancer [editorial]. Br J Ind Med 46:289–291, 1989.
46. McLaughlin JK, Chen J-Q, Dosemeci M, et al: A nested case-control study of lung cancer among silica exposed workers in China. Br J Ind Med 49:167–171, 1992.

47. Merlo F, Fontana L, Reggiardo G, et al: Mortality from lung cancer among 515 Genoa, Italy silicotics: Results from the follow-up period 1961–1987. Scand J Work Environ Health 21(Suppl 2):77–80, 1995.

48. Miller AB, Scarpelli D, Weiss NS: Report to the Workers' Compensation Board on the Ontario Gold Mining Industry of the Scientific Panel on Mortality from Cancer Among Ontario Gold Miners 1955–1977. Toronto, Industrial Disease Standards Panel, Ontario Ministry of Labour, 1987.

49. Mirer F, Silverstein M, Maizlish N, et al: Dust measurements and cancer mortality at a ferrous foundry. In Goldsmith DF, Winn DM, Shy CM (eds): Silica, Silicosis, and Cancer: Controversy in Occupational Medicine. New York, Praeger, 1986, pp 29–44.

50. Muhle H, Takenaka S, Mohr U, et al: Lung tumor induction upon long-term low-level inhalation of crystalline silica. Am J Ind Med 15:343–346, 1989.

51. Neuberger M, Kundi M, Westphal G, Grundorfer W: The Viennese dusty worker study. In Goldsmith DF, Winn DM, Shy CM (eds): Silica, Silicosis, and Cancer: Controversy in Occupational Medicine. New York, Praeger, 1986, pp 415–422.

52. Ng PN, Chan SL, Lee J: Mortality of a cohort of men in a silicosis register: Further evidence of an association with lung cancer. Am J Ind Med 17:163–171, 1990.

53. Pairon JC, Brochard P, Jaurand MC, Bignon J: Silica and lung cancer: A controversial issue. Eur Respir J 4:730–744, 1991.

54. Proposition 65: Chemicals known to the State (of California) to cause cancer or reproductive toxicity. Scientific Advisory Board, Proposition 65, State of California Safe Drinking Water and Toxic Enforcement Act of 1986, 1988.

55. Redmond CK, Weiand HS, Rockette HE, et al: Long-term Mortality Experience of Steelworkers. Cincinnati, U.S. Department of Health and Human Services, Public Health Service, Centers for Disease Control, National Institute for Occupational Health, 1981.

56. Rice CH, Harris RL, Checkoway H, Symons MJ: Dose-response relationships for silicosis from a case-controls study of North Carolina dusty trades workers. In Goldsmith DF, Winn DM, Shy CM (eds): Silica, Silicosis, and Cancer: Controversy in Occupational Medicine. New York, Praeger, 1986, pp 77–86.

57. Saffiotti U: The pathology induced by silica in relation to fibrogenesis and carcinogenesis. In Goldsmith DF, Winn DM, Shy CM (eds): Silica, Silicosis, and Cancer: Controversy in Occupational Medicine. New York, Praeger, 1986, pp 287–307.

58. Saffiotti U, Daniel LH, Mao Y, et al: Biological studies on the carcinogenic mechanisms of quartz. In Guthrie GD, Mossman BT (eds): Health Effects of Mineral Dusts. Washington, DC, Mineralogical Society of America, 1993, pp 523–544.

59. Saffiotti U, Stinson SF: Lung cancer induction by crystalline silica: Relationships to granulomatous reactions and host factors. J Environ Sci Health 6:197–222, 1988.

60. Saffiotti U, Williams AO, Daniel LN, et al: Carcinogenesis by crystalline silica: Animal, cellular, and molecular studies. In Castranova V, Vallyathan V, Wallace WE (eds): Silica and Silica-Induced Diseases: Current Concerns. Boca Raton, FL, CRC Press, 1995, p 345.

61. Selikoff IJ: Carcinogenic potential of silica compounds. In Benz G, Lindquist I (eds): Biochemistry of Silicon and Related Problems. New York, Plenum, 1978, pp 311–336.

62. Simonato L, Fletcher AC, Saracci R, Thomas TL (eds): Occupational Exposure to Silica and Cancer Risk. Lyon, France, International Agency for Research on Cancer, 1990, p 124.

63. Smith AH, Lopipera PA, Barroga VR: Meta-analysis of studies of lung cancer among silicotics. Epidemiology 6:617–624, 1995.

64. Spietoff A, Wesch H, Wegener K, Klimisch H: The effects of thoratrast and quartz on the induction of lung tumors in rats. Health Physics 63:101–110, 1992.

65. Steenland K, Brown DP: Mortality study of goldminers exposed to silica and nonasbestiform amphibole minerals: An update. Am J Ind Med 27:217–229, 1995.

66. Steenland K, Goldsmith DF: Silica exposure and auto-immune diseases. Am J Ind Med 28:603–608, 1995.

67. U.S. Department of Health and Human Services: The Health Consequences of Smoking: Cancer. A Report of the Surgeon General. Rockville, MD, Department of Health and Human Services, Public Health Service, Office of the Assistant Secretary for Health, Office on Smoking and Health, 1982.

68. U.S. Department of Health: Smoking and Health. Washington, DC, U.S. Public Health Service, Office of Surgeon General, 1964.

69. Wagner MMF, Wagner JC, Davies R, Griffiths DM: Silica-induced malignant histiocytic lymphoma: Incidence linked with strain of rat and type of silica. Br J Cancer 41:908–917, 1980.

70. Wagoner JK, Miller RW, Lundin FE, et al: Unusual cancer mortality among a group of underground metal miners. N Engl J Med 269:284–289, 1963.

71. Weisenfeld SL, Perotta DM, Abraham JL: Epidemic of accelerated silicosis in West Texas sand-blasters. In Second International Symposium on Silica, Silicosis, and Cancer, 1993, San Francisco. Western Consortium for Public Health.

72. Williams AO, Saffiotti U: Transforming growth factor beta 1, ras and p53 in silica-induced fibrogenesis and carcinogenesis. Scand J Work Environ Health 21(Suppl 2):30–34, 1995.

73. Winter PD, Gardner MJ, Fletcher AC, Jones RD: A mortality follow-up study of pottery workers: Preliminary findings on lung cancer. In Simonato L, Fletcher AC, Saracci R, Thomas TL (eds): Occupational Exposure to Silica and Cancer Risk. Lyon, France, International Agency for Research on Cancer, 1990, pp 83–94.

74. Wyndham CH, Bezuidenhout BN, Greenacre MJ, Sluis-Cremer GK: Mortality of middle aged white South African gold miners. Br J Ind Med 43:677–684, 1986.

75. Zambon P, Simonato L, Mastrangelo G, et al: A mortality study of workers compensated for silicosis during 1959 to 1963 in the Veneto region of Italy. Scand J Work Environ Health 13:118–123, 1987.

76. Ziskind M, Jones RN, Weill H: Silicosis—Sate of the art review. Am Rev Respir Dis 113:643–665, 1976.

MICHAEL D. ATTFIELD, PhD
GREGORY R. WAGNER, MD

CHRONIC OCCUPATIONAL RESPIRATORY DISEASE

From the Division of Respiratory
  Disease Studies
National Institute for Occupational
  Safety and Health
Morgantown, West Virginia

Reprint requests to:
Michael D. Attfield, PhD
Divison of Respiratory Disease
  Studies
NIOSH, Room 234
1095 Willowdale Road
Morgantown, WV 26505-2888

Epidemiology is an effort to learn the determinants of diseases through the study of human populations. Factors conferring or ameliorating risk are explored through investigation of the distribution of disease in defined groups. In occupational epidemiology, relationships are sought between workplace exposures and human health responses. This chapter considers methodologic issues relevant to epidemiologic investigations of chronic occupational lung diseases. Such studies pose a range of challenges: exposures are often mixed; disease outcomes may be uniquely occupational (e.g., pneumoconioses) or quite nonspecific (e.g., chronic airway dysfunction); and potential subjects available for study move in and out of the workforce, in part depending on health status.

These and other challenges have been met, and at times overcome, in path-breaking efforts to relate coal mine dust exposure to respiratory health effects in miners. The most basic tools of occupational lung disease epidemiology have been used: employment histories, particle counts and mass measurement to estimate exposure; questionnaires, chest radiographs, and spirometry to assess health response.

Each section below discusses a particular methodologic issue pertinent to epidemiologic study of chronic occupational lung disease. Examples to illustrate both problems inherent in chronic occupational lung disease epidemiology and approaches to surmounting them have been selected from the extensive literature on coal miners' lung diseases. Coal miners are probably the most epidemiologically studied group of all workers, and there is a wide variety of types of study from which to draw examples. Although there is a large amount of information concerning other groups of workers (e.g., workers exposed to silica and asbestos), a focus on one disease facilitates comparison among methods. Coal mining was one of the first industries to be studied epidemiologically; early investigations incorporated many novel approaches and techniques, many of which were used much later in the history of epidemiology and remain pertinent today. The rich diversity of information and examples relating to coal miners should compensate for the omission of studies of workers from other industries.

DESCRIPTION OF STUDIES

By 1952 it had become apparent that chronic respiratory disease was an endemic problem among underground coal miners in most coal mining regions of Great Britain. Based on this knowledge and following state takeover of ownership of coal mines, the British National Coal Board initiated an epidemiologic investigation of dust exposure and respiratory disease.[19] The objective was to "determine how much and what kinds of dust cause pneumoconiosis and to establish what environmental conditions should be maintained if mine workers are not to be disabled by the dust that they breathe during the course of their work." Accordingly, a large-scale prospective study, entitled the Pneumoconiosis Field Research (PFR), was begun in 1952. Beginning, as it did, in the early days of epidemiologic inquiry, without the experience that has subsequently developed, the investigation required the development of new procedures to cope with the methodologic problems that were encountered. Medical surveys in the PFR continued until 1986, permitting a wide range of cross-sectional, longitudinal, and other analyses to be undertaken.

In 1945, researchers at the Pneumoconiosis Research Unit (PRU), a branch of the Medical Research Council of Great Britain, had also started conducting epidemiologic studies of respiratory disease in coal miners. They undertook a number of separate studies of various industries, including coal mining,[13,14] in different regions of Great Britain. Their study designs differed somewhat in nature from those of the PFR. Whereas the PFR was mine-based, incorporated exposure measurement as an intrinsic part of the study design, and involved repeated surveys at the same locations, the PRU studies tended to be population-based (and thus included ex-miners and comparison groups of workers from other industries), had little or no exposure data apart from surrogate measures, and involved one or at most two surveys at the same locations.

Although various epidemiologic studies had taken place earlier in different locations in the United States, large-scale, prospective epidemiologic research into miners' respiratory disease in the United States began in 1969, prompted by the passage of the Federal Coal Mine Health and Safety Act of 1969.[5] The American research was patterned broadly after the PFR, although dust concentration was assessed by compliance samples obtained by coal mine operators rather than by the study team. The research, entitled the National Study of Coal Workers' Pneumoconiosis, consisted of three cross-sectional studies at basically the same set of mines, and one follow-up survey of selected study participants from the first two surveys.[5]

More limited studies of coal miners have been undertaken in other countries, but only in Germany has much research been done on exposure-response relationships—and that research has not been undertaken under the auspices of one consistent program. Nevertheless, German researchers have contributed novel analyses, which are included below.

METHODOLOGIC ISSUES

Sample Selection

It is rare for occupational epidemiologic studies to include simple random samples of the general population of workers in an industry. Rather, workers are selected by cluster, e.g., at a specific mine or factory. Such clusters should be selected with a view to the eventual objectives of the study. If the object is to derive absolute measures of disease prevalence for the whole industry, the selection strategy should provide the most efficient estimate. If, however, the objective is to study exposure-response, a different strategy is called for—a strategy in which clusters with widely different exposure levels may be preferentially selected.

In neither the PFR nor the NSCWP were the cohorts representative of all working miners. In fact, the mines in the PFR were specifically selected to fulfill a quasi-experimental design rather than to be representative of all miners. This design encompassed a range of exposures and types of dust, according to four factors at two levels each in a two[4] pattern. Eventually, the sixteen mines selected to fit these criteria were supplemented by another nine to ensure regional representation.[19] In this study and in the NSCWP, larger mines and mines with a long life expectancy were selected preferentially to minimize project costs and to ensure that mines would be in operation for later surveys. As a result, it is likely that disease prevalence estimates from these studies furnished biased estimates for the whole population of miners in their respective countries. However, it is unlikely that this bias greatly affected the estimation of exposure-response.

Study Design

This section concentrates on issues relating to type of study design. Three types are considered: cross-sectional, longitudinal, and case-control.

CROSS-SECTIONAL STUDY

Cross-sectional studies consist of snapshots of the workforce employed at the facilities visited during the short period of the medical surveys. They often do not reflect accurately features of workers ever exposed to the contaminant of concern. Affected workers may have died, left the industry, or sought work in areas of the industry with low exposure, leaving the unusually hardy or healthy to remain at highest risk. Furthermore, they may have been healthier than the average population initially in order to seek or be selected for work in dusty or unpleasant conditions. Smokers may have given up smoking in response to the effects of both dust and tobacco smoke. Exposure estimation for cross-sectional studies is often difficult because of the frequent paucity of prior industrial hygiene data; in addition, work histories have to be drawn from worker interviews.

The PFR and NSCWP both started as cross-sectional medical surveys at groups of mines, at which all employed miners were eligible for examination. Subsequently, the mines were revisited at roughly five-year intervals for further cross-sectional surveys. Various analyses were undertaken on the basis of these surveys. For example, the first round of medical surveys in the NSCWP provided the data for important investigations of exposure-response of CWP prevalence[8] and of ventilatory function level.[6] Cumulative exposures for the period from starting work to the medical survey were computed using self-reported work histories and dust concentration information collected a few years before and after the medical survey.[9] Some evidence of healthy worker selection is seen in the NSCWP first-round results. For example, a nine-year mortality follow-up of the first-round survey miners found that an upward trend in mortality with dust exposure level ceased and reversed at very high exposures.[30] A similar tendency was observed with CWP prevalence and dust exposure. These findings are consistent with the concept that miners must be super hardy to remain at work after suffering lengthy high exposures.

Cross-sectional analyses of data from various rounds of the PFR were also undertaken. In most of these, however, the researchers did not use the complete cross-sectional data set but instead analyzed a subset of miners who had participated in a previous cross-sectional study. For instance, the first epidemiologic evidence of an association between dust exposure and ventilatory function in coal miners was obtained from a cross-sectional analysis of PFR round-three data from miners who had participated previously in the first round of research.[43] This approach had the significant advantage of providing measured exposure data for the ten-year period between the two medical surveys. Another example of the quasi-cross-sectional method is the study of exposure-response for ventilatory function in the PFR, which used data from the fifth round, for miners who had attended the first, third, and fifth rounds of the PFR.[48] Of the 33 years' average tenure for the miners, dust exposure information was available for the last 20 years from the routine sampling undertaken by the study at the mines.

The potential for survivor bias in excess of that of the pure cross-sectional study seems likely, in this quasi-cross-sectional approach, because workers had to be fit enough to work the full inter-survey period. Nevertheless, despite this fear, the findings by Soutar et al. were almost identical to results reported for U.S. miners based on a single cross-sectional study.[6]

LONGITUDINAL STUDY

Longitudinal studies have advantages and disadvantages compared with cross-sectional studies. In the cross-sectional study, the medical status of a study participant is known at only one point in time, and it is often difficult or impossible to determine how he or she developed that condition. For instance, a person with lower than expected lung function may have started work that way or suffered abnormal declines due to toxic exposures at work or elsewhere. They may have changed jobs or stopped smoking because of perceived changes in health, but none of this information is available to the investigator. In contrast, the longitudinal study permits examination of temporal factors related to both exposure and outcome, because the same individuals are observed over time. Moreover, prospective longitudinal studies have the potential for exposure assessment during the study interval and thus provide exposure data of much better quality than is typically available for cross-sectional studies.

Longitudinal studies have limitations, however. If they are based solely on employed workers, they suffer from the potential for bias due to healthy worker selection, because workers who are affected by exposure and leave the industry are not in the group studied. This bias may be greater than that intrinsic to cross-sectional studies, especially with lengthy follow-up periods. In addition, longitudinal studies can be complicated and difficult to analyze compared with cross-sectional study. Whereas the cross-sectional study provides single variables (e.g., one statement concerning cough, one measurement of the forced expiratory volume in one second [FEV_1]), the longitudinal study has repeated measures of each variable. Deciding on the appropriate way to summarize and model these variables can be perplexing. The method of longitudinal analysis seems attractive, because each worker acts as his own control, thereby removing inter-person variation from the analysis and apparently eliminating the need for adjustment. In reality, the perceived potential advantages are not always realized, and adjustment may still be required. In addition, because the outcome variable in longitudinal analyses often involves some measure of change and thus depends on multiple measurements, it may be less reliable than single-point outcome variables. For example, change in ventilatory function derived from two endpoints suffers from twice the degree of measurement variation (equipment plus day-to-day) compared with cross-sectional analyses. Finally, a substantial disturbing factor in longitudinal analysis may be the presence of survey effects. Apparently random factors may cause all data points to be shifted from one survey to another. Potential causes include differences among technicians, interviewers, equipment, and season, although it is often difficult or impossible to determine the cause. These effects severely affect the analysis of longitudinal change in health status.

One of the most significant analyses of longitudinal data in the PFR concerned a ten-year study of CWP incidence and progression. Findings from this study were used by legislators in the setting of both British and U.S. compliance limits for underground miners. Apart from its historical interest, the study was noteworthy for its innovative use of the Markov probabilistic approach to extrapolate from the 10-year incidence and progression to 35-year working-life estimates of CWP prevalence.[26] Another longitudinal PFR study involved research into factors associated with the development of the severe form of CWP: progressive massive fibrosis (PMF). Investigators pooled together information collected over 24 years in six cross-sectional surveys of British coal miners. Within this composite group, data for all miners who were examined at successive medical surveys were identified, and the incidence and progression of CWP were determined. The resulting information was used to obtain 40-year predictions of risk, again using the Markov approach. The study had the advantage of maximizing the amount of information for analysis, which is desirable for reliable estimation of some categories of CWP, although the pooling of possibly somewhat heterogeneous data collected over a wide period does have potential problems.[23]

Both the PFR and the NSCWP included miners actively employed at the work site in their initial rounds of medical surveys. Concentration on working coal miners meant that there was no non-miner group with whom the miners could be compared. This lack of comparison is somewhat of a problem, but it is not a major defect. It is difficult to evaluate absolute measures of certain outcomes, such as ventilatory function variables, in terms of occupational effects. To cite an artificial example, an overall 55-ml decline in FEV_1 per year among miners may be thought to be excessive. But without a comparison group it is difficult to know whether this is a real effect of exposure or due to one or more extraneous factors, such as methodologic effects (e.g., systematic variation in measurement from survey to survey) or a general tendency for high rates of lung function decline in the region in which the miners lived. With good exposure measures, this problem is largely mitigated, however, for then it is possible to study relative effects. For instance, it may be found that miners with high dust exposures suffered a 65-ml decline, whereas miners working on the surface area had only 45-ml declines. Hence, it is likely that exposure to coal mine dust causes about a 20-ml additional decrement in annual decline. This excess may be compared with estimates of typical annual decline widely available in the literature for the general population.*[1]

Longitudinal analysis was also made of ventilatory function changes in several studies by examining change over two points in time.[32,46] Despite expectations that the longitudinal approach may be a more powerful method for assessment of dust exposure effects, the findings on exposure-response were less clear than the findings obtained from corresponding cross-sectional studies. Probable reasons were the extra random error inherent in using a response variable dependent on two measurements (initial and final), possible survey effects, and the small range of dust concentration levels encountered during the longitudinal period in the NSCWP study compared with the much wider range in the cross-sectional analysis.

Recent German longitudinal investigations involving assessment of exposure-response for CWP have used a different approach from all previous British and U.S. studies. The researchers took advantage of the fact that about 10 sequential radiographs were available for the miners for a period of 20 years. Hence, they were able to use an adaption of survival analysis, in which the outcome was development of CWP (small opacities).[36] Careful parameterization of the model enabled them to estimate a threshold limit value and also an influence limit value (an exposure above which the response does not increase).

CASE-CONTROL STUDY

Case-control methods are typically applied in situations in which the outcome is rare. They provide a powerful and efficient approach and have been used extensively in studies of cancer outcomes. They have been used infrequently in studies of chronic respiratory disease in coal miners, generally because most of the outcome variables studied (e.g., CWP or chest symptoms) are common. Another reason for their disfavor is the difficulty in identifying appropriate comparison groups. In many coal mining areas there are few industries other than the coal mines; if other indutries exist, they, too, are dusty (e.g., steel making). There is the danger, then, that individuals who choose not to go into mining or other dusty jobs may be less healthy; therefore, their inclusion as controls would lead to bias in the findings.

In one of the few case-control studies of coal mine lung disease, a group of 245 miners who developed the severe form of CWP over about 11 years were compared with controls.[33] The intent was to discover the relationship between PMF development and a range of environmental and medical factors. Case-control methods were

---

* Oddly enough, it is for CWP that a comparison or baseline estimate of prevalence may be useful. One would expect that CWP would be found only in workers exposed to coal mine dust and that zero prevalence logically would be found in a non-exposed group. The problem arises, however, because the ILO classification of pneumoconiosis used worldwide to categorize chest radiographs is based on the detection of small opacities on the x-ray.[25] These small opacities may or may not actually coincide with the dust deposits and nodules of CWP. As a result, the prevalence of small opacities is probably not zero in individuals unexposed to coal mine dust and probably rises with age. Hence, in an exposed group, the increasing prevalence of small opacities (often equated with CWP) corresponds to the effects of both dust exposure and a general background level. As a consequence, the availability of a comparison group could help to isolate the two effects, permitting better estimation of the dust exposure factor alone. Other methods, such as the inclusion of an age effect in modeling, are less satisfactory, because the effect of dust exposure on disease development may vary with age (consistent with either more susceptibility with age or, conversely, the loss of susceptible individuals from the work place) or perhaps age reflects inadequacies in the estimated exposures, among other things.

useful because of the wide variety of variables of interest to be explored. The study reported that certain factors, such as body shape and presence of chest symptoms, appeared to be related to PMF development, although it failed to reveal any obvious effects of dust composition or particle size apart from residence time in the lungs. Another case-control study, currently continuing, is designed to elucidate information about causes of rapid lung function decline in U.S. miners. Analysis of existing data is to be followed by new, detailed medical examinations of cases and controls.[51]

Selection Issues

With two exceptions, the data gathered during the PFR and NSCWP were collected from working coal miners. The study results may be biased, because only workers fit enough to continue in the mines are included in the cohorts. The investigators for both studies accepted this point and took steps to include ex-miners in additional studies. In analyses that included ex-miners,[10,34,46,48] the findings revealed that ex-miners had more lung disease and abnormality than current workers. This finding prompted the question as to whether workers who had developed disease and had left mining were more susceptible to dust. However, little evidence was found that ex-miners and current miners differed in terms of their exposure-response relationship for CWP and dust exposure. Hence, it appeared that greater exposure rather than susceptibility was responsible for the elevated levels of abnormality in the ex-workers, and the reality of a survivor effect on the remaining working population was confirmed.

Another selection issue concerns workers who choose not to participate in epidemiologic studies. Nonparticipants may refuse to take part in a study for various reasons. In some instances, less healthy workers may be concerned, despite assurances to the contrary, that their medical status may be reported to the company, with the fear that they might then lose their job. They would then choose not to be examined. The concern for the epidemiologist is not only that this trend would lead to biased prevalence figures, but also that estimates of exposure-response may be biased. Alternatively, workers who perceive themselves to be unhealthy may be more likely to avail themselves of a free medical examination. This issue was examined in two studies of coal miners. In the first, prior data were analyzed according to whether the miners chose or chose not to be examined in medical surveys held about ten years later.[20] In most respects (e.g., age, height, smoking status) the two groups were similar. Nonparticipants, however, had slightly lower initial ventilatory function despite lower cumulative exposures to dust. This finding prompted the question as to whether nonparticipants were more susceptible to the effects of dust. Upon analysis, however, this was not found to be the case. A study of U.S. coal miners[39] did a similar analysis, although without the benefit of dust exposures. Findings again suggested that ventilatory function was lower in nonparticipants to a small degree, although prevalence of CWP was actually less. Perhaps contrary to the British study, there was a suggestion that nonparticipants were more susceptible to exposure to coal mine dust, but because the surrogate years underground rather than measured exposure had to be used, it is not possible to be certain.

ESTIMATING EXPOSURE-RESPONSE

Exposure Metrics

Cumulative exposure is probably the most appropriate exposure metric for use in connection with chronic occupational respiratory disease. Chronic diseases usually develop slowly and may require the accumulated effects of years of exposure to become manifest. For the pneumoconioses, in particular CWP, disease development is determined to a large extent by the slow deposition and accumulation of particles in the lung. For this reason, cumulative exposure, derived as the sum of products of time and dust concentration, has been the primary exposure metric evaluated in many British and U.S. studies of health effects in coal miners. Researchers have demonstrated links with CWP,[8,28] respiratory symptoms,[40,45] and ventilatory function.[6,43]

Cumulative exposure, although a useful indicator of risk, clearly has its potential drawbacks. It does not, for example, take intensity of exposure (peak effects) into account very well. A large cumulative exposure may have been due either to high dust concentrations for a short period or to low exposures for a lengthy period. One may reasonably suspect that different exposure patterns would have different implications for disease causation and development. Slow, low exposures provide the opportunity for the body to clear the particles, whereas high exposures may overwhelm the defense mechanisms. Neither does cumulative exposure account for the time the dust remains in the lungs, that is, the so-called residence time effect.

These and other exposure metrics have been examined in coal mining to some extent. Peak exposures were investigated in one German study.[41] The results suggested that workers with greater peak exposures for given cumulative exposure had a higher risk of contracting CWP. The same researchers also looked at residence time through use of an exposure metric based on summing the products of exposure level and time from first exposure to medical examination.[41] The results suggested that younger miners should be especially protected from high exposures. In one study,[22] dust level and exposure time were entered separately to a logistic model using the form:

$$\alpha \log (\text{mean dust concentration}) + \beta \log (\text{exposure duration})$$

where α and β are the regression coefficients for dust concentration and exposure duration. This approach permits separate weights to be estimated for exposure level and duration and is equivalent to a power of cumulative exposure if α and β are similar in magnitude. Thus use of (duration of exposure)^2 rather than simple duration may be more appropriate. The authors commented that this approach may imply a dust residence time effect. Overall, however, the respective superiority or validity of different exposure metrics has not been fully investigated. An approach was recently suggested for fitting a generalized model that takes into account both exposure level and exposure time.[47] As special cases it included cumulative exposure, mean exposure, mean time worked, and residence time. The method was applied to two medical outcomes among coal miners with mixed results.

There are countless ways to measure dust exposure. Methods to assess worker exposures in coal mining have changed as knowledge increased and new techniques became available. Much of the early sampling was based on particle counts (e.g., impingers in the U.S.[11] and thermal precipitators in the U.K.[19]). Early experience with application of such data to health outcomes revealed, however, that the better correlate with CWP incidence was not particle count but particle weight.[27] As a result, gravimetric assessment of dust concentrations is now customary in most countries where coal is mined.

The PFR investigation included regular sampling and analysis for silica and other minerals in the airborne mine dust. The measurements were used to derive cumulative exposures and were applied to a number of exposure-response analyses, in addition to cumulative mixed mine dust exposures.[21,22,28,50] Overall, however, evidence repeatedly suggested that the main factor determining CWP incidence and progression was mixed mine dust. Silica dust appeared to play a lesser role, except in high concentrations.[35,44] There was also an indication that the prevalence and incidence of CWP were lower in mines in which the level of clay dust (e.g., kaolin and mica) was high.[50] (This observation prompted an investigation of particles using a novel approach involving electron microscopy, which indicates that clays may occlude silica particles, thereby preventing activity in the lungs.[49]) Coal rank, a measure related to the degree of coal metamorphosis by heat and pressure, has also been found to be an important determinant of CWP occurrence.[8,42,50]

Despite the fact that dust exposure is an excellent predictor of CWP prevalence and incidence, substantial unexplained variation exists from mine to mine.[16] This finding has led to exploration of other potentially important exposure characteristics such as particle composition and particle size.

Much of the early epidemiologic work relating to coal miners was directed toward elucidating the relationship between dust exposure and CWP. Thus researchers concentrated on the dust metric thought to be most pertinent to CWP causation, i.e., respirable dust, which is defined by a curve representing the proportion of particles of different size that deposit deep into the lung (alveolar region).[29] Sampling instruments were devised to simulate this pattern of size selection.[29] Later—and of necessity, because no other data were available—the same exposure metrics were used to investigate exposure-response for nonpneumoconiotic outcomes, such as ventilatory function and symptoms. It was acknowledged[40,43] that respirable dust may not be the index most relevant to the causation of such diseases; rather, thoracic dust may be more appropriate, because obstructive lung disease and bronchitis (for instance) develop higher in the respiratory tract and in a region where larger-sized particles preferentially deposit. To date, however, the few attempts to develop and use dust exposures pertinent to thoracic or other upper respiratory tract regions have not demonstrated significant superiority over the original metrics based on respirable dust.

Exposure-Response Models

Apart from mortality studies, two main modeling approaches have dominated epidemiologic investigations of lung disease in coal miners: the linear regression approach, used extensively in studies of ventilatory function, and the logistic model, used for much of the exposure-response modeling for CWP. Mention has already been made of a related topic, the choice of exposure metric, but obviously the selection of model form is also critical to the outcome of the analysis. Various model forms can be considered for CWP: the threshold model, the zero risk at zero exposure model, and the non-zero risk at zero exposure model. The first approach was intrinsic to the first major exposure-response analysis of CWP in underground coal miners.[28] Undertaken on 10-year incidence data for British miners, it used the arcsine square root transformation of the binomial response to stabilize the variance. This method leads to an S-shaped exposure-response curve, similar to that of the probit or logistic functions. Unlike the probit or logit curves, however, the exposure-response curve can touch zero response at a non-zero exposure, thereby allowing for a threshold. The actual analysis indicated zero response at an exposure close to 2 mg/m^3 (for a 35-year working life). Later British studies used the logistic model.[21,22] The use of logarithms of dust level and exposure period (as discussed earlier) with the logistic model constrained the predicted risk to be zero at either zero dust concentration or zero exposure time and non-zero elsewhere. Hence, this approach embodied a different perspective from the threshold model used earlier. It also implies a different viewpoint in the use of age and untransformed cumulative exposure adopted in U.S. studies.[8,10] This model takes into account the problem of a background of apparent abnormality. It permits the predicted prevalence of abnormality to be non-zero at zero dust exposure and allows the prevalence to rise with increasing age as well as increasing exposure. Other approaches are, of course, possible but have not been exhaustively explored.

One problem inherent in complex modeling of disease outcomes with regard to exposure involves the potential for interference by worker selection effects. For example, loss of affected individuals from the study group would result in lower observed prevalences of disease at the highest exposure levels than actually existed among all miners and ex-miners. Models fitted to such data, therefore, would be pulled downward at higher exposure levels. The pivoting effect around the mean thereby created would cause overestimates for predicted prevalences at lower concentrations, thus disturbing the observed exposure-response relationship in that area, a region of exposure in which threshold and related effects normally would be sought for application to risk assessment and standard setting.

Choice of Outcome Variable

In studies of pneumoconiosis a wide variety of methods have been used to condense the available information into concise yet meaningful outcome variables. The International Labour Office (ILO) classification for the pneumoconioses provides a 12-point scale of abnormality, thus offering potentially 12 different outcome variables. The ILO categories represent ordinal scores rather than measured ratio variables. Moreover, since x-ray reading is a somewhat subjective process, most studies include readings by several readers. This strategy, of course, provides even more choice of analytic approach.

Early in the history of epidemiologic analysis of coal miner data, an attempt was made to derive a linearizing transformation for x-ray scores.[53] This approach was based on the concept that each category in the ILO classification is not equally spaced along a continuum in the true development of the disease. It was argued that the difference between categories 0 and 1 represents a much longer period of disease development than the interval between categories 1 and 2 or 2 and 3. This argument has credence in terms of observed disease incidence, because progression rates of disease tend to be much higher than corresponding incidence rates for the same exposure level. However, after some initial use, the transformation fell into disfavor.

In one PFR analysis, the 12-point ILO categories were converted to integer values, and the resulting scores were averaged over all readers, converted back to the 12-point scale, and then dichotomized for analysis as a proportion.[28] An alternative technique for averaging across readers is to take consensus or median readings. In the first approach, the final determination is based on agreement by two or more readers as to the profusion category (on either the 4-point or 12-point scale). If agreement does not exist between the readers, further readings have to be obtained. The second approach is simpler, relying on the simple median of the available ILO scores. No method is entirely satisfactory. The arithmetic mean approach ignores the fact that the data are not measurements but rather represent unequal stages on a continuum of disease. The median method gets into minor difficulties when the number of available readings is even and the true median does not lie exactly within one of the available categories. In this case, an arbitrary decision must be made to round down or up to the next available category. An alternative to the summarization methods noted above is to undertake exposure-response model fitting to the data from each x-ray reader separately and then to summarize the resulting information from the fitted curves. There are several ways in which this can be done. One is to average the coefficients across models.[22] Another is to take some type of average of the predicted values from the individual models.

Another issue concerns type of opacity. In the past, convention called for examination of rounded opacities for the coal- and silica-related pneumoconioses and irregular opacities for asbestos- and other fiber-related pneumoconioses. Indeed, until 1980 the ILO classification scheme was set up to elicit separately information about the profusion of opacities of each type.[24] However, it became clear that the distinction between rounded and irregular types was somewhat artificial. Not only were irregular types evident and related to dust exposure in coal miners,[15] but it was frequently found that readers could disagree among themselves on the type of opacity on the radiograph. The most recent version of the ILO classification[25] changes the main reading focus from type of opacity to profusion and thus goes some way to alleviating the problem. However, there remains much controversy about the significance of irregular opacities, particularly with regard to smoking.[12,17,52]

Most ventilatory function variables (e.g., FEV_1, forced vital capacity [FVC], flow rates) are measured on a continuous scale. Three approaches are generally used in their analysis: direct modeling based on the observed values, analysis of observed/predicted ratios, and analysis of derived dichotomous variables according to some health-based criterion (e.g., <80% of predicted). Overall, the first approach is considered the most powerful and valid, when data are sufficient, and the objective is to model exposure-response. Use of observed/predicted ratios has its limitations in this situation, because the population from which the predicted equation was obtained may not be strictly applicable to the worker group. This would lead to spurious conclusions. Lastly, analysis based on dichotomous variables may be less powerful than analysis of the continuous variables themselves.

Use of average values of ventilatory function variables as summary measures of overall effect has been questioned.[38] It has been argued that small decrements due to coal mine dust exposure observed among the majority give rise to an average effect that may be similar to the combination of a large decrement in a minority with no change in the remainder, corresponding to the effects of cigarette exposure. As a consequence, what may appear to be similar average effects of coal mine dust exposure and cigarette smoking overall conceal important differences in actual abnormality. However, an analysis that looked into the distribution of FEV_1 values in coal miners failed to confirm this hypothesis.[7]

Exposure Estimation for Epidemiologic Analysis

Exposure estimation is critical; unfortunately, it is often the weakest part of epidemiologic studies. All too often, insufficient resources are allocated, or the information available is severely limited. In addition, when environmental samples are taken, they are not collected in a manner that is clearly linked with the objectives and hypotheses of the epidemiologic analysis. Generally an optimal sampling strategy for epidemiologic studies differs from the strategy used to assess compliance with dust standards.

A prospective study with simultaneous collection of environmental and health information provides the opportunity for a well-controlled investigation. This was the case for the PFR.[19] When the study was begun, industrial hygienists were stationed at the mines permanently to collect daily dust exposure measurements. As a result, many thousands of measurements were made, furnishing probably the best database on coal miner exposures in the world.

The PFR went even further, however, incorporating many novel approaches and procedures, some of which were rediscovered and publicized much later. Realizing that industrial hygiene assessment of the mining environment was not a separate task distinct from the eventual epidemiologic analysis but a task that must be intrinsically connected to the ultimate hypotheses to be examined, the researchers devised a scheme for optimal allocation of sampling effort to the measurement of dust concentrations.[2] Only recently have these issues been revisited.

Noting that the total effort that could be allocated to environmental characterization was limited by available funds and personnel, the researchers set out to identify a criterion for best allocation and to isolate factors that impinged on attainment of that criterion. They decided that the overall objective would be to minimize the average variance of the workers' cumulative exposure estimates (or, alternatively, to minimize the sum of the variances over all workers). Observing that cumulative exposures are derived as sums of products of dust concentrations and time spent in jobs, they derived an expression for the variance of any worker's cumulative exposure in terms of the innate variation of the dust concentrations for that job, the numbers of workers who normally work in that job, and the time normally spent in the job. The resulting formula told the hygienists how to allocate their sampling effort. In general, jobs with higher intrinsic variation, more workers, or higher exposure times received the greater attention. It should be noted, however, that the adopted criterion, although logical, is only one of a number that could be selected. In a sense it is generic and not directed toward any particular statistical analysis of exposure-response.

Fundamental to the assessment of worker exposures was the adoption of the concept of occupational groups. Realizing that separate assessment of exposures for each worker by use of personal sampling was far beyond the means available to the study, the researchers developed the idea of occupational groups. Workers with similar dust exposures would be placed together in groups and the group mean concentration applied to each miner who worked in the group. To ensure that the group mean was applicable to each miner, the industrial hygienist was told to select a miner at random from the pool of workers in the group and to sample him for one shift. This concept was reinvented some time later, and discussions of related issues continue in the literature.

DATA VALIDITY AND RELIABILITY

Although methods for standardization of spirometry have been well established,[1] use of questionnaires and radiographs as well as exposure measurement pose particular problems for assurance of data reliability. The PFR addressed many of these problems.

Data collected for epidemiologic study should be as reproducible and valid as possible. Pains should be taken to minimize variation caused by interviewers, technicians, equipment, or badly worded questionnaires. Reported data should reflect the actual abnormality outcomes under investigation.

Because it was a large study and employed a large number of technicians, many of whom worked at some distance from each other, the PFR was in danger of suffering from poor data due to by inter-technician and inter-interviewer differences and variation. For example, assessment of dust concentrations required manual examination of glass slides for particle counting, and technicians were employed in various regions of Britain for this task.[19] Similarly, different field teams surveyed different coal fields, with the potential for systematic variation in responses to questionnaires and to pulmonary function tests arising from methodologic causes, including personal characteristics (e.g., sex, age, manner, appearance) of the team staff.

To monitor and correct traits associated with inter-technician differences, an extensive and continuing series of procedures was put into place. Often, these procedures required special trials or studies at regular intervals, at which the different personnel would undertake repeat operations on the same entities (e.g., count the same slides). The results from the different technicians were compared, and if differences of note were found, remedial action was taken (retraining, for instance).

Details from a series of trials of questionnaires interviewing clerks illustrate the hazards to data quality that may be encountered in epidemiologic studies involving respiratory symptoms questionnaires. The different interviewers were brought together and employed on the same medical survey. (They interviewed separate groups of miners and did not do repeat interviews because of the possibility that the interviewee would remember previous replies.) During some of the interviews, a supervisor sat nearby and listened to the interviews. Comparison of the percentages of positive responses to each question obtained by each interviewer revealed systematic differences for some questions. Sometimes such differences persisted despite retraining. Various reasons were found for interviewer differences. One interviewer was reformulating questions (perhaps believing that the question was poorly worded and needed improvement or perhaps simply to alleviate boredom). Sometimes an interviewer would force answers instead of sticking to the protocol that an ambiguous answer would be taken as a "no." Although these variations in interviewing behavior naturally affected the overall responses, some differences in responses could not be explained by observable technique.

Chest radiographs are commonly used in epidemiologic studies of chronic occupational respiratory disease, because many dusts cause radiologic abnormality of one kind or another. Multiple readers (typically three or more) must be employed, because x-rays readers differ among themselves, despite persistent attempts to achieve consistency. The PFR set up a system to monitor the performance of the different readers.[19] Because it had been shown that the B-reader certification program for x-ray readers in the U.S.[31] had not been totally successful in eliminating major discrepancies among readers,[4,18] a strategy designed to minimize reader disagreement was used in a recent study of exposure-response for CWP. Readers were selected from a pool of experienced interpreters who had been engaged in reading radiographs for a large surveillance program of coal miners, according to their relative prevalence ranking.[3] It was hoped that this strategy would result in readings that reflected typical levels among all B-readers and thus give rise to generally representative findings.

CONCLUSION

Numerous methodologic issues have been recognized and substantially overcome in epidemiologic investigations of chronic occupational respiratory diseases in coal miners. The extensive literature reporting findings from these efforts provides substantial guidance relevant to the design of investigations of other occupational groups and industries.

REFERENCES

1. American Thoracic Society Statement: Standardization of Spirometry–1994 Update. Am J Respir Crit Care Med 152:1107–1136, 1995.
2. Ashford JR: The design of a long-term sampling programme to measure the hazard associated with an industrial environment. J R Statist Soc A 121:333–347, 1958.

3. Attfield MD, Althouse RB: Surveillance data on U.S. coal miners' pneumoconiosis, 1970 to 1986. Am J Public Health 82:971-977, 1992.

4. Attfield MD, Althouse RB, Reger RB: An investigation of inter-reader variability among X-ray readers employed in the underground coal miner surveillance program. Ann Am Conf Gov Ind Hyg 14:401–409, 1986.

5. Attfield MD, Castellan RM: Epidemiological data on U.S. coal miners' pneumoconiosis, 1960 to 1988. Am J Public Health 82:964–970, 1992.

6. Attfield MD, Hodous TK: Pulmonary function of U.S. coal miners related to dust exposure estimates. Am Rev Respir Dis 14:605–609, 1992.

7. Attfield MD, Hodous TK: Does regression analysis of lung function data obtained from occupational epidemiologic studies lead to misleading inferences regarding the true effect of smoking? Am J Ind Med 27:281–291, 1995.

8. Attfield MD, Morring K: An investigation into the relationship between coal workers' pneumoconiosis and dust exposure in U.S. coal miners. Am Ind Hyg Assoc J 53:486–492, 1992.

9. Attfield MD, Morring K: The derivation of estimated dust exposures for U.S. coal miners working before 1970. Am Ind Hyg Assoc J 53:248–255, 1992.

10. Attfield MD, Seixas NS: Prevalence of pneumoconiosis and its relationship to dust exposure in a cohort of U.S. bituminous coal miners and ex-miners. Am J Ind Med 27:137–151, 1995.

11. Baier EJ, Diakun R: Comparison of dust exposures in Pennsylvania anthracite and bituminous coal mines. Am Ind Hyg Assoc J 25:476–480, 1964.

12. Blanc PD: Cigarette smoking and pneumoconiosis: Structuring the debate [editorial]. Am J Ind Med 16:1–4, 1989.

13. Cochrane AL: The attack rate of progressive massive fibrosis: Br J Ind Med 19:52–64, 1962.

14. Cochrane AL, Higgins ITT, Thomas J: Pulmonary ventilatory functions of coalminers in various areas in relation to the X-ray category of pneumoconiosis. Br J Prev Soc Med 15:1–11, 1961.

15. Collins HPR, Dick JA, Bennett JG, et al: Irregularly shaped small shadows on chest radiographs, dust exposure, and lung function in coalworkers' pneumoconiosis. Br J Ind Med 45:43–55, 1988.

16. Crawford NP, Bodsworth FL, Dodgson J: A study of the apparent anomalies between dust levels and pneumoconiosis at several British collieries. In Walton WH (ed): Inhaled Particles V. Pergamon Press, Oxford, 1982, pp 725–744.

17. Dick JA, Morgan WKC, Muir DCF, et al: The significance of irregular opacities on the chest roentgenogram. Chest 102:251–260, 1992.

18. Ducatman AM, Yang WN, Forman SA: 'B-readers' and asbestos medical surveillance: J Occup Med 30:644–647, 1988.

19. Fay JWJ, Rae S: The Pneumoconiosis Field Research of the National Coal Board. Ann Occup Hyg 1:149–161, 1959.

20. Gauld SJ, Hurley JF, Miller BG: Differences between long-term participants and non-responders in a study of coalminers' respiratory health and exposure to dust. Ann Occup Hyg 32:545–551, 1988.

21. Hurley JF, Alexander WP, Hazledine DJ, et al: Exposure to respirable coalmine dust and incidence of progressive massive fibrosis. Br J Ind Med 44:661–672, 1987.

22. Hurley JF, Burns J, Copland L, et al: Coalworkers' simple pneumoconiosis and exposure to dust at 10 British coalmines. Br J Ind Med 39:120–127, 1982.

23. Hurley JF, Maclaren WM: Dust-related Risks of Radiological Changes in Coalminers over a 40-Year Working Life: Report TM/87/09. Edinburgh, Institute of Occupational Medicine, 1987.

24. International Labour Office: ILO U/C International Classification of Radiographs of Pneumoconioses 1971. Occupational Safety and Health, Series no. 22 (Rev). Geneva, International Labour Office, 1972.

25. International Labour Office: Guidelines for the Use of ILO International Classification of Radiographs of Pneumoconioses [abstract]. Genva, International Labour Office, 1980.

26. Jacobsen M: Effects of some approximations in analyses of radiological response to coalmine dust exposure. In Proceedings of International Symposium on Recent Advances in the Assessment of the Health Effects of Environmental Pollution, Paris, 24–28 June, 1974, vol. I. Luxembourg, CEC, 1975, pp 211–229.

27. Jacobsen M, Rae S, Walton WH, Rogan JM: New dust standards for British coal mines. Nature 227:445–447, 1970.

28. Jacobsen M, Rae S, Walton WH, Rogan JM: The relation between pneumoconiosis and dust exposure in British coal mines. In Walton WH (ed): Inhaled Particles III. Old Woking, England, Unwin Brothers, 1971, pp 903–919.

29. Jacobson M: Respirable dust in bituminous coal mines in the U.S. In Walton WH (ed): Inhaled Particles III. Old Woking, England, Unwin Brothers, 1971, pp 745–756.

30. Kuempel ED, Stayner LT, Attfield MD, Buncher CR: Exposure-response analysis of mortality among coal miners in the United States. Am J Ind Med 28:167–184, 1995.
31. Liddell FDK, Morgan WKC: Methods for assessing serial films of the pneumoconioses: A review. J Soc Occup Med 28:6–15, 1978.
32. Love RG, Miller BG: Longitudinal study of lung function in coal-miners. Thorax 37:193–197, 1982.
33. Maclaren WM, Hurley JF, Collins HPR, Cowie AJ: Factors associated with the development of progressive massive fibrosis in British coalminers: A case-control study: Br J Ind Med 46:597–607, 1989.
34. Maclaren WM, Soutar CA: Progressive massive fibrosis and simple pneumoconiosis in ex-miners. Br J Ind Med 42:734–740, 1985.
35. Miller BG, Addison J, Brown GM, et al: The effects of quartz in coalmine dust—a synthesis of results from research in the British coal industry. In Hurych J, Lesage M, David A (eds): Proceedings of the Eighth International Conference on Occupational Lung Diseases, September, 1992, Prague, vol. 2. Prague, Czech Medical Society, 1993, pp 594–602.
36. Morfeld P, Rohleder F, Vautrin H-J, et al: An epidemiological approach in estimating a threshold limit value for respirable dust in German hard coal mining. Ann Occup Hyg 38(Suppl 1): 799–803, 1994.
37. Morgan RH: Proficiency examination of physicians for classifying pneumoconiosis chest films. A J R 132:803–808, 1979.
38. Morgan WKC: Industrial bronchitis. Br J Ind Med 35:285–291, 1978.
39. Petersen M, Attfield M: Estimates of bias in a longitudinal coal study. J Occup Med 23:44–48, 1981.
40. Rae S, Walker DD, Attfield MD: Chronic bronchitis and dust exposure in British coalminers. In Walton WH (ed): Inhaled Particles III. Old Woking, England, Unwin Bros, 1971, pp 883–896.
41. Reisner MTR: Results of epidemiological studies of pneumoconiosis in West German coal mines[asbstract]. II:921, 1971.
42. Reisner MTR, Robock K: Results of epidemiological, mineralogical, and cytotoxicogical studies on the pathogenicity of coal-mine dusts. In Walton WH (ed): Inhaled Particles IV. Oxford, Pergamon Press, 1977, pp 703–716.
43. Rogan JM, Attfield MD, Jacobsen M, et al: Role of dust in the working environment in development of chronic bronchitis in British coal miners. Br J Ind Med 30:217–226, 1973.
44. Seaton A, Dodgson J, Dick JA, Jacobsen M: Quartz and pneumoconiosis in coalminers. Lancet 1272–1275, 1981.
45. Seixas NS, Robins TG, Attfield MD, Moulton LH: Exposure-response relationships for coal mine dust and obstructive lung disease following enactment of the Federal Coal Mine Health and Safety Act of 1969. Am J Ind Med 21:715–734, 1992.
46. Seixas NS, Robins TG, Attfield MD, Moulton LH: Longitudinal and cross sectional analyses of exposure to coal mine dust and pulmonary function in new miners. Br J Ind Med 50:929–937, 1993.
47. Seixas NS, Robins TG, Becker M: A novel approach to the characterization of cumulative exposure for the study of chronic occupational disease. Am J Epidemiol 137:463–471, 1993.
48. Soutar CA, Hurley JF: Relation between dust exposure and lung function in miners and ex-miners. Br J Ind Med 43:307–320, 1986.
49. Wallace WE, Harrison JC, Grayson RL, et al: Aluminosilicate surface contamination of respirable quartz particles from coal mine dusts and from clay works dusts. Ann Occup Hyg 1994.
50. Walton WH, Dodgson J, Hadden GG, Jacobsen M: The effect of quartz and other non-coal dusts in coalworkers' pneumoconiosis. In Walton WH (ed): Inhaled Particles IV, vol 2. Oxford, Pergamon Press, 1977, pp 669–689.
51. Wang ML, Petsonk EL, Attfield MD, et al: Miners with clinically important declines in FEV_1: Analysis of data from the U.S. National Coal Study. App Occup Env Hyg 1996 [in press].
52. Weiss W: State of the art. Cigarette smoke, asbestos, and small irregular opacities. Am Rev Respir Dis 130:293–301, 1984.
53. Wise ME, Oldham PD: Effect of radiographic technique on readings of categories of simple pneumoconiosis. Br J Industr Med 20:145–153, 1963.

KI MOON BANG, PhD, MPH

EPIDEMIOLOGY OF OCCUPATIONAL CANCER

From the Division of Respiratory
Disease Studies
National Institute for Occupational
Safety and Health
Morgantown, West Virginia

Reprint requests to:
Ki Moon Bang, PhD, MPH
Division of Respiratory Disease
Studies
NIOSH-Room 234
1095 Willowdale Road
Morgantown, WV 26505-2888

Cancer is a major cause of morbidity and mortality worldwide. Occupational carcinogens were among the first human carcinogens to be identified, and the causal relationship between occupational exposures and some human cancers has been established. Occupational carcinogens include chemical substances, physical agents, and microbiological agents that are present in the workplace. Occupational carcinogens may cause a significant increase in a particular type of cancer in the exposed working population. Although the number of known occupational carcinogens to humans are limited so far, the prevention of occupational cancer and the protection of workers against exposure to carcinogens are needed. This chapter provides an up-to-date review of the occurrence and causes of occupational cancer based on epidemiologic studies in humans, characteristics of occupational cancer, research priorities, and cancer surveillance.

MAGNITUDE OF OCCUPATIONAL CANCER

Cancer is the second leading cause of death in the United States.[94] The American Cancer Society estimated 1,359,000 new cancer cases in 1996 based on data from the Surveillance, Epidemiology, and End Results (SEER) program of the National Cancer Institute.[6] A recent report showed that age-adjusted incidence rates for all cancers combined increased by 18.6% among males and 12.4% among females from 1975–1979 to 1987–1991, due to large increases in prostate cancer incidence rates in men and for breast and lung cancer in women.[17]

More than half of a million deaths due to cancer, with an annual age-adjusted cancer mortality of 133.1 per 100,000 population in 1992, were reported.[94,95] About 30–40% of Americans will develop cancer during their lifetimes.[25] Cancer mortality is increasing, and occupational exposures appear to account for at least part of the pattern.

The proportion of occupational cancer to exposure is difficult to precisely calculate. Adequate data that allow calculations of the number of exposed individuals or levels of exposure are not available. Two possible approaches to calculate the proportion of cancer due to occupation[33] include the following:

1. Calculation based on exposure to occupational factors. In this case, it is necessary to know (a) the total population exposed to the hazard, (b) the duration and level of exposure, (c) confounding variables, and (d) the increased relative risk associated with exposure at different dose levels.

2. Calculation based on evaluating the cause of cancer at each site. It is probably more appropriate to examine cancers at each site and to calculate the proportion due to defined or suspected factors. From such calculations, it may be possible to establish the upper limits of the proportion of cancers that could be predominantly due to occupational factors.

An investigation in the United Kingdom showed that only 6% of cancers might be occupationally related to exposures in the workplace, while 88% are due to other lifestyle factors.[33] In 1991, Vineis and Simonato evaluated the proportion of cancers attributable to occupation.[104] The proportion ranged from 1–5% when considering only exposure to asbestos and 40% for subjects exposed to ionizing radiation. Three quarters of occupational cancers among men are found in the lungs.[18] Between 13–27% of lung cancers are attributable to some form of occupational exposure and, in particular, asbestos exposure.[47] Up to 25% of bladder cancer cases in the general population can be attributed to occupational exposure.[83,103,104] These estimates were determined by the prevalence of exposed individuals within the general population and the proportion of individuals actually exposed within the group under consideration. Doll and Peto have estimated that about 4% of all cancer deaths can be attributed to occupational exposures.[18] Recently, Leigh and coworkers estimated that 6–10% of all cancers have occupational origins.[50] In the United States, this would represent 80,897–134,828 new cancer cases and 33,018–55,030 deaths due to occupational exposures in 1996 (Tables 1 and 2).

TABLE 1.   Estimated Incidence of Occupational Cancer, United States, 1996

	Estimated Number of New Cases*		Percentage Due to Occupation†	Estimated Number of Cases Due to Occupation
	All Ages	25 Years & Older		
All sites	1,359,150	1,348,277	6–10	80,897–134,828
Lung	177,000	176,929	10	17,693
Prostate	317,100	314,563	1	3,146
Leukemia	27,600	25,723	7	1,801
Bladder	52,900	52,879	7	3,702
Skin	38,300	37,994	6	2,280

* Estimated by the American Cancer Society, 1996.
† Estimated by Richard Doll and Richard Peto, 1981.

TABLE 2.   Estimated Number of Deaths Due to Occupational Cancer, United States, 1996

Cancer Site	Estimated Number of Deaths*		Percentage Due to Occupation†	Estimated Number of Deaths Due to Occupation
	All Ages	25 Years & Older		
All sites	554,740	550,302	6–10	33,018–55,030
Lung	158,700	158,636	10	15,864
Prostate	41,400	41,069	1	411
Leukemia	21,000	19,572	7	1,370
Bladder	11,700	11,606	7	812
Skin	7,300	7,242	6	434

* Estimated by the American Cancer Society, 1996.
† Estimated by Richard Doll and Richard Peto, 1981.

HISTORY OF OCCUPATIONAL CANCER

An occupational carcinogen was first reported more than 200 years ago. In 1775, Sir Percival Pott reported the first occupational cancer, scrotal skin cancer, among chimney sweeps in England who were heavily exposed to soot.[68] In 1822, Paris reported excess scrotal cancer among Cornish smelter workers.[65] Over the years, other chemicals were found to cause cancer after occupational exposures, including aromatic amines, asbestos, arsenic, benzene, vinyl chloride, and various radioactive materials. In 1879, Haerting and Hesse identified cancer of the lung.[31] Prior to 1950, the association between lung cancer and cigarette smoking was not well established. Currently, about 85–90% of all lung cancer cases are estimated to be caused by cigarette smoking.[18] Since 1973, various occupational exposures were reported to be associated with lung cancer. In 1973, Figueroa reported an excess lung cancer among chloromethyl methyl ether workers.[24]

Other occupational cancers recognized before 1950 were bladder cancer in Geman dyestuff workers,[71] bone cancer in American radium dial painters,[55,56] and leukemia in Italian workers exposed to benzene.[102] Since 1950, various occupations have been evaluated in many case-control and prospective studies. Because of the importance of occupational cancer and the protection of workers against cancer in the workplace, the International Labor Conference in 1973 and 1974 recommended prevention and control methods of occupational hazards caused by carcinogenic substances and agents.[42]

In 1977, a working group of the International Agency for Research on Cancer (IARC) reviewed and standardized the evaluations of evidence for carcinogenic activity from both human and animal studies, and a scheme for categorizing degrees of evidence for carcinogenicity was developed. They categorized the agents as sufficient, limited, inadequate, and lacking evidence for carcinogenicity.[100]

The history of federal regulation of carcinogens has been summarized by Yodaiken et al.[110] A precursor to the National Cancer Institute (NCI) was established in 1937. The National Cancer Act was signed in 1971, and it established the national cancer program. The NCI is responsible for a comprehensive research program that includes prevention, diagnosis, and treatment. The next step was the control of the workplace safety and health. In 1970, the Occupational Safety and Health Act established the Occupational Safety and Health Administration and the National Institute for Occupational Safety and Health. Both NIOSH and the Environmental Protection

TABLE 3. Occupational Carcinogens Regulated by OSHA

Section	Carcinogen
1910.1001	Asbestos
1910.1001	4-Nitrobiphenyl
1910.1004	Alpha-Naphthylamine
1910.1006	Methyl chloromethyl ether
1910.1007	3,3'-Dichlorobenzidine
1910.1008	bis-Chrolomethyl ether
1910.1009	beta-Naphthylamine
1910.1010	Benzidine
1910.1011	4-Aminodiphenyl
1910.1012	Ethyleneimine
1910.1013	beta-Propiolactone
1910.1014	2-Acetylaminofluorene
1910.1015	4-Dimethylaminoazobenzene
1910.1016	N-Nitrosodimethylamine
1910.1017	Vinyl chloride
1910.1018	Inorganic arsenic
1910.1027	Cadmium
1910.1028	Benzene
1910.1029	Coke oven emissions
1910.1044	1,2-dibromo-3-chloropropane
1910.1045	Acrylonitrile
1910.1047	Ethylene oxide
1910.1048	Formaldehyde
1910.1050	Methylenedianline

From 29 CFR, Part 1910—Occupational Safety and Health Standards, July 1995.

Agency prepared publications that provided information on possible carcinogens and methods for controls.[110] NIOSH especially recommended exposure limits and appropriate preventive measures that were designed to reduce adverse health effects of occupational chemicals in accordance with the OSHA rulemaking process.[69] OSHA has issued regulations for occupational carcinogens in the workplace (Table 3).[64]

CHARACTERISTICS OF OCCUPATIONAL CANCER

Latency Period

The latency period is the interval between the first exposure to the responsible agents and the first appearance of the manifestation of the tumor. It is a summation of the times required for the initiation of the malignant change and for the growth of the tumor to a size that permits recognition and diagnosis. Cancer does not usually develop within months after exposure. The minimum latency period is usually 5 years for noncutaneous cancers, with a large proportion of cases appearing 10–30 years after first exposure. For humans, the latency period varies from a minimum of 6 years for radiation-induced leukemia to 40 or more years for some cases of asbestos-induced mesothelioma. For most tumors, the interval is 12–25 years.[26]

Occupational skin cancers exhibit a wide span of latent periods—from less than 1 year to more than 50 years.[32,82] In general, the higher the dose the more likely the latency will be shorter. The latency period has an important impact on the design of epidemiologic studies of occupational groups exposed to potential or known carcinogens. In a relatively short follow-up study, if the workers are young, the cancer incidence may not occur within the time limitations of the study.

Dose-Response Relationship

Although thresholds may not exist, there is strong evidence for a dose-relationship for most carcinogens that have been adequately studied. The degree of exposure has been used to indicate relative concentrations such as high, medium, and low. An increasing risk with increasing exposures is generally observed. Both experimental studies in animals and epidemiologic reports in humans support this concept. For example, dose-response relationships have been shown for lung cancer associated with asbestos[22,57] and coke oven emissions.[52]

Threshold Limit Values

The threshold limit value is the time-weighted average concentration that may safely be inhaled over an 8-hour working day. However, the TLV is a controversial issue. No one knows if a "safe" level for carcinogens exists. Since a single mutation in a single cell can theoretically give rise to a malignancy, it has been argued that there is no safe level of exposure in terms of cancer development. However, other arguments have shown support for establishing thresholds. Those who favor the threshold theory believe that defense mechanisms operate to inhibit or inactivate carcinogenic agents.[30] The assumption is that as long as a healthy immune defense system exists, there will be a threshold. Still, there is no way of knowing the adequacy of each individual's defense mechanism.

In epidemiologic studies in humans, no safe threshold for carcinogen exposure has been demonstrated with certainty. Currently, there is insufficient evidence to prove the existence of a threshold for carcinogens. While it is impossible to prove the existence of thresholds for carcinogens, some recent studies in animals indicate that a threshold mechanism exists.[21,28] A recent study on the relationship between saccharin and bladder cancer reported that a threshold effect exists in male rats, but a carcinogenic effect on the human urothelium is unlikely at even the highest levels of human consumption of saccharin.[21] If a threshold does exist for saccharin bladder tumor promotion that is above the saccharin consumption level of all humans, the risk is zero.[28] In the absence of a safe dose for a carcinogen, a dose-response curve for each carcinogen can estimate the risk at low levels of exposure. With this information, one can evaluate the risks that are probable in the workplace.[30]

Histologic Types

Cancers developing from the same anatomic site may differ widely in histologic properties and in factors of causation. For some sites, such differences may be associated with well-defined dissimilarities in the microscopic appearance of the neoplasms. For example, patients with various cell types of leukemia differ in regard to clinical characteristics. Some occupational cancers also show different histologic types. For example, angiosarcoma is the particular cell type of liver cancer associated with vinyl chloride.[86] In primary bronchial carcinoma, a number of microscopic types have been identified; some differ in their clinical characteristics as well as in their association with occupational or environmental factors such as cigarette smoking. For lung cancer associated with bischloromethyl ether, arsenic, and radiation, the histologic cell types are predominantly small cell, undifferentiated carcinomas.[24,63,76]

Demographic Variables

The age at diagnosis of cancer is related to the age at first exposure. People older than 50 and younger than 15 are more sensitive to carcinogens.[30] Occupational cancers are still manifested after age 65 among individuals who have retired from hazardous industries. For example, increased lung cancer has been observed among retirees who worked at asbestos plants.[22]

Gender is another variable being evaluated to determine cancer frequency. The incidence of lung cancer is generally much higher for males than females due to confounding variables (i.e., smoking) and occupational exposures.[104]

OCCUPATIONAL CARCINOGENS IN HUMANS

The International Agency for Research on Cancer categorizes four groups of carcinogenicity based on the amount of evidence:[40] group 1 is sufficient evidence of carcinogenicity in humans; group 2 is limited evidence, group 3 is insufficient evidence, and group 4 is lack of evidence of carcinogenicity. Group 1 includes chemicals and processes established as human carcinogens based on epidemiologic studies in humans. Table 4 summarizes group 1 occupational carcinogens.

Known lung carcinogens are asbestos, arsenic, chloromethyl ethers, chromium, mustard gas, nickel compounds, radon, and polychlorinated aromatic hydrocarbons including coke production.[4,40] These carcinogens are classified as occupational carcinogens based on sufficient evidence from various human epidemiologic studies.

Skin cancer is associated with arsenic, coal tars, coke production, mineral oils, shale oils, and soots. Mineral oils are a complex class of materials ranging from crude petroleum through various fractions produced at refineries to products used as coolants and lubricants in various industries. But not all mineral oils cause cancer of the skin. Extraction and refining of oil from Scottish shale oil has been associated with skin cancer among workers exposed to certain fractions of unrefined oils.[40]

Liver cancer is associated with aflatoxins and vinyl chloride; bladder cancer is caused by benzidine and beta-naphthylamine.

Occupational cancer epidemiology requires valid research methods depending on the research objectives. The primary objective in epidemiologic studies of occupational cancer is to study cancer morbidity and mortality in working populations and to investigate the distribution of causal factors. The evidence required for establishing carcinogenicity from epidemiologic studies is a positive association between exposure and disease in groups of individuals with known exposures that (1) are not explicable by bias in recording or detection, confounding or chance, (2) vary with dose and time after exposure, and (3) are observed repeatedly in different circumstances. There are two types of epidemiologic studies of cancer: descriptive and analytic studies. Descriptive epidemiologic studies are usually concerned with the collection of cancer incidence, prevalence, and mortality in the working population. These studies are used to test hypotheses that a particular segment of the population, for instance an occupational group or a group of employees in specific work settings, are subject to an increased risk of cancer. In such studies, national or regional rates of cancer mortality or cancer incidence are normally used as reference values. Descriptive cancer epidemiology is of great importance in occupational health. It would be impossible to set up effective

TABLE 4. Occupational Carcinogens in Humans*

Carcinogen	Cancer Site	Exposure	Industry/Occupation
Aflatoxin	Liver, lung	Ingestion of contaminated food	Grains, peanuts
4-Aminobiphenyl	Bladder	Inhalation; skin absorption	Dye manufacture, dye intermediate, rubber antioxidant
Arsenic and arsenic compounds	Lung, skin	Inhalation; skin absorption; ingestion	Copper and cobalt smelters, glass production, wood treatment, pesticides, wool fiber production, mining of gold-bearing ores containing arsenic
Asbestos	Lung, mesothelioma	Inhalation	Asbestos industry, insulation, buildings, brake and shoes workers, shipyard workers, sheet-metal workers, asbestos cement industry, plumbers and pipe-fitters
Benzene	Leukemia	Inhalation; skin absorption	Petroleum, coking industry, rubber and petrochemical workers
Benzidine	Bladder	Skin absorption; inhalation	Dye manufacture, rubber, plastic, cable industries, chemical industries
Bis(chloromethyl) ether	Lung	Inhalation; skin absorption	Ion-exchange resin production, chemical intermediate, contaminant of chloromethyl methyl ether, electronic, chemical, ceramic, mining industries
Chromium	Lung, nasal cavity	Inhalation	Chromium production, plants, chromate pigment industry, plating, painters, jewelers
Coal tar and coal tar pitches	Skin, lung, bladder	Inhalation; skin contact	Paving and roofing, steel industries, patent-fuel workers, coal gasification, coke production, tar-distilling, optical lens workers
Mineral oils	Skin	Inhalation; skin contact	Solvents in printing, lubricant in metal-working
Mustard gas	Lung	Inhalation; skin contact	Manufacture of mustard gas, poison gas manufacture
Beta-naphthylamine	Bladder	Dye industry	(No longer in commercial use)
Nickel compounds	Lung, nasal cavity	Inhalation	Nickel refining and smelting industries
Radon	Lung	Inhalation	Underground miners, uranium mining, iron mining
Shale oils	Skin	Skin contact	Oil shale industry, cotton-textile workers
Soots	Skin, lung	Skin contact	Chimney sweepers
Vinyl chloride	Liver (angiosarcoma)	Inhalation	Polyvinyl plastic production workers, polyvinyl chloride resins production industry

* Sufficient evidence for carcinogenicity to humans, according to evaluation by the International Agency for Research on Cancer.

cancer control programs for working populations in the absence of such data. In analytical epidemiologic studies, specific hypotheses concerning association between factors in the working environment and the occurrence of cancer are examined.

The number of well-established occupational carcinogens and associated cancers are relatively small (see Table 4). Some carcinogens and related cancers that are reviewed using epidemiologic study results are described below.

Asbestos and Respiratory Diseases:
Lung Cancer, Mesothelioma, Asbestosis

There is sufficient evidence for the carcinogenicity of asbestos in humans.[40,80,81] Occupational exposure to asbestos has been associated with three important diseases: lung cancer, malignant mesothelioma, and asbestosis. There are four commercially important forms of asbestos: chrysotile, amosite, anthophyllite, and crocidolite. Asbestos is used in roofing products, friction products, asbestos cement, and gaskets.[96] Asbestos, which is not a single mineral, has two natural forms: amphiboles, which are chain silicates and have straight fibers, and serpentine forms, which have a short structure and fibers arranged to produce hollow, tube-like spirals. The two common varieties of the amphiboles are crocidolite (blue asbestos) and amosite (brown asbestos). The serpentine form is known as chrysotile (white asbestos), which is currently used almost exclusively in industry.

The major industrial use of asbestos is restricted to chrysotile in the manufacture of piping, roofing, insulation, and friction materials. The lung cancer mortality of occupationally exposed chrysotile miners in Quebec has been well documented by McDonald.[58] Occupational exposures to chrysotile, amosite, anthophyllite, and mixed fibers containing crocidolite have also resulted in a high incidence of lung cancer.

Malignant mesothelioma is a rare cancer associated with asbestos exposure. In 1960 the first case, which was reported by Wagner, was associated with crocidolite exposure in South Africa.[105] The importance of the amphiboles in pathogenesis was further demonstrated by Newhouse and Thompson in 1965.[62] The incidence of mesothelioma has increased over the years, with an annual incidence for adults in North America of 2–3 cases per million for men and 0.7 per million for women.[25] In 1994, the OSHA permissible exposure limit (PEL) for asbestos fibers in the workplace was changed from an 8-hour time weighted average of 0.2 f/cc to 0.1 f/cc.[99] This exposure standard requires personal protective equipment, training, medical surveillance, and engineering controls.[96]

Aromatic Amines: Bladder Cancer

Several chemicals within aromatic amines, including 2-naphthylamine and 4-aminobiphenyl benzidine, have been reported as the cause of bladder cancer.[43] The first occupational bladder cancer was associated with the German dyestuff industry.[71] 2-naphthylamine was used mainly as an intermediate in the manufacture of dyes and as an antioxidant in the rubber industry. However, it was not produced for commercial use in the United States.[96] Benzidine has been used for more than 60 years as an intermediate in the production of azo dyes, sulfur dyes, fast color salts, naphthols, and other dyeing compounds.[96] The primary routes of potential human exposure to benzidine are inhalation, ingestion, and dermal contact.

A survey of workers with dyestuff intermediates revealed that a large number of bladder cancer cases over 30 years were associated with benzidine and naphthylamines.[79] This result was confirmed in numerous studies.[13,27] In addition to benzidine and 2-naphthylamine, a number of other aromatic amines have been suspected of bladder carcinogenicity. Melick et al. reported that there was an increased risk of bladder cancer associated with exposure to 4-aminobiphenyl, which was used in the North American rubber industry.[58,59] Two other aromatic amines, including N-phenyl-2-naphthylamine and N,N-bis (2-chloroethyl-2-naphthlamine), have been reported as possible human carcinogens.[36]

Alkylating Agents: Lung Cancer and Leukemia

Alkylating agents are of interest from the point of view of cancer induction because the alkylation of nucleic acids is thought to be an important mechanism in carcinogenesis. Of all known alkylating agents, bis-chloromethyl ether is known to be a carcinogen that causes lung cancer in humans. BCME occurs as a contaminant in the production of chloromethyl methyl ether, which is used as a chloromethylating agent in the manufacture of ion exchange resins. BCME also has been used in dental restorative materials. The primary routes of potential human exposure to BCME are inhalation and dermal contact. Evidence for the carcinogenicity of BCME has come from studies conducted in the Federal Republic of Germany,[89] Japan,[77] and the United States.[24] In all cases, BCME was associated with oat-cell carcinomas.

Ethylene oxide is one of the epoxide alkylating agents with a three-numbered ring that readily opens even under mild conditions. Ethylene oxide is primarily used as intermediate in the production of several industrial chemicals, most notably, ethylene glycol. It also has been used as a sterilant and fumigant in health products and flame retardants. Human studies associated with exposure to ethylene oxide have been inconclusive. However, Scandinavian studies have reported increased risk of leukemia in a small group of workers using ethylene oxide as a sterilant.[35] In a study of ethylene oxide in the United States, no excess mortality was found, and a cohort study of the chronic effects of this chemical in the U.S. workers showed no adverse hematologic findings.[16]

Benzene: Myelogenous Leukemia

Benzene is an integral component of petrochemical feed stocks and is present in gasoline in the United States in the range of 1.0–1.5%. Benzene is also formed during coke oven operations. Benzene is a major raw material used extensively as a solvent in the chemical and drug industries. It is a useful intermediate in organic synthesis and is frequently used in research and commercial laboratories. The primary routes of potential human exposure to benzene are inhalation and dermal contact. Benzene is associated with acute and chronic myelogenic leukemia.[1–3,37,38] A causal relationship has been established through epidemiologic research.[48] The form of leukemia associated with benzene is usually myeloid, occasionally monocytic, but never lymphatic. The most recent mortality study of 74,828 benzene-exposed workers in China reported significantly increased risk of myelogenous leukemia.[109]

In 1977, after NIOSH identified a group of rubber workers with a fivefold increased risk of acute myelogenous leukemia, OSHA attempted to lower the workplace standard for benzene to 1 ppm. In 1987, OSHA established the 1 ppm TWA (time-weighted average) standard for benzene based on the rubber workers cohort.[72]

Polycyclic Aromatic Hydrocarbons: Scrotal Cancer and Lung Cancer

Polycyclic aromatic hydrocarbons are a large group of chemicals. In industry, their main sources are soots, tars, and mineral oils, and the primary routes of potential exposure are inhalation, ingestion, and dermal contact. There is sufficient evidence for the carcinogenicity of soots, coal tars, and mineral oils in humans.[40] In the 18th century, Percival Pott reported that scrotal cancer in chimney sweeps was caused by soots. An increased number of skin and scrotal causes have been found in workers operating aromatic lathes who are exposed to the fine mists of cutting oils.[49,106] Although scrotal and skin cancer remain a problem in a number of industries due to the exposure to polycyclic aromatic hydrocarbons, there is an increasing recognition that other sites of cancer are associated with these materials.

Evidence of an increased risk of lung cancer has been found in workers exposed to coal and tar gas.[45] Foundry workers also are at risk from exposure to polycyclic aromatic hydrocarbons; an increased risk of lung cancer was particularly associated with iron and steel foundries.[29,61,88] Several studies in Finland showed a high excess of lung cancers in foundry workers, and molders were the group apparently at highest risk. In these studies, occupations were classified according to their exposure to benzo-(a)-pyrene, and higher exposures were more common among cases than controls, which suggested that exposure to polycyclic compounds may be a causative factor.

Vinyl Chloride: Angiosarcoma

Vinyl chloride is a colorless gas but is usually handled as a liquid under pressure. It is used for production of vinyl chloride resins, production of methyl chlorform, and as a component of propellant mixtures. The primary cancer site associated with human exposure to vinyl chloride is the liver. This association has been confirmed in many studies since 1974.[9,10,27,107] More than 30 cases of angiosarcoma of the liver have been reported among vinyl chloride polymerization workers in the United States and in nine other nations.[14,23] Because this tumor is extremely rare, the occurrence of these cases suggests a causal relationship to a specific phase of vinyl chloride production. However, after reviewing the epidemiologic studies conducted in the United States and United Kingdom, Doll concluded that the evidence that vinyl chloride is a human lung carcinogen is weak.[19]

Although the latency period from first exposure to diagnosis varies considerably, in most cases it is between 15–24 years from first exposure, with a median latency of 15–19 years.[36] In 1994, the Environmental Protection Agency and the Food and Drug Administration banned the use of vinyl chloride as an aerosol propellant, eliminating the potential vinyl chloride exposure of 1 million-5 million people annually.[96] OSHA has adopted a permissible exposure limit of 1 ppm for vinyl chloride as an 8-hr TWA, with a 5-ppm ceiling for any 15-minute period. OSHA also requires medical surveillance and the use of protective clothing and respirators in the workplace.

Metals: Lung Cancer and Skin Cancer

The association between chromates and lung cancer has been confirmed in several studies on the chromate production industry.[5,53] The first report of an increased risk of respiratory cancer among nickel workers came from Wales, and the association was confirmed by studies in other countries.[88] The risk was generally attributed to nickel carbonyl, a gas that is produced when nickel reacts with carbon monoxide. Nickel carbonyl has been found to be carcinogenic in experimental studies in animals, and epidemiologic studies of workers exposed to other nickel compounds have shown an excess of lung and other respiratory tract cancers.[66] In 1987, IARC concluded that long-term occupational exposure to cadmium also may contribute to lung cancer.[40]

Arsenic was widely used as a herbicide and fungicide, and it is still extensively used in wood treatment. The carcinogenic properties of arsenic have been suspected since the 1820s, but the first clear association between arsenic exposure and cancer was demonstrated by Hill and Faming in 1948.[34] There is sufficient evidence for the carcinogenicity of inorganic arsenic compounds in humans.[40] Skin cancer was the original cancer associated with arsenic, and the relationship has been well documented.[7] Epidemiologic studies on smelter workers have indicated a synergistic effect between arsenic exposure and cigarette smoking in the induction of lung cancer.[12]

Cadmium, which is broadly distributed in the environment, has many industrial applications, including electroplating, pigment production, and additives for plastics, especially polyvinyl chloride.[67] Although information on the carcinogenicity of cadmium is incomplete, recent epidemiologic studies have provided evidence that cadmium is carcinogenic in the lung but not in the prostate. In 1987, IARC concluded that long-term occupational exposures to cadmium may contribute to lung cancer.[40]

Metalworking Fluids: Cancers of the Stomach, Bladder, Pancreas, Larynx, Skin, and Other Sites

Metalworking fluids (MWF) have been used in various industries and encompass a diverse group of agents. Rather than describing a specific chemical composition, the term machine fluids describes a function, that of cooling and lubricating surfaces in machining operations. Suspected carcinogens contained in various types of machining fluid as additives or contaminants include polyaromatic hydrocarbons, nitrosoamines, sulfur-containing compounds, formaldehyde-releasing biocides, and certain metals.[90] The route of exposure to MWFs is generally through dermal contact or inhalation. Large sizes of many airborne particles can lead to gastrointestinal exposure.

Many studies suggest an association between MWF exposure and various cancers, including the stomach, bladder, pancreas, larynx, skin, and esophagus. Specific classes of MWFs may be associated with cancer at certain sites. Straight oil exposure has been associated with an increased risk of laryngeal cancer and rectal cancer, while synthetic oil exposure has been associated with an elevated risk of pancreatic cancer. For stomach cancer, several studies reported that MWF exposure is associated with a significantly elevated risk.[73,84] Soluble oil exposure may be associated with an increased risk of stomach cancer.[84] A number of MWF-exposed cohorts were reported to have an increased risk of bladder cancer.[84,101] Based on case-control studies, other MWF-exposed populations have been found to have an increased risk of bladder cancer. Mortality studies have found an excess of pancreatic cancer among workers exposed to soluble oils.[90] The risk of pancreatic cancer mortality was increased among workers who were employed 10 or more years as grinders at ball bearing manufacturing plants.[84] For laryngeal cancer, several studies of MWF-exposed cohorts reported significantly elevated risk of laryngeal cancer.[90,101] Specifically, study groups were exposed to straight oils. For skin cancer, a cohort study[44] and a population-based case-control study have found an increased risk of skin cancer among MWF-exposed workers.[74] A recent mortality study in England reported that significantly elevated proportional mortality ratios of scrotal cancer were found in metal machinists exposed to cutting oils.[15]

OCCUPATIONAL CANCER SURVEILLANCE

Occupational cancer surveillance monitors cancer incidence, mortality, and exposure to workplace hazards. The ultimate purpose of occupational cancer surveillance is to provide useful information for planning cancer control programs that are directly linked to preventive action. The surveillance efforts include data collection through surveillance systems and surveillance activities such as disease-based surveillance, exposure-based surveillance, and medical screening.

Mortality Data

The National Center for Health Statistic codes each of the 2 million deaths in the United States that are reported to vital registration offices annually. The data for each decedent include underlying and contributing causes of death, age, sex, race, and residence. Since 1985, the usual occupation and industry of each decedent have been available for about 25 states. Since 1985, these mortality data have provided valuable information on relationships between cancer and occupation. In 1976, a comprehensive analysis of occupation and cause of death for the state of Washington was completed.[60] In England and Wales,[70] similar data have been available for analysis every 10 years.

Cancer Survey Data

As part of the Third National Cancer Survey in the United States, occupational histories were obtained on a random sample of incident cases. The data were analyzed to evaluate associations between specific cancer sites and various occupations.[108] The Third National Health and Nutrition Examination Survey (NHANES III) conducted by the National Center for Health Statistics collected information on skin cancer and occupation as a part of its survey components during 1988–1994.[97] The NHANES III is a 6-year survey measuring the health and nutritional status of the civilian noninstitutionalized U.S. population aged 2 months and older. Revision of the Bureau of Labor Statistics Annual Survey beginning in 1992 allowed identification of numbers of specific diseases that were considered serious. According to this 1992 survey, among the serious cases, employers reported 103 employees with occupational cancer.[91]

Cancer Registries

In 1994, the NCI expanded the SEER program, which is a network of nine population-based cancer incidence registries located in selected areas of the country and covering about 10% of the U.S. population. Currently, the cancer files maintain about 1.7 million cancer cases, and about 120,000 are added each year.[17] Unfortunately, this registry does not contain information on occupational history. To be useful for occupational surveillance in the future, it would need to collect the usual occupational information in certain types of cancer on the SEER registry system. In Europe, the European Cancer Registry-Based Study of Survival and Care of Cancer Working Group collected data on cancer survival from 30 cancer registries in 11 countries and established a database that covered about 800,000 cancer patients who were diagnosed in 1978–1985 and followed to the end of 1990.[41]

Type of Occupational Cancer Surveillance

DISEASE-BASED SURVEILLANCE

Disease-based surveillance includes case reports on the occurrence of cancer in a person with a specified occupation. Evaluation of routinely collected data on occupation and persons with cancers may lead to the identification of unrecognized occupational hazards. A formalization and generalization of case reports is known as the sentinel health event.[75] The occurrence of diseases known to be associated with occupational exposure can lead to identification of currently uncontrolled exposures. The SEER program is an example of disease-based surveillance, but it does not contain occupational information. The next level of disease-based surveillance is the conduct of formal case-control studies. Case-control studies are useful in finding new occupational causes of cancer. The advantages of disease-based surveillance of possible occupationally related cancer are that specific cancers can be targeted for evaluation and that a wide variety of occupations can be related to the occurrence of cancer.

EXPOSURE-BASED SURVEILLANCE

Exposure-based surveillance is usually based on cohort or follow-up studies in which persons with an occupation of concern are identified and followed in order to measure the rate of occurrence of cancer. If follow-up is prospective, exposure can be measured with greater accuracy. In a retrospective study, it is difficult to measure the exposure level, and an approximation is possible. Researchers conducting retrospective cohort studies should consider the issues of what, whom, where, and how to study. Levine and Eisenbud have identified more than 20 industrial populations that could potentially be studied retrospectively.[89] Some of these populations include persons with exposure to known human carcinogens, including benzene and chromates.

Through prospective studies, exposure can be quantified with accuracy and exposed persons followed according to adverse health outcomes. A disadvantage of these studies is that many years of follow up are required for appropriate evaluation of possible associations between exposure and the occurrence of cancer.

NIOSH conducted the National Occupational Exposure Survey in 1981–1983.[98] It consisted of an on-site exposure survey in a sample of 4,490 establishments that had been selected to represent most sectors of the American workforce covered by the Occupational Safety and Health Act of 1970.

MEDICAL SCREENING

Medical screening programs are used to detect early signs of disease. In general, ideal programs should be simple, inexpensive, and accurate in testing a population with a high prevalence of a certain disease. Furthermore, intervention should be available for those who are found to have a positive sign of disease. Occupational medical screening is one of the most complex processes in medical practice. In designing a medical screening program, practitioners should be familiar with clinical medicine and toxicology and understand a standardized approach to data collection.[8] Medical surveillance of populations at high risk of cancer is only effective in the following situations: (1) if the screening test is easy to perform and sensitive, (2) if it detects premalignant abnormalities or tumors at an early stage, and (3) if there is an effective intervention that reduces morbidity and mortality when applied to early tumors.[25]

Cancer surveillance in occupational settings has been explored for bladder cancer among workers exposed to beta-naphthylamine and for benzidine exposures and lung cancers. For bladder cancer screening, two methods have been used: urinalysis for microscopic hematuria and urine cytology. Hematuria is relatively sensitive in detecting superficial and invasive bladder cancer, but it may result in a high false-positive rate. Urine cytology has good sensitivity and specificity for invasive bladder cancer, but no survival advantage has been demonstrated with this technique. However, in 1989, the International Conference on Bladder Cancer Screening in High-Risk Groups concluded that urinalysis and cytology might be appropriate.[78]

Lung cancer surveillance includes chest radiography or sputum cytology. These methods have been evaluated at several academic institutions in the 1970s. Medical screening for lung cancer was comprehensively reviewed by Marfin and Schenker in 1991.[54] The results from these approaches showed a significant increase in lung cancer detection, but there was no significant decrease in lung cancer mortality. With these results and other data, no routine surveillance for lung cancer was recommended, even to high-risk populations.[87] Other medical surveillance for occupational cancers includes Pap tests for cervical cancer, fecal occult blood testing and sigmoidoscopy for colorectal cancer, and mammography for breast cancer. Some form of medical surveillance is required by the OSHA standard for asbestos, arsenic, benzene, and a variety of other carcinogens[85] (see Table 3).

PRIORITIES FOR OCCUPATIONAL CANCER RESEARCH

Priorities for occupational cancer research should be considered in relation to occupational carcinogenic hazards. Several papers have suggested the importance of priorities for future occupational cancer research.[20,39] In 1996, the National Occupational Research Agenda includes occupational cancer research methods as one of the 21 research priorities identified by NIOSH.[93] The NORA emphasizes the importance of molecular biology as a powerful new research tool that may lead to information that could be used to take protective measures before workers suffer the consequences of exposures to various potential carcinogens. Advances in understanding the mechanisms of cancer causation are beginning to improve the ability of scientists to use laboratory research to evaluate the carcinogenic potential of a substance and to describe the hazard to humans with accuracy. More research is needed on comparative mechanisms of toxicity and on the development of rapid and inexpensive tests to complement or modify traditional animal toxicity tests. Advanced techniques of molecular biology are needed to understand interactions of chemicals with critical target genes and to develop more accurate and less expensive methods to estimate worker exposure to potential carcinogens.

Numerous factors need to be considered when hypothesizing that an occupational cancer exists in a given occupation: (1) the level of significance of the possible association between occupation and types of cancers, (2) the possibility of confounding factors such as smoking, (3) the number of cancers sites with which the occupation is associated, (4) the likelihood of occupational exposure levels, (5) the degree to which the occupation-cancer association is supported by other epidemiologic studies, and (6) whether occupations with similar exposures have an excess of the cancer of interest due to known or suspected carcinogenic agents.

Dubrow and Wegman recommended five working groups for further study:[20]

Asbestos Workers. Asbestos is a well-known occupational carcinogen that is associated with cancers of the lung, larynx, esophagus, stomach, and other sites.[40] The association between asbestos exposure and lung cancers or mesotheliomas among asbestos insulation workers and shipyard workers are particularly well established.[11,46,80,81] Additional work is needed to characterize level of exposure and cancer risk and to establish a safe dose level at the workplace. The problem of asbestos exposure has been widely recognized and has occupational and public health significance. Therefore, a national program for prevention of asbestos exposure is needed.

Motor Vehicle Operators. The United States had more than 3.9 million commercial motor vehicle operators in 1995.[92] Cancers of the lung and larynx have been reported among motor vehicle operators. As risk factors for these cancers, smoking, diesel exhaust and gasoline should be studied.

Machinists and Related Occupations. There were more than 2.8 million machinists and related workers in the United States in 1995.[92] In particular, tool makers were reported to have excess cancers of the large intestine and bladder. Potential carcinogenic agents include synthetic abrasives and cutting fluids.

Electric Workers.   The United States had more than a half million electric workers in 1995.[92] Electricians were reported to have an excess of lymphoma and cancers of the bladder and brain. Potential carcinogenic exposure includes nonionizing radiation.

Metal Molders.   There were more than 100,000 metal molders in the United States in 1995.[92] Metal molders had a high risk of lung cancer. Potential carcinogenic exposures include polycyclic aromatic hydrocarbons, metal dusts, fumes, and oxides.

A panel from IARC developed 10 criteria for selecting occupational exposures in epidemiologic studies.[39] These criteria, which are related to the issues of potential public health importance, include (1) the number of workers exposed, (2) level of exposure to workers, (3) quality of exposure data, (4) carcinogenic potential, (5) evidence of human carcinogenicity, (6) ongoing exposure to known carcinogens at permissible levels of exposure, (7) trends in exposure, (8) control of confounding factors, (9) cases potentially attributable to exposure, and (10) length of time since first exposure.

For epidemiologic approaches in occupational cancer, the epidemiologist develops hypotheses from clinical observations or from statistical associations between specific forms of cancer and population characteristics that are derived from an analysis of population morbidity or mortality statistics. By means of such statistics, the cancer epidemiologist seeks to discover and to exploit variations in the occurrence of cancer. Such variations are recognized by making comparisons, for example, between different times between groups of people living in different areas, or perhaps between groups of people living closely but who differ in such characteristics as sex, age, occupation, or habits such as smoking. For comparisons of cancer occurrence to be valid, the following requirements must be fulfilled: (1) the diagnosis of cancer must be clearly and uniformly defined, (2) a uniform procedure must exist for selecting the recognized cases of cancer that will be used to obtain an estimate of cancer occurrence; and (3) the population groups themselves and the group characteristics must be adequately defined. All epidemiologic data should be integrated with experimental and clinical data, and the epidemiologist should attempt to derive inferences from these data regarding etiologic factors. The methods have general applications, but each method is not equally applicable to all sites. For example, cancer of the skin, which has a low fatality rate, cannot be studied through mortality data, and prospective inquiries are seldom suitable unless the incidence of the cancer under study is relatively high.

CONCLUSION

Occupational cancer differs from other occupational diseases in several ways: (1) no safe level of exposure to carcinogens has been determined; (2) cancer develops many years after exposure; (3) many different sites of cancer exist; and (4) most cancers are preventable. The risk of cancer in humans is increased by a variety of occupational/environmental factors, ranging from exposure to an identified agent to exposures through lifestyle factors such as smoking or socioeconomic conditions. Occupation may contribute to the development of cancer if there is an exposure to certain carcinogenic agents, such as certain metals, dyes, organic and inorganic dusts, solvents, and pesticides. Since carcinogenesis is a multisequential process, reductions in exposures to carcinogens at the workplace are necessary to maximize the effectiveness of cancer prevention in the workplace. Prophylactic intervention is also possible for some known risk factors associated with certain cancer sites. Cancer prevention and control intervention in the workplace must include (1) primary prevention programs that emphasize avoiding potential exposures and use of proper education; (2) secondary prevention programs that emphasize increasing medical screening practices; and (3) appropriate surveillance programs. The prevention of occupational cancer requires the participation of various federal and state agencies and the development of good practice. At present, fewer than 20 known carcinogenic agents have been evaluated based on studies in humans and animals. Furthermore, exciting developments in epidemiologic and animal studies will contribute to the identification of additional carcinogenic agents in the workplace. New biologic markers of exposures and cancer-related outcomes need to be identified and integrated into epidemiologic studies. Because epidemiologic data regarding the carcinogenicity of many exposures are not available, research methods to evaluate and improve the predictive value of animal and in vitro systems must be developed. A more complete understanding of occupational cancer trends will require further research on occupational cancer risks and means of prevention. Finally, ultimate prevention of occupational cancer could be effectively accomplished when health administrators, epidemiologists, industrial hygienists, occupational physicians, toxicologists, and safety engineers work together as a team to provide proper guidelines for preventive strategies and controls.

REFERENCES

 1. Aksoy M, Erdem S, Dincol G: Leukemia in shoe workers exposed chronically to benzene. Blood 44:837–847, 1974.
 2. Aksoy M, Erdem S, Dincol G: Types of leukemia in benzene poisoning: A study in thirty-four patients. Acta Haematol 56:65–72, 1976.
 3. Aksoy M, Dincol K, Erdem S, Dincol G: Acute leukemia due to exposure to benzene. Am J Med 52:160–166, 1992.
 4. Alderson M: Occupational Cancer. Butterworths, London, 1986.
 5. Alderson MR, Rattan NS, Bidstrup L: Health of workmen in the chromate producing industry in Britain. Br J Ind Med 38:117–124, 1981.
 6. American Cancer Society: Cancer Facts and Figures. Atlanta, American Cancer Society, 1996.
 7. Axelson O: Arsenic compounds and cancer. In Vainio H, Grosa M, Hemminki K (eds): Occupational Cancer and Carcinogenesis. Washington, Hemisphere Publishing, 1980, pp 309–315.
 8. Baker, EL, Honchar PA, Fine LJ: Surveillance is occupational illness and injury: Concepts and content. Am J Public Health 79(suppl):9–11, 1989.
 9. Baxter PJ, Anthony PP, Mac Sween RNM, Scheuer PJ: Angiosarcoma of the liver in Great Britain, 1963–73. BMJ 11:919–921, 1977.
10. Baxter PJ, Anthony PP, Mac Sween RNM, Scheuer PJ: Angiosarcoma of the liver: Annual occurrence and aetiology in Great Britain. Br J Ind Med 37:213–221, 1980.
11. Blot WJ, Harrington JM, Toledo A, et al: Lung cancer after employment in shipyards during World War II. N Engl J Med 299:620–624, 1978.
12. Cahow K: The cancer conundrum. Environ Health Perspect 103:998–1004, 1995.
13. Case RAM, Hosker MED: Tumor of the urinary bladder as an occupational disease in the rubber industry in England and Wales. Br J Prev Social Med 8:39–50, 1957.
14. Creech JL, Johnson MN: Angiosarcoma of liver in the manufacture of polyvinyl chloride. J Occup Med 16:150–151, 1974.
15. Coggon D, Inskip H, Winter P, Pannett B: Mortality from scrotal cancer in metal machinists in England and Wales, 1979–80 and 1982–90. Occup Med 46:69–70, 1996.
16. Currier MF, Carlo GC, Poston PL, Ledford WE: A cross-sectional study of employees with potential exposure to ethylene oxide. Br J Ind Med 41:492–498, 1984.
17. Devesa SS, Blot WJ, Stone BJ, et al: Recent cancer trends in the United States. J Natl Cancer Inst 87:175–182, 1995.
18. Doll R, Peto R: The Cause of Cancer. Oxford, Oxford University Press, 1981.

19. Doll R: Effects of exposure to vinyl chloride. Scand J Work Environ Health. 14:61–78, 1988.
20. Dubrow R, Wegman DH: Setting priorities for occupational cancer research and control: Synthesis of the results of occupational disease surveillance studies. J Natl Cancer Inst 71:1123–1142, 1983.
21. Ellwein LB, Cohen SM: The health risks of saccharin revisited. Crit Rev Toxicol 20:311–326, 1990.
22. Enterline P, Decoufle P, Henderson V: Respiratory cancer in relation to occupational exposures among retired asbestos workers. Br J Ind Med 30:162–166, 1973.
23. Falk H, Creech JL, Heath CW, et al: Hepatic disease among workers at a vinyl chloride polymerization plant. JAMA 230:59–63, 1974.
24. Figueroa WG, Raskowski R, Weiss W: Lung cancer in chloromethyl ether workers. N Engl J Med 288:1096–1097, 1973.
25. Fishman ML, Cadman EC, Desmond S: Occupational Cancer. In LaDou J (ed): Occupational Medicine. Norwalk, CT, Appleton and Lange, 1990, pp 182–207.
26. Fox AJ, Lindars DC, Owen R: A survey of occupational cancer in the rubber and cable-making industries: The result of five-year analysis, 1967–71. Br J Ind Med 31:140–151, 1974.
27. Fox AJ, Collier PF: Mortality experience of workers exposed to vinyl chloride monomer in the manufacture of polyvinyl chloride in Great Britain. Br J Ind Med 34:1–10, 1977.
28. Gaylor DW, Kadlubar FF, West RW: Estimates of the risk of bladder tumor promotion by sacchrin in rats. Regul Toxicol Pharmacol 8:467–470, 1988.
29. Gibson ES, Martin RH, Lockington JN: Lung cancer mortality in a steel foundry. J Occup Med 19:807–812, 1978.
30. Groth DH: Identifying carcinogens. In Lewis RJ (ed): Carcinogenically Active Chemicals: A Reference Guide. New York, Van Nostrand Reinhold, 1991.
31. Haerting FH, Hesse W: Der Lungenknebs, die Bergkrankheit in den Schneeberger Gruben, Vierteljahresschr. Gerichtl Med Oeff 30, 296–313, 1879.
32. Henry SA: Occupational cutaneous cancer attributable to certain chemicals in inudstry. Br Med Bull 4:389–401, 1947.
33. Higginson J: Proportion of cancer due to occupation. Prev Med 9:180–188, 1980.
34. Hill AB, Faming EL: Studies in the incidence of cancer in a factory handling inorganic compounds of arsenic. 1. Mortality experienced in the factory. Br J Ind Med 5:1–6, 1948.
35. Hogstedt C, Malmqvist N, Wadman B: Leukemia in workers exposed to ethylene oxide. JAMA 241:1132–1133, 1979.
36. Howard JK: Occupationally related cancer. In Howard JK, Tyrer FH (ed): Textbook of Occupational Medicine. London, Churchill Livingstone, 1987, pp 167–194.
37. Infante PF, Rinsky RA, Wagoner JK, Young RJ: Leukemia in benzene workers. Lancet 2:76–78, 1977.
38. Infante PF, Rinsky RA, Wagoner JK, Young RJ: Leukemia in benzene workers. J Environ Pathol Toxicol 2:251–257, 1979.
39. International Agency for Research on Cancer: Priorities in Occupational Cancer Epidemiology. Lyon, IARC, 1986, Joint IARC/CEC Working Group report 86/004.
40. International Agency for Research on Cancer: IARC monographs on the evaluation of carcinogenic risks to humans, Suppl 7. Overall Evaluations of Carcinogenicity: An Updating of IARC Monographs. Vol 1-42. Lyon, IARC, 1987.
41. International Agency for Research on Cancer: Survival of cancer patients in Europe: The European study. Lyon, IARC 1995, scientific publication 132.
42. International Labor Office: Occupational Cancer: Prevention and Control. 2nd ed. Geneva, International Labor Office, 1988.
43. Jackson CD, Baetcke KP: Causative agents in the induction of bladder cancer. Ann Clin Lab Sci 6:223–232, 1976.
44. Jarvholm B, Fast K, Lavenius B, Tomsic P: Exposure to cutting oils and its relation to skin tumors and premalignant skin lesions on the hands and forearms. Scand J Work Environ Health 11:365–369, 1985.
45. Kennaway EL, Kennaway NM: Further study of the incidence of cancer of the lung and larynx. Br J Cancer 1:260–298, 1947.
46. Kolonel LN, Yoshizawa CN, Hirohata T, Myers BC: Cancer occurrence in shipyard workers exposed to asbestos in Hawaii. Cancer Res 45:3924–3928, 1985.
47. Kvale G, Bjelke E, Heuch I: Occupational exposure and lung cancer risk. Int J Cancer 37:185–193, 1986.
48. Laskin S, Goldstein BD: Benzene toxicity, a clinical evaluation. J Toxicol Environ Health 2:(suppl 2) 23–36, 1977.
49. Lee WR, Alderson MR, Downs J: Scrotal cancer in the north west of England 1962-1968. Br J Ind Med 29:188–195, 1972.
50. Leigh JP, Markowitz S, Fah M, et al: Costs of occupational injuries and illnesses in 1992: Final NIOSH report for cooperative agreement with ERC, Inc. 1996.

51. Levine RJ, Eisenbud M: Have we overlooked important cohorts for follow-up studies? Report of the Chemical Industry Institute of Toxicology Conference of World War II-era industrial health specialists. J Occup Med 30:655–660, 1988.

52. Lloyd JW: Long-term mortality study of steelworkers. V. Respiratory cancer in coke plant workers. J Occup Med 13:53–68, 1971.

53. Machle W, Gregorius F: Cancer of the respiratory system in the United States chromate producing industry. Public Health Rep 63:1114–1127, 1948.

54. Marfin AA, Schenker M: Screening for lung cancer: Effective tests awaiting effective treatment. Occup Med State Art Rev 6:111–131, 1991.

55. Martland HS, Humphries RE: Osteogenic sarcoma in dial painters using luminous paint. Arch Pathol 7:406–417, 1929.

56. Martland HS: The occurrence of malignancy in radioactive persons. Am J Cancer 15:2435–2516, 1931.

57. McDonald AD, McDonald JC: Malignant mesothelioma in North America. Cancer 46:1650–1656, 1980.

58. Melick WF, Escue HM, Narayka JJ, et al: The first reported human bladder tumors due to a new carcinogen-xenylamine. J Urol 74:760–766, 1955.

59. Melick WF, Naryka JJ, Kelly RE: Bladder cancer due to exposure to para-aminobiphenyl: A 17-year follow up. J Urol 106:220–226, 1971.

60. Milham S: Occupational mortality in Washington State, 1950–1971. Vol 1-3. Cincinnati, National Institute for Occupational Safety and Health, 1976, publication 76-175.

61. Morrison SL: Occupational mortality in Scotland. Br J Ind Med 14:130–132, 1957.

62. Newhouse ML, Thompson H: Mesothelioma of pleura and peritoneum following exposure to asbestos in the London area. Br J Ind Med 22:261–269, 1965.

63. Newman JA, Archer VE, Saccomanno G: Histologic types of bronchogenic carcinoma among members of copper-mining and smelting communities. Ann N Y Acad Sci 271:260–268, 1976.

64. Office of the Federal Register National Archives and Records Administration: Code of Federal Regulations, 29 Part 1910: Occupational Safety and Health Standards, July 1995.

65. Paris JA: Pharmacologia. Vol. 2. 5th ed. London, W. Phillips, 1822.

66. Pedersen E, Hogetveit AC, Andersen A: Cancer of the respiratory organs among workers at a nickel refinery in Norway. Int J Cancer 12:32–41, 1973.

67. Pier SM, Bang KM: The role of heavy metals in human health. In Trieff NM (ed): Environment and Health. Ann Arbor, MI, Ann Arbor Science Publishers, 1980, pp 367–409.

68. Pott P: Chronological Observations Relative to the Cataract, the Polypus of the Nose, the Cancer of the Scrotum, the Different Kinds of Ruptures, and the Mortification of the Toes and Feet. London, Clarke and Collins, 1775.

69. Proctor NH: Chemical hazards of the workplace: Appendix 1. NIOSH Recommendations for Occupational Safety and Health Standards (August 1988). New York, Van Nostrand Reinhold, 1991.

70. Registrar General's Decennial Supplement, England and Wales 1990–72. Occupational Mortality Series DS No. 1. London, Her Majesty's Stationery Office, 1978.

71. Rehn L: Blasengeschwulste bei Fuchsin-Arbeitern. Arch Klin Chir 50:588, 1895.

72. Rinsky RA, Young RJ, Smith AB: Leukemia in benzene workers. Am J Ind Med 2:217–245, 1981.

73. Rotini C, Austin H, Delzell E, et al: Retrospective follow-up study of foundry and engine plant workers. Am J Ind Med 24:485–498, 1993.

74. Roush GC, Kelly J, Meigs JW, Flannery JT: Scrotal carcinoma in Connecticut metal workers. Am J Epidem 116:76–85, 1982.

75. Rutstein DD, Mullan RJ, Frazier TM, et al: Sentinel health events (occupational): A basis for physician recognition and public health surveillance. Arch Environ Health 39:159–168, 1983.

76. Saccomanno G, Archer VE: Histologic types of lung cancer among uranium miners. Cancer 7:515–523, 1971.

77. Sakabe H: Lung cancer due to exposure to bis (chloromethyl) ether. Ind Health 11:145–147, 1973.

78. Schulte P, Halperin W, Ward E: Final discussion: Where do we go from here? J Occup Med 32:936–945, 1990.

79. Scott TS: The incidence of bladder toumors in a dye stuff factory. Br J Ind Med 9:127–132, 1952.

80. Selikoff IJ, Hammond EC, Seidman H: Mortality experience of insulation workers in the United States and Canada, 1943–1976. Ann N Y Acad Sci 330:91, 1979.

81. Selikoff IJ, Churg J, Hammond EC: Relation between exposure to asbestos and mesothelioma. N Engl J Med 272:560–565, 1965.

82. Sexton RJ: The hazards to health in the dehydrogenation of coal. IV. The control program and the clinical effects. Arch Environ Health 1:208–231, 1960.

83. Silverman DT, Levin LI, Hoover RN, Hartge P: Occupational risks of bladder cancer in the United States: I. White men. J Natl Cancer Inst 81:1472–1480, 1989.

84. Silverstein M, Park R, Marmar M, et al: Mortality among beating plant workers exposed to metalworking fluids and abrasives. J Occup Med 30:706–714, 1988.

85. Silverstein M: Analysis of medical screening and surveillance in 21 occupational safety and health administration standards: Support for a generic medical surveillance standard. Am J Ind Med 26:283–295, 1994.

86. Spirtas R, Kaminski RJ: Angiosarcoma of the liver in vinyl chloride/polyvinyl chloride workers. J Occup Med 20:427–429, 1978.

87. Strauss GM, Gleason RE, Sugarbaker DJ: Screening for lung cancer re-examined. A reinterpretation of the Mayo Lung Project randomized trial on lung cancer screening. Chest 103:337S, 1993.

88. Sunderman FW Jr: A review of the carcinogenicities of nickel, chromium and arsenic compounds in man and animals. Prev Med 5:279–294, 1976.

89. Thiess AM, Hey W, Zellar H: Zur toxikologie von dichdor dimethyl ather: Verdacht out kenkerogenic wirkung auch beim menschen. Zentralbl Arbeitsmedizin 23:97–102, 1973.

90. Tolbert P, Eisen E, Pothier LJ, et al: Mortality studies of machinery-fluid exposure in the automobile industry. II. Risks associated with specific fluid types. Scand J Work Environ Health 18:351–360, 1992.

91. U.S. Bureau of Labor Statistics: Occupational injuries and illnesses: Counts, rates, and characteristics, 1992. Washington, DC, U.S. Dept. of Labor, April 1995, bulletin 2455.

92. U.S. Department of Labor, Bureau of Labor Statistics: Employment and Earnings. Vol 43 (No.1). Washington, DC, U.S. Dept. of Labor, January 1996.

93. U.S. Department of Health and Human Services, National Institute for Occupational Safety and Health: National occupational research agenda. Cincinnati, NIOSH, 1996, publication 96-115.

94. U.S. Department of Health and Human Services: Health United States 1994. Washington, DC, National Center for Health Statistics, 1995, publication PHS 95-1232.

95. U.S. Department of Health and Human Services: Vital Statistics of the United States 1991, Volume II—Mortality part A. Washington, DC, National Center for Health Statistics, 1995, publication PHS 95-1101.

96. U.S. Department of Health and Human Services: National Toxicology Program: Seventh Annual Report on Carcinogens 1994. Washington, DC, DHHS, 1994.

97. U.S. Department of Health and Human Services: Plan and Operation of the Third National Health and Nutrition Examinations Survey, 1988–94. Washington, DC, National Center for Health Statistics, 1994, publication PHS 94-1308.

98. U.S. Department of Health and Human Services, National Institute for Occupational Safety and Health: National occupational exposure survey: Analysis of management interview responses. Cincinnati, NIOSH, 1988, publication 89-103.

99. U.S. Department of Labor, Occupational Safety and Health Administration: Federal Register, 29 CFR Parts 90: Occupational exposure to asbestos; Final Rule, August 1994.

100. Vainio H, Wilbourn J: Identification of carcinogens within the UARC monograph program. Scand J Work Environ Health 18:64–73, 1992.

101. Vena J., Sultz HA, Fiedler RC, Barnes RE: Mortality of workers in an automobile engine and parts manufacturing complex. Br J Ind Med 42:85–93, 1985.

102. Vigliani EC, Saita G: Benzene and leukemia. N Engl J Med 271:872, 1964.

103. Vineis P, Simonato L: Estimation of the proportion of bladder cancers attributable to occupation. Scand J Work Enviorn Health 12:55–60, 1986.

104. Vineis P, Simonato L: Proportion of lung and bladder cancers in males resulting from occupation: A systematic approach. Arch Environ Health 46:6–15, 1991.

105. Wagner JC, Sleggs CA, Marchand P: Diffuse pleural mesotheliomas and asbestos exposure in the north western cape province. Br J Ind Med 17:260–271, 1960.

106. Waterhouse JAH: Cutting oils and cancer. Ann Occup Hyg 124:161–170, 1971.

107. Waxweiler RJ, Stringer W, Wagoner JK, Jones J: Neoplastic risk among workers exposed to vinyl chloride. Ann N Y Acad Sci 271:40, 1976.

108. Williams RR, Stegens NL, Goldsmith JR: Associations of cancer site and type with occupation and industry from the Third National Cancer Survey interview. J Natl Cancer Inst 59:1147–1185, 1977.

109. Yin SN, Hayes RB, Linet MS, et al: A cohort study of cancer among benzene-exposed workers in China: Overall results. Am J Ind Med 29:227–235, 1996.

110. Yodaiken RE, Jones E, Spolnicki HG, Deitchman S: Regulators and workplace carcinogens. Occup Med State Art Rev 2:197–206, 1987.

AVIMA M. RUDER, PhD

EPIDEMIOLOGY OF OCCUPATIONAL CARCINOGENS AND MUTAGENS

From the Industrywide Studies
Branch
Division of Surveillance, Hazard
Evaluation, and Field Studies
National Institute for Occupational
Safety and Health
Cincinnati, Ohio

Reprint requests to:
Avima Ruder, PhD
NIOSH Taft Labs MS R-16
4676 Columbia Parkway
Cincinnati, OH 45226

Associations between occupational exposure and carcinogenesis have been recognized since 1775.[75,76] From a public health perspective, confirming occupational exposures to individual substances or mixtures as carcinogenic would support the development of recommendations for reducing those exposures. Epidemiologic studies of occupational risk may require a large sample and a long follow-up to demonstrate clearly an effect, if it exists. Meanwhile, exposures may continue. The International Agency for Research on Cancer evaluates study design as well as results when it reviews epidemiologic studies to determine carcinogenicity.[42] In general, the IARC requires solid epidemiologic evidence (several well-designed studies with consistent results) of carcinogenicity before identifying chemicals as belonging in group 1. For chemicals classified in groups 2A and 2B, IARC regards the epidemiologic evidence for carcinogenicity as insufficient or inconsistent.[42]

Scientists have long sought ways to predict human carcinogenicity. Studies in animals are one well-established approach,[33,41] but the dose levels, usually relatively higher than occupational exposures, and species differences in various toxicokinetic factors[36,40] (and *vide* saccharin studies) have kept animal studies from becoming the "gold standard" that can convince both scientists and nonscientists. It also has been argued that the high doses given to experimental animals induce cell proliferation and that it is this, rather than a specific effect of the chemicals, that leads to carcinogenesis.[2] Beginning in the 1970s, the emergence of molecular biology held the promise of elucidating the cellular mechanisms leading to

OCCUPATIONAL MEDICINE: State of the Art Reviews—
Vol. 11, No. 3, July–September 1996. Philadelphia, Hanley & Belfus, Inc.   **487**

carcinogenesis—the sequence of events between exposure and the emergence of the tumor. In addition, new in vitro assays[4] were to be the gold standard for mutagenesis, which in vivo could lead to health effects other than cancer. The chain of evidence from specific exposure to disease is still incomplete for nearly all occupational exposures. In some cases, the carcinogenic agent(s) has not been defined, because multiple simultaneous exposures exist, e.g., in iron foundry workers[66] or workers exposed to diesel exhaust.[82] For others, the mechanism by which cancer arises is not well understood but is thought to be epigenetic rather than genetic (e.g., for tetrachloroethylene[17,34]). Although every known mutagen of eukaryotic cells in vivo could be considered a potential carcinogen, a number of carcinogens, including asbestos and cadmium, do not appear to have any mutagenic activity.[46]

A number of questions regarding what exactly constitutes occupational carcinogens and mutagens need to be explored. It is clear that not all carcinogens are mutagens, as defined as a substance that interacts with deoxyribonucleic acid, leading to a heritable change in DNA, in either somatic or germ-line cells. Some nonmutagenic carcinogens increase cell proliferation; an increase in the number of replication cycles is associated with an increased risk of random mutation,[85] of mutation fixation, the incorporation of a mutation into the genomes of daughter cells when a cell divides, and of carcinogenesis.[5]

The development of a spectrum of in vitro and in vivo mutagenicity tests raises another question. What is the gold standard for declaring a substance or mixture mutagenic? Although IARC monographs and supplements review data on mutagenicity,[42–46] the substances are not classified as to the strength of the evidence on mutagenicity.

METHODS
To explore the relationship between carcinogenesis and mutagenesis, we evaluated all the substances or exposures for which IARC evaluations have been done and for which we could obtain some estimate of numbers of exposed workers in the United States. A search was done in the Registry of Toxic Effects of Chemical Substances database in TOXNET, the National Library of Medicine's on-line retrieval Toxicology Information Program,[64] for substances having both IARC reviews (1,275 citations) and estimates of numbers of workers potentially exposed from the National Occupational Exposure Survey (NOES) conducted in the early 1980s[84] (4613 citations). A total of 614 substances had both IARC reviews and NOES estimates. When estimates from the National Occupational Hazard Survey (NOHS)[70] conducted in the early 1970s (5043 citations), as well as NOES citations, were allowed, 654 substances had both IARC reviews and estimates of numbers of potentially exposed workers. In NOES and NOHS, potential exposure is based on survey data, not on sampling for the substance, and estimates of numbers of workers are extrapolated from a sample that excluded certain sectors of the workforce.

A Medical Literature Analysis and Retrieval System bibliography covering 1966–1996, generated by searching on "(occupational exposure AND (carcinogenicity OR mutagenicity))," provided citations to supplement the IARC summaries. Information from the citations was used to summarize the tests relevant to mutagenicity (Table 1).

All IARC group 1 (sufficient evidence of carcinogenicity in humans) industrial and agricultural chemicals are included in Table 2. Tables 3 and 4 present group 2A probable carcinogens and group 2B possible carcinogens. IARC group 3 chemicals (not classifiable as to their carcinogenicity in humans) to which more than 10,000 U.S. workers are potentially exposed are included in Table 5. Other chemicals of interest for which the number of exposed workers is not available (but which in most cases is presumed to be large) were added to Tables 2–5.

OCCUPATIONAL CARCINOGENS AND IN VITRO MUTAGENS

The IARC rating system is considered by many in the scientific community as a gold standard for carcinogens.[38,98] To date, IARC has categorized the carcinogenicity of more than 1,000 chemicals of the millions known and tens of thousands in common use.[38] It is clear that the pace of human studies is inadequate to evaluate definitively even the most commonly used chemicals. Occupational cohort studies are often criticized because critical lifestyle information, such as smoking history, is unavailable. For many cancer sites, smoking is the predominant risk factor. However, methods have been developed to adjust for the lack of data on smoking for the entire cohort.[12,92] In occupational cohort mortality studies, workers may be characterized as having been diagnosed with cancer on the basis of the death certificate. Cancers in remission at the time of death may not even be listed as "other significant conditions." Occupational mortality studies may be unable to detect increases in cancers with high survival rates, such as bladder, breast, and prostate cancer. Hospital- or population-based case-control studies and death certificate studies may not have sufficient work-history data to characterize exposures. However, despite their faults, epidemiologic studies have established many widely used chemicals as carcinogenic. And even if a single study, considered alone, may not be definitive, evidence accumulates as more and more studies are done.

In vitro assays are quicker and cheaper than epidemiologic studies or rodent bioassays but raise the question of whether they reflect human carcinogenicity. In the original bacterial mutagenicity assay, a *Salmonella typhimurium* strain requiring histidine for growth was raised on histidine-negative medium on which only mutant revertants to wild type survived.[3] Plates to which various substances had been added were scored against control plates.[3] Since spontaneous mutations occur in every individual in every species, what is being tested is always relative mutagenicity. The relevant question is: Does exposure to this substance significantly increase the mutation rate over the background mutation rate?

Modifications of the Ames method, such as incubation with liver extract to facilitate the formation of mutagenic metabolites from a nonmutagenic parent compound,[4] and incubation with β-glucuronidase to convert glucuronide-conjugated arylamines to mutagenic metabolites,[86] enhanced its applicability to the study of human exposure to mutagens. Ames test assays of known animal carcinogens show that the majority are mutagenic; when McCann and Ames tested 175 carcinogens, 90% were mutagenic.[62] Another large survey found 60% of 230 carcinogens to be mutagenic and 61% of 44 noncarcinogens to be nonmutagenic.[20] The predictability of the Ames test varied by chemical class from 73% for hydrocarbon carcinogens to 23% for alcohol carcinogens.[20] Bacterial assays also are not consistent for metal carcinogens.[93] As the mutagenicity assay results presented in Tables 2–5 show, bacterial mutagenicity is not a consistent predictor of mammalian mutagenicity.

Determination of mutagenicity is important because of the link to carcinogenicity, but also in and of itself. There is a spectrum of effects due to mutagens, from adduct formation to sperm lethality.[27] Nonlethal de novo mutations in the germ line may be transmitted for generations.[101] Somatic mutations could cause other disease outcomes as well as cancer.

A battery of mutagenicity tests has been developed in the past quarter century (Table 1), comprising direct evidence of mutagenicity (revertant mutants, mutations in vivo and in vitro), indirect evidence (chromosome aberrations; micronuclei; increased unscheduled DNA synthesis; DNA adducts, alkylation, single-strand breaks, and crosslinks; sister chromatid exchanges), and evidence of body burden (protein adducts, protein alkylation).

When urine or other specimens of exposed workers and referents, rather than the original chemical, are used as the putative mutagen in in vitro Ames tests,[86,103] metabolites of the suspected parent compound are captured. Such tests also are useful when the specific suspect compound is not known or there are multiple suspect chemicals.[28,53] However, if the compound or metabolites are not detectable or are inactivated in urine, saliva, or other specimens,[28,77,82] these assays may fail to show a difference between exposed and unexposed individuals. In addition, an increase in in vitro mutations after incubation with body fluid does not establish the presence of the parent compound or metabolites in the presumed target organ.[61,68]

Another group of mutagenicity tests uses human cells as the substrate: most often, peripheral lymphocytes.[29] Levels of chromosome aberrations,[27,59] SCEs,[73] DNA damage,[25,30,38,100] and DNA repair[10,50] are compared between exposed and unexposed individuals. In the gamma-ray challenge,[10] cells of exposed and unexposed workers are dosed with gamma-rays to test the hypothesis that exposure has compromised the ability of the cells of exposed workers to repair an additional environmental insult.

A drawback of any of these tests comparing specimens from exposed and unexposed individuals is that exposure must have occurred in the former group. An ideal test would predict mutagenicity or carcinogenicity in humans without anyone having to be exposed.

There are other questions to consider in evaluating the relevance of a human-specimen-based in vitro test to the possibility of human carcinogenesis. Because of the multiple effects of cigarette smoke,[11] it is important to control for smoking. Since these tests require a biologic specimen from each individual, smoking habits could be asked about or cotinine testing done on urine, with permission. Information about other potential risk factors or confounders (medicines, radiation, chemotherapy, other occupational exposures) could be obtained by collecting a complete medical, work, and lifestyle-exposure history.

It should be made clear whether the level of mutagenicity (% mutated cells) in exposed workers' specimens is being compared to that in the general population, to that in a referent group,[19] or to that in the same workers, prior to the exposure. The last comparison would control for confounding exposures, as well as individual variations such as whether the worker was a slow or fast acetylator.[86] Slow acetylators have a higher N-oxidated arylamine/N-acetylated arylamine ratio[15] and apparently metabolize aromatic amines such as 2-naphthylamine an order of magnitude more slowly than do fast acetylators.[49] When exposed to aromatic amines, slow acetylators are at greater risk of bladder cancer. Studies of the acetylator status of bladder cancer patients have shown a significant excess of slow acetylators among those whose bladder cancer is associated with aromatic amine exposure.[60] A number of other genetic polymorphisms affect the response to occupational and environmental carcinogens.

Some, but not all, of the studies in human populations cited in Tables 2–5 control for these confounders. Clearly, the development of a standard checklist of major possible confounders would aid both the researchers conducting these studies and those considering the results in risk assessments.

A final consideration in comparing tests of mutagenesis is their utility in mass screening, including considerations of ease of administration, cost, and implications for the worker tested.[14,37]

The existence of multiple possible tests raises another difficulty—that a substance may be mutagenic in one assay system but not others. If results for one test are positive and for another are ambiguous or negative, how is the chemical to be classified as to mutagenicity? In Tables 2–5 we have tallied test results as interpreted by the authors of the articles or the IARC reviewers. It is clear that some substances are mutagenic in every system tested (e.g., vinyl chloride, 2-naphthylamine, sulfur mustard, which are all group 1 carcinogens). However, even among the group 1 carcinogens there is some ambiguity in mutagenicity test results (e.g., nickel, coke production) and some apparent nonmutagens (e.g., cadmium, asbestos). It is also clear from the gaps in Tables 2–5 that there has been no systematic attempt to evaluate the mutagenicity of IARC-categorized "probable" and "possible" carcinogens to which hundreds of thousands of workers are currently exposed.

The effort to relate mutagenicity to potential carcinogenicity is being pursued by the National Toxicology Program. Prediction of unlikely, possible, or probable carcinogenicity, with a genotoxic or nongenotoxic mechanism, is based on a compound's structural similarity to known carcinogens, and results of bacterial assays and short-term (90 day) subchronic experimental animal toxicity tests.[94] These predictions have been compared to the results of 2-year animal studies: 3 of 16 compounds predicted to be noncarcinogenic were animal carcinogens and 7 of 24 predicted to be carcinogens were noncarcinogenic,[9] making 25% of the predictions discordant. The goal is a standard battery of in vitro tests and an algorithm that predicts rodent (and possibly human) carcinogenicity accurately enough to make long-term animal studies unnecessary.[9] Without a standard battery of tests,[8] predictability will not improve.

DISCUSSION

The development of in vitro assays for mutagenicity more than 25 years ago raised expectations of rapid, reliable, relatively inexpensive tests that would obviate the need for animal tumor studies and occupational cohort cancer studies. That has not happened yet. In 1995, the National Institute for Environmental Health Sciences hosted a meeting, "Mechanism-Based Toxicity in Cancer Risk Assessment," to consider ways of shortening the testing period for compounds being evaluated by NTP, by reaching a consensus on which in vitro assays and short-term animal tests could predict human carcinogenicity with near certainty, but consensus is not yet possible. In addition to their relevance to carcinogenity, mutagens can cause birth defects and other problems.[27] Many exposure standards are based on whether a compound is a toxin or irritant, not on potential mutagenicity or carcinogenicity. Agreement ultimately will be reached on what level of response in which in vitro assay(s) best predicts human mutagenicity and carcinogenicity, and how to predict the possible carcinogenicity of nonmutagens.[20,95] Until then, exposure recommendations relative to carcinogenicity will continue to be based on experimental animal and human epidemiology studies.

What are the definitive tests? Results from tests using bacterial cells are difficult to relate to human disease. Adding liver extract to the Ames test induces formation of metabolites. In vivo, however, humans are polymorphic for a number of enzymes. The addition of standard S9 enzymes may mask the difference between those who in vivo do convert the parent compound to a mutagen (and therefore are at higher risk) and those who are deficient in the relevant enzyme in vivo and do not make the conversion. The most relevant tests appear to be those using human cells, especially from exposed individuals. Each biomarker test focuses on one stage between exposure and disease, providing high or low statistical probability of an association, but not definitive evidence connecting exposure and disease. Furthermore, by the time markers of disease are evident, biomarkers of exposure such as urine or serum levels of a compound or its metabolite(s) may no longer be evident. Prospective studies monitoring workers to document body burden during the period of exposure, followed by periodic monitoring for effects of exposure and early markers of disease, would link exposure and disease in the same individuals.

Millions of workers in the United States alone are potentially exposed to chemicals already evaluated by IARC as being carcinogenic in humans, and millions more to probable and possible carcinogens. With thousands of unevaluated chemicals already in use, and with newly synthesized chemicals being put into commercial production at the rate of thousands yearly, clearly there is an urgent need for rapid evaluation of the risk of mutagenicity and carcinogenicity. There also is a need for additional epidemiologic studies focusing on chemicals currently classified by IARC in groups 2A and 2B, for which IARC has judged the epidemiologic evidence to date as insufficient or inconsistent[42] and to which large numbers of workers are currently exposed.

ACKNOWLEDGMENT

Thanks to Glenn Talaska of the University of Cincinnati and Elizabeth Ward and Tom Reid of NIOSH for helpful suggestions.

REFERENCES

1. al-Sabti K, Lloyd DC, Edwards AA, Stegnar P: A survey of lymphocyte chromosomal damage in Slovenian workers exposed to occupational clastogens. Mutat Res 280:215–223, 1992.
2. Ames BN: Mutagenesis and carcinogenesis: Endogenous and exogenous factors. Environ Mol Mutagen 14 Suppl 16:66–77, 1989.
3. Ames BN: Carcinogens are mutagens: Their detection and classification. Environ Health Perspect 6:115–118, 1973.
4. Ames BN, McCann J, Yamasaki E: Methods for detecting carcinogens and mutagens with the Salmonella mammalian microsome mutagenicity test. Mutat Res 31:347–64, 1975.
5. Ames BN, Shigegaga MK, Gold LS: DNA lesions, inducible DNA repair, and cell division: Three key factors in mutagenesis and carcinogenesis. Environ Health Perspect 101(suppl 5):34–44, 1993.
6. Anwar WA, Shamy MY: Chromosomal aberrations and micronuclei in reinforced plastics workers exposed to styrene. Mutat Res 327:41–47, 1995.
7. Apostoli P, Leone R, Porru S, et al: Urinary mutagenicity tests in lead-exposed workers. Mutat Res 222:245–251, 1989.
8. Ashby J, Richardson CR: Tabulation and assessment of 113 human surveillance cytogenetic studies conducted between 1965 and 1984. Mutat Res 154:111–133, 1985.
9. Ashby J, Tennant RW: Prediction of rodent carcinogenicity for 44 chemicals: Results. Mutagenesis 9:7–15, 1994.
10. Au WW, Bechtold WE, Whorton EB Jr, Legator MS: Chromosome aberrations and response to gamma-ray challenge in lymphocytes of workers exposed to 1,3-butadiene. Mutat Res 334:125–130, 1995.
11. Au WW, Ramanujam VMS, Ward JB Jr., Legator MS: Chromosome aberrations in lymphocytes of mice after sub-acute low-level inhalation exposure to benzene. Mutat Res 260:219–224, 1991.
12. Axelson O, Steenland K: Indirect methods of assessing the effects of tobacco use in occupational studies. Am J Ind Med 13:105–118, 1988.
13. Bagwe AN, Bhisey RA: Occupational exposure to unburnt bidi tobacco elevates mutagenic burden among tobacco processors. Carcinogenesis 16:1095–1099, 1995.
14. Baker EL: Role of medical screening in the prevention of occupational disease. J Occup Med 32:787–788, 1990.

15. Beland FA, Kadlubar FF: Factors involved in the induction of urinary bladder cancer by aromatic amines. Banbury Report 23:315–326, 1986.

16. Bos RP, Jongeneelen FJ, Theuws JL, Henderson PT: Exposure to mutagenic aromatic hydrocarbons of workers creosoting wood. IARC Sci Publ 59:279–288, 1984.

17. Bronzelli G, Bauer C, Corsi C, et al: Genetic and biochemical studies on perchloroethylene 'in vitro' and 'in vivo'. Mutat Res 116:323–331, 1983.

18. Carstensen U, Alexandrie AK, Hogstedt B, et al: B- and T-lymphocyte micronuclei in chimney sweeps with respect to genetic polymorphism for CYP1A1 and GST1 (class Mu). Mutat Res 289:187–195, 1993.

19. Choi BC, Connolly JG, Zhou RH: Application of urinary mutagen testing to detect workplace hazardous exposure and bladder cancer. Mutat Res 341:207–216, 1995.

20. Claxton LD, Stead AG, Walsh D: An analysis by chemical class of Salmonella mutagenicity tests as predictors of animal carcinogenicity. Mutat Res 205:197–225, 1988.

21. Clonfero E, Granella M, Marchioro M, et al: Urinary excretion of mutagens in coke oven workers. Carcinogenesis 16:547–554, 1995.

22. Compton-Quintana PJ, Jensen RH, Bigbee WL, et al: Use of the glycophorin A human mutation assay to study workers exposed to styrene. Environ Health Perspect 99:297–301, 1993.

23. Di Giorgio C, De Meo MP, Laget M, et al: The micronucleus assay in human lymphocytes: Screening for inter-individual variability and application to biomonitoring. Carcinogenesis 15:313–317, 1994.

24. Dubeau H, Zazi W, Baron C, Messing K: Effects of lymphocyte subpopulations on the clonal assay of HPRT mutants: Occupational exposure to cytostatic drugs. Mutat Res 321:147–157, 1994.

25. Ehrenberg L, Osterman-Golkar S: Alkylation of macromolecules for detecting mutagenic agents. Teratog Carcinog Mutag 1:105–127, 1980.

26. Elovaara E, Heikkila P, Pyy L, Mutanen P, Riihimaki V: Significance of dermal and respiratory uptake in creosote workers: Exposure to polycyclic aromatic hydrocarbons and urinary excretion of 1-hydroxypyrene. Occup Environ Med 52:196–203, 1995.

27. Fabricant JD, Legator MS: Etiology, role and detection of chromosomal aberrations in man. J Occup Med 23:617–625, 1981.

28. Falck K: Biological monitoring of occupational exposure to mutagenic chemicals in the rubber industry. Use of the bacterial urinary mutagenicity assay. Scand J Work Environ Health 9:39–42, 1983.

29. Forni A, Bertazzi PA: Epidemiology in protection and prevention against environmental mutagens/carcinogens. Examples from occupational medicine. Mutat Res 181:289–297, 1987.

30. Fuchs J, Burg J, Hengstler JG, et al: DNA damage in mononuclear blood cells of metal workers exposed to N- nitrosodiethanolamine in synthetic cutting fluids. Mutat Res 342:95–102, 1995.

31. Fučić A, Garaj-Vrhovac V, Barković D, Kubelka D: The sensitivity of the micronucleus assay for the detection of occupational exposure to vinyl chloride monomer. Mutat Res 325:53–56, 1994.

32. Fučić A, Garaj-Vrhovac V, Dimitrović B, Škara M: The persistence of sister-chromatid exchange frequencies in men occupationally exposed to vinyl chloride monomer. Mutat Res 281:129–132, 1992.

33. Gold LS, Manley NB, Slone TH, et al: Sixth plot of the Carcinogenic Potency Database: Results of animal bioassays published in the general literature 1989 to 1990 and by the National Toxicology Program 1990 to 1993. Environ Health Perspect 103(suppl 8):3–123, 1995.

34. Goldsworthy TL, Lyght O, Burnett VL, Popp JA: Potential role of α-2μ-globulin, protein droplet accumulation, and cell replication in the renal carcinogenicity of rats exposed to trichloroethylene, perchloroethylene, and pentachloroethane. Toxicol Appl Pharmacol 96:367–379, 1988.

35. Granella M, Clonfero E: The mutagenic activity and polycyclic aromatic hydrocarbon content of mineral oils. Int Arch Occup Environ Health 63:149–153, 1991.

36. Green T: Species differences in carcinogenicity: The role of metabolism in human risk evaluation. Teratog Carcinog Mutag 10:103–113, 1990.

37. Halperin WE, Ratcliffe J, Frazier TM, et al: Medical screening in the workplace: Proposed principles. J Occup Med 28:547–552, 1986.

38. Hemminki K, Sorsa M, Vainio H: Genetic risks caused by occupational chemicals: Use of experimental methods and occupational risk group monitoring in the detection of environmental chemicals causing mutations, cancer and malformations. Scand J Work Environ Health 5:307–327, 1979.

39. Herskowitz IH: Principles of Genetics. 2nd ed. New York, Macmillian, 1977.

40. Hoel DG, Haseman JK, Hogan MD, et al: The impact of toxicity on carcinogenicity studies: Implications for risk assessment. Carcinogenesis 9:2045–2052, 1988.

41. Huff J: Chemicals and cancer in humans: First evidence in experimental animals. Environ Health Perspect 100:201–210, 1993.

42. International Agency for Research on Cancer: Some Industrial Chemicals. IARC Monogr Eval Carcinog Risks Hum 60: 1994.
43. International Agency for Research on Cancer: Solar and Ultraviolet Radiation. IARC Monogr Eval Carcinog Risks Hum 55: 1992.
44. International Agency for Research on Cancer: Occupational Exposures to Mists and Vapours from Strong Inorganic Acids; and Other Industrial Chemicals. IARC Monogr Eval Carcinog Risks Hum 54: 1992.
45. International Agency for Research on Cancer: Some Organic Solvents, Resin Monomers and Related Compounds, Pigments and Occupational Exposures in Paint Manufacture and Painting. IARC Monogr Eval Carcinog Risks Hum 47: 1989.
46. International Agency for Research on Cancer: Overall Evaluations of Carcinogenicity: An Updating of IARC Mongraphs Volumes 1 to 42. IARC Monogr Eval Carcinog Risks Hum Suppl 7: 1987.
47. Joksic G, Markovic B: [Cytogenetic changes in persons exposed to polychlorinated biphenyls] Arh Hig Rada Toksikol 43:29 35, 1992.
48. Karelova J, Jablonicka A, Gavora J, Hano L: Chromosome and sister-chromatid exchange analysis in peripheral lymphocytes, and mutagenicity of urine in anesthesiology personnel. Int Arch Occup Environ Health 64:303–306, 1992.
49. Kirlin WG, Trinidad A, Yerokum T, et al: Polymorphic expression of acetyl coenzyme A-dependent arylamine N-acetyltransferase and acetyl coenzyme A-dependent O-acetyltransferase-mediated activation of N-hydroxyarylamines by human bladder cytosol. Cancer Res 49:2448–2454, 1989.
50. Knudsen LE, Boisen T, Christensen JM, et al: Biomonitoring of genotoxic exposure among stainless steel welders. Mutat Res 279:129–143, 1992.
51. Knudsen LE, Sorsa M: Human biological monitoring of occupational genotoxic exposures. Pharmacol Toxicol 72:86–92, 1993.
52. Krøkje A, Schmid R, Zahlsen K: Liver, lung and kidney homogenates used as an activation system in mutagenicity studies of airborne particles and of expectorate and urine samples from exposed workers in a coke plant. Mutat Res 259:49–65, 1991.
53. Krøkje A, Tiltnes A, Mylius E, Gullvag B: Testing for mutagens in an aluminium plant. The results of Salmonella typhimurium tests on expectorates from exposed workers. Mutat Res 156:147–152, 1985.
54. Kučerová M, Zhurkov VS, Polívková Z, Ivanova JE: Mutagenic effect of epichlorohydrin. II. Analysis of chromosomal aberrations in lymphocytes of persons occupationally exposed to epichlorohydrin. Mutat Res 48:355–360, 1977.
55. Latt SA: Sister chromatid exchanges, indices of human chromosome damage and repair. Proc Natl Acad Sci U S A 71:3162–3166, 1974.
56. Lauwerys RR, Hoet P: Industrial Chemical Exposure Guidelines for Biological Monitoring. 2nd ed. Boca Raton, FL, Lewis Publishers, 1993.
57. Legator MS, Au WW, Ammenheuser M, Ward JB Jr: Elevated somatic cell mutant frequencies and altered DNA repair responses in nonsmoking workers exposed to 1,3-butadiene. IARC Sci Publ 127:253–263, 1993.
58. Lin X, Sugiyama M, Costa M: Differences in the effect of vitamin E on nickel sulfide or nickel chloride-induced chromosomal aberrations in mammalian cells. Mutat Res 260:159–164, 1991.
59. Loomis DP, Shy CM, Allen JW, Saccomanno G: Micronuclei in epithelial cells from sputum of uranium workers. Scand J Work Environ Health 16:355–362, 1990.
60. Lower GM: Arylamines and bladder cancer causality: Application of conceptual and operational criteria. Clin Pharmacol Ther 34:129–135, 1983.
61. Ma XF, Babish JG, Scarlett JM, et al: Mutagens in urine sampled repetitively from municipal refuse incinerator workers and water treatment workers. J Toxicol Environ Health 37:483–494, 1992.
62. McCann J, Ames B: Detection of carcinogens as mutagens in the Salmonella/microsome test. Assay of 300 chemicals. Proc Natl Acad Sci U S A 73:950–954, 1976.
63. Migliore L, Parrini M, Sbrana I, et al: Micronucleated lymphocytes in people occupationally exposed to potential environmental contaminants: the age effect. Mutat Res 256:13–20, 1991.
64. National Library of Medicine: Toxicology Information Program. Bethesda, MD, National Library of Medicine, 1990.
65. Norppa H, Hirvonen A, Järventaus H, et al: Role of GSTT1 and GSTM1 genotypes in determining individual sensitivity to sister chromatid exchange induction by diepoxybutane in cultured human lymphocytes. Carcinogenesis 15:1261–1264, 1995.
66. Omland O, Sherson D, Hansen AM, et al: Exposure of iron foundry workers to polycyclic aromatic hydrocarbons: benzo(a)pyrene-albumin adducts and 1-hydroxypyrene as biomarkers for exposure. Occup Environ Med 51:513–518, 1994.

67. Osterman-Golkar SM, Bond JA, Ward JB Jr, Legator MS: Use of haemoglobin adducts for biomonitoring exposure to 1,3-butadiene. IARC Sci Publ 127:127–134, 1993.

68. Pasquini R, Monarca S, Sforzolini GS, et al: Mutagenicity studies and D-glucaric acid determination in urine of workers exposed to mineral oils. Int Arch Occup Environ Health 56:275–284, 1985.

69. Pasquini R, Monarca S, Sforzolini GS, et al: Mutagens in urine of carbon electrode workers. Int Arch Occup Environ Health 50:387–395, 1982.

70. Pederson DH, Young RO, Sundin DS: A model for the identification of high-risk occupational groups using RTECS and NOHS Data. Cincinnati, National Institute for Occupational Safety and Health, 1983, publication 83-117.

71. Perera FP, Dickey C, Santella R, et al: Carcinogen-DNA adducts and gene mutation in foundry workers with low- level exposure to polycyclic aromatic hydrocarbons. Carcinogenesis 15:2905–2910, 1994.

72. Perera FP, Tang DL, O'Neill JP, et al: HPRT and glycophorin A mutations in foundry workers: Relationship to PAH exposure and to PAH-DNA adducts. Carcinogenesis 14:969–973, 1993.

73. Perry P, Evans HJ: Cytological detection of mutagen-carcinogen exposure by sister chromatid exchanges. Nature 258:121–125, 1975.

74. Popp W, Vahrenholz C, Goch S, et al: [Experiences with alkaline filter elution for the detection of DNA damage by genotoxic compounds]. Zentralbl Hyg Umweltmed 193:140–149, 1992.

75. Pott P: Chirurgical Observations. London, Hawes, Clarke and Collins, 1775. Cited in Checkoway H, Pearce NE, Crawford-Brown DJ: Research Methods in Occupational Epidemiology. New York, Oxford University Press, 1989.

76. Rehn L: Blasengeschwülste bei fuchsinarbeitern. Verhandl Deut Ges Chir pt 1:240–252, 1895. Cited in Hueper WC Occupational and Environmental Cancers of the Urinary System. New Haven, CT, Yale University Press, 1969.

77. Reuterwall C, Aringer L, Elinder CG, et al: Assessment of genotoxic exposure in Swedish coke-oven work by different methods of biological monitoring. Scand J Work Environ Health 17:123–132, 1991.

78. Santella RM, Hemminki K, Tang DL, et al: Polycyclic aromatic hydrocarbon-DNA adducts in white blood cells and urinary 1-hydroxypyrene in foundry workers. Cancer Epidemiol Biomarkers Prev 2:59–62, 1993.

79. Sasiadek M: Sister-chromatid exchanges and cell-cycle kinetics in the lymphocytes of workers occupationally exposed to a chemical mixture in the tyre industry. Mutat Res 302:197–200, 1993.

80. Sbrana I, Caretto S, Battaglia A: Chromosomal aberration analysis of workers in tannery industries. Mutat Res 260:331–336, 1991.

81. Sbrana I, Caretto S, Lascialfari D, et al: Chromosomal monitoring of chromium-exposed workers. Mutat Res 242:305–312, 1990.

82. Schenker MB, Kado NY, Hammond SK, et al: Urinary mutagenic activity in workers exposed to diesel exhaust. Environ Res 57:133–148, 1992.

83. Schenker MB, Samuels SJ, Kado NY, et al: Markers of exposure to diesel exhaust in railroad workers. Res Rep Health Eff Inst 33:1–51, 1990.

84. Seta JA, Sundin DS, Pedersen DH: National occupational exposure survey field guidelines. Cincinnati, National Institute for Occupational Safety and Health, 1988, pp 88–106.

85. Shields PG, Harris CC: Molecular epidemiology and the genetics of environmental cancer. JAMA 266:681–687, 1991.

86. Sinues B, Perez J, Bernal ML, et al: Urinary mutagenicity and N-acetylation phenotype in textile industry workers exposed to arylamines. Cancer Res 52:4885–4889, 1992.

87. Sinues B, Sanz A, Bernal ML, et al: Sister chromatid exchanges, proliferating rate index, and micronuclei in biomonitoring of internal exposure to vinyl chloride monomer in plastic industry workers. Toxicol Appl Pharmacol 108:37–45, 1991.

88. Skipper PL, Tannenbaum SR: Protein adducts in the molecular dosimetry of chemical carcinogens. Carcinogenesis 11:507–518, 1990.

89. Sobti RC, Bhardwaj DK: Cytogenetic damage and occupational exposure. I. Exposure to stone dust. Environ Res 56:25–30, 1991.

90. Sorsa M, Autio K, Demopoulos NA, et al: Human cytogenetic biomonitoring of occupational exposure to 1,3-butadiene. Mutat Res 309:321–326, 1994.

91. Sorsa M, Falck K, Maki-Paakkanen J, Vainio H: Genotoxic hazards in the rubber industry. Scand J Work Environ Health 9:103–107, 1983.

92. Steenland K, Beaumont J, Halperin W: Methods of control for smoking in occupational cohort mortality studies. Scand J Work Environ Health 10:143–149, 1984.

93. Sunderman FW Jr: Recent advances in metal carcinogenesis. Ann Clin Lab Sci 14:93–122, 1984.

94. Tennant RW, Spalding J, Stasiewicz S, Ashby J: Prediction of the outcome of rodent carcinogenicity bioassays currently being conducted on 44 chemicals by the National Toxicology Program. Mutagenesis 5:3–14, 1990.

95. Tennant RW, Zeiger E: Genetic toxicity: Current status of methods of carcinogen identification. Environ Health Perspect 100:307–315, 1993.

96. Tomanin R, Ballarin C, Bartolucci GB, et al: Chromosome aberrations and micronuclei in lymphocytes of workers exposed to low and medium levels of styrene. Int Arch Occup Environ Health 64:209–215, 1992.

97. Tompa A, Sapi E: Detection of 6-thioguanine resistance in human peripheral blood lymphocytes (PBL) of industrial workers and lung cancer patients. Mutat Res 210:345–351, 1989.

98. Vaino H, Hemminki K: Use of exposure information and animal cancer data in the prevention of environmental and occupational cancer. Cancer Detect Prevent 15:7–16, 1991.

99. Van Hummelen P, Severi M, Pauwels W, et al: Cytogenetic analysis of lymphocytes from fiberglass-reinforced plastics workers occupationally exposed to styrene. Mutat Res 310:157–165, 1994.

100. van Schooten FJ, Jongeneelen FJ, Hillebrand MJ, et al: Polycyclic aromatic hydrocarbon-DNA adducts in white blood cell DNA and 1-hydroxypyrene in the urine from aluminum workers: Relation with job category and synergistic effect of smoking. Cancer Epidemiol Biomarkers Prev 4:69 77, 1995.

101. Vogel F, Motulsky AG: Human Genetics. New York, Springer-Verlag, 1979.

102. Willems MI, de Raat WK, Wesstra JA, et al: Urinary and faecal mutagenicity in car mechanics exposed to diesel exhaust and in unexposed office workers. Mutat Res 222:375–391, 1989.

103. Yamasaki E, Ames BN: Concentration of mutagens from urine by adsorption with the non-polar resin XAD-2; cigarette smokers have mutagenic urine. Proc Natl Acad Sci U S A 74:3555-3559, 1977.

KEY FOR TABLES 1–5

Nonhuman mutagenicity

A[L]	Substance increases mutations in bacteria in Ames test [with liver enzymes]
DNA[A,AK,B,X]	DNA of exposed animals or in vitro [has adducts, is alkylated, has strand breaks, is cross-linked]
M[B,C,F,V]	Substance increases mutations in [bacteria, animal cells in vitro, fungi, animals in vivo]
SCE	Substance induces sister chromatid exchanges in cultured mammalian cells

Human mutagenicity

Alb[A]	Albumin of exposed workers [has adducts]
E[GPA,μ]	Erythrocytes of workers [have lost glycophorin A gene, have micronuclei]
FA[L]	Feces of exposed workers increase mutations in bacteria in Ames test [with liver enzymes]
Hb[A,AK]	Hemoglobin of exposed workers [has adducts, is alkylated]
PL[C,μ,SCE,γ]	Peripheral lymphocytes of workers have increased [chromosomal aberrations, micronuclei, sister chromatid exchanges, deficiency of DNA repair after γ-ray challenge]
PL[HPRT, UDS]	Peripheral lymphocytes of workers show [hypoxanthine-guanine-phosphoribosyl transferase deficiency and 6-thioguanine resistance, unscheduled DNA synthesis]
SA[L]	Saliva of exposed workers increases mutations in bacteria in Ames test [with liver enzymes]
SE[μ]	Exfoliated cells from saliva of workers have micronuclei
UA[β,L]	Urine of exposed workers increases mutations in bacteria in Ames test [incubated with β-glucuronidase, with liver enzymes]
WDNA[A,AK,B]	DNA of exposed workers [has adducts, is alkylated, has strand breaks]

TABLE 1. Cytological Tests and Their Relevance to Mutagenicity

Test Code	Name of test	What It Tests	Relevance to Mutagenicity	Reference
A,FA,UA, SA [B,L]	Ames test	# of revertant bacterial colonies induced by actual chemical or body fluid (urine, feces, saliva) of exposed (and unexposed) individuals. Liver extract may be added so metabolites form. Incubation with β-glucuronidase will convert glucuronide-conjugated arylamines to mutagenic metabolites.	Only revertant colonies survive on the medium. Number of revertants on treated vs. control plates is a measure of mutagenicity over background. Test can be tailored to specific types of mutation (base-pair substitution, frame shift).	4,28,86
DNA^A, WNDA^A, DNA^AK	adduct formation with DNA; DNA alkylation	Binding of substance or metabolite to DNA of lab animals; DNA from cells of exposed workers has adducts bound to it; alkyl group or radical becomes attached to a DNA base by substituting for a hydrogen. Immunoassays using fluorescent antibodies to the substance detect level of adduct formation.	Adducts can lead to errors in DNA replication and thus permanent changes in DNA (changes in base sequence, deletions). These errors may change genes or suppress or permit gene transcription. Adducts can also cause mistakes during DNA transcription to RNA. Some changes in DNA or RNA prevent the RNA from leaving the nucleus for translation. Others affect the protein translation, causing deletions (if 3, 6, etc. bases were deleted from the DNA or not transcribed), frame-shift mutations (if any other multiple of bases was deleted from DNA or not transcribed), or premature terminations of translation. Any change in the amino acid sequence may affect the life or activity of the protein.	25,38,39,71.72
DNA^B, WDNA^B	strand breaks	Single strand breaks in DNA in cultured cells or in DNA from peripheral lymphocytes or other cells of exposed workers.	A measure of genotoxic burden. Broken strands are useful to detect combined effects of a number of chemicals. If single-strand breaks are not repaired they can lead to errors in DNA replication or RNA transcription.	30
DNA^X	crosslinks	Formation of physical link between two bases in same or opposite DNA strands, often by a chemical molecule linking to both bases.	Interstrand links can prevent DNA replication or transcription in the area of the link. Intrastrand links can cause replication or transcription errors. Repair of the link can also cause errors.	39,74
E^GPA	glycophorin A	Flow cytometry records #s of cells with/without M and N cell surface proteins using erythrocytes of workers with MN blood type (50% of population). Normal MN cells fluoresce red (anti-M antibody) and green (anti-N antibody). Cells fluorescing green or red only would presumably no longer produce the corresponding protein.	Cells with cell surface proteins are presumed to be normal and cells without cell surface proteins, mutants. Detects mutations of several types (chromosome-wide events as well as mitotic recombination).	22,72,101
E^μ, PI^μ, SE^μ	micronuclei	Levels of micronuclei in erythrocytes, peripheral lymphocytes, exfoliated cells from saliva of exposed workers. Micronuclei form from chromosome fragments not incorporated in daughter nuclei during cell division.	# micronuclei a measure of both chromosome breaks and chromosome loss. Scoring rapid and needs little expertise.	23,59

TABLE 1. Cytological Tests and Their Relevance to Mutagenicity *(Cont.)*

Test Code	Name of test	What It Tests	Relevance to Mutagenicity	Reference
Hb^A, Alb^A, Hb^{AK}	adduct formation with protein; hemoglobin alkylation	Binding to hemoglobin, albumin, or other protein. Alkylation is preferentially of the terminal valine and of cysteine and histidine.	Monitoring protein adducts might assess exposure to a chemical, indicate the possibility of polymorphisms in processing the chemical, or, by extrapolation, estimate the possible extent of DNA alkylation. Reactivity of proteins toward alkylating agents higher than reactivity of DNA. More protein than DNA available for analyses.	25,56,67,88
PL^C	chromosomal aberrations	Include chromatid and isochromatid deletions, chromatid gaps, acentric and dicentric chromosome fragments, chromatid exchanges, SCEs	Estimate of extent of genetic damage. Deletions can eliminate genes or controls of gene expression such as tumor suppressors. Germ cell mutations or somatic cell mutations in the developing embryo and fetus can lead to increased rates of infertility, spontaneous abortion, stillbirth, birth defects.	6,27
PL^γ	γ-ray challenge	Cells from exposed and unexposed workers dosed with γ rays at G1 phase; chromosome aberrations in first post-irradiation metaphase are scored.	Measure of deficiencies in DNA repair (due to the chemical exposure).	10
PL^{HPRT}	HPRT	Rate of hypoxanthine-guanine-phosphoribosyl transferase (HPRT) deficiency and 6-thioguanine (6TG) resistance in cells tested on 6TG medium which kills nonmutant cells.	Demonstrates a mutation event. If there are more resistant cells at higher doses (measured by conventional monitoring or level or urinary metabolites), the evidence for mutagenicity due to a particular exposure is stronger.	24,57
PL^{SCE}	sister chromatid exchange	Rate of sister chromatid exchanges in peripheral lymphocytes of exposed (and unexposed) individuals during mitosis.	Less persistent than chromosomal aberrations so possibly useful in assessing short-term increase or decrease in exposure. There is a strong effect of smoking on SCE, so smoking status should be known	29,55,73
SCE	sister chromatid exchange	Number of SCEs induced in cultured mammalian cells dosed with test chemical	SCE is symmetrical exchange at one locus, detectable with autoradiography, 5-bromodeoxyuridine treatment, fluorescent staining. SCE induction rate parallels induction rate of gross chromosomal aberrations.	73
UDS	unscheduled DNA synthesis	Cells incubated with chemical X, then with [³H]thymidine in chemical X-free medium. Thymidine uptake rate compared with that of control cells.	Measure of overall DNA repair. Repair capacity defined as UDS rate/binding of chemical X to DNA.	50

For mutagenicity test codes, see Key for Tables 1-5

TABLE 2. IARC Group I * Industrial and Agricultural Chemicals, with Any Evidence of Mutagenicity

Chemical Name or Industry	Est. Minimum No. of Workers†	Cytological Test [agent or job title tested] (Effect Seen in Exposed?)	Reference
Coal-tars	3,380,000	PL^C (Y), A^L (Y)	46
Nickel & nickel compounds^N	1,000,000	PL^C (Y), PL^{SCE} (N), M^V (Q), M^C (Y), M^B (N), M^C (Y)	46 58
Aluminum production	1,100,000	PL^{SCE} (N), PL^C (N), UA^L (Q), DNA^A [PAH] (Y), SA^L (Y)	46 100 53
Mineral oils, untreated & mildly-treated oils	1,100,000	PL^C (Y), UA^L (Y), A^L (Y), A^L (Y)	46 35
Hexavalent chromium compounds (chromic acid)^N	850,000	PL^C (Q), M^C (Y), M^V (Y), M^F (Y), M^B (Y)	46
Sulfuric acid/ strong inorganic acid mists containing sulfuric acid	750,000	PL^{SCE} (Y), PI^μ (Y), PL^C (Y)	44
Furniture & cabinet making (wood)	500,000	A^L [beechwood dust] (Y)	46
Cadmium & cadmium compounds^{N,O}	500,000	PL^C (N), M^V (N), M^F (N), M^B (N)	46
Asbestos^{N,O}	500,000	PL^{SCE} (Q), DNA^B (N), M^B (N), M^C (N), M^V (N)	46
Iron & steel founding	350,000	$WDNA^A$ [benzo[a]pyrene] (Y), DNA^A [PAH, aromatics] (Y, Y), PL^{HPRT} (Y), DNA^A [PAH] (Y), Alb^A (N)	46 71,72 78 66
Benzene^{N,O}	250,000	M^C (Y), M^V (Y), PL^C (Q), M^V (Y)	46 11
Ethylene oxide^{N,O}	250,000	PL^{SCE} (Y), PL^C (Y), E^μ (Y), Hb^A (Y), PI^μ (Q), M^V (Y), M^C (Y), DNA^X (Y), DNA^B (N)	46 42 74

TABLE 2. IARC Group 1* Industrial and Agricultural Chemicals, with Any Evidence of Mutagenicity *(Cont.)*

Chemical Name or Industry	Est. Minimum No. of Workers†	Cytological Test [agent or job title tested] (Effect Seen in Exposed?)	Reference
Rubber industry	200,000	PL^{SCE} (Y), UA^L (Y), PL^C [weighers,mixers] (Y) PL^C (Y), PL^{SCE})Y) UA^L (Y) PL^{SCE} (N), UA^L [tire bldrs,vulcanizers] (N)	91 79 28 46
Painter (occupational exposure as a)	130,000	PI^μ (Y) PL^{SCE} (N)	23 45
Coke production (coke dust)^{N,O}	130,000	PL^{SCE} (Y), UA^L (Y) $WDNA^A$ [benzo[a]pyrene] (Y) UA^L [PAH] (Q) UA^L (N), PI^μ (N), PL^C (N), PL^{SCE} (N)	46 46 21 77
Vinyl chloride^{N,O}	80,000	PL^C (Y), PL^{SCE} (Y) PI^μ (Y) PL^{SCE} (Y) PL^{SCE} (Y), PI^μ (Y) PL^{HPRT} (Y)	46 31 32 87 97
Arsenic & arsenic compounds^{N,O}	60,000	PL^C (Q), PL^{SCE} (Q)	46
Beryllium & beryllium compounds	40,000	M^C (Q), M^B (Q)	46
Boot & shoe manufacture & repair	30,000	DNA^B (Y), DNA^X (N)	74
Cyclophosphamide	30,000	SCE (Q), M^C (Q) M^Y (Y), M^B (Y)	73 46
Coal-tar pitches^N	15,000	A^L (Y), M^C (Y), DNA^B (N)	46
Benzidine^{N,O}	15,000	DNA^A (Y), M^C (Y), M^F (N), M^B (Y)	46
Magenta, manufacture of	10,000	M^B (Y), M^C (N), M^F (N)	46
Talc containing asbestiform fibers	4,000	M^Y (N), M^C (N), M^F (N), M^B (N)	46
Auramine, manufacture of	700	M^Y (N), M^C (Y), M^F (Y), M^B (Y)	46
Shale-oils (crude)	300	M^Y (Q), M^C (Q)	46
2-Naphthylamine^{N,O}	275	M^Y (Y), M^C (Y), M^F (Y), M^B (Y)	46

TABLE 2. IARC Group 1* Industrial and Agricultural Chemicals, with Any Evidence of Mutagenicity *(Cont.)*

Chemical Name or Industry	Est. Minimum No. of Workers†	Cytological Test [agent or job title tested] (Effect Seen in Exposed?)	Reference
Bis-chloromethyl ether[N,O] and/or chloromethyl methyl ether[N,O]		PL^C (Y), M^V (N), M^C (Y), M^B (Y)	46
4-Aminobiphenyl[N]	n/a	M^V (Y), M^C (Y), M^B (Y)	46
Aflatoxins (grain/nut processing)	n/a	M^C (Y), M^V (Y), M^B (Y)	46
Erionite (mineral fiber)	n/a	M^V (Y), M^C (Y)	46
Underground hematite mining with exposure to radon	n/a	M^C (N)	46
Mustard gas (sulfur mustard)	n/a	$DNA^{A,K}$ (Y), M^C (Y), M^V (Y), M^F (Y), M^B (Y)	46
Radon & its decay products	n/a	Se^U (N), PL^{SCE} (Y) PL^{SCE} (Y)	59 / 1
Solar radiation	n/a	DNA^B (Y), M^C (Y)	43
Soots	n/a	A (Y), A^L (Y), M^C (Y) PI^U (N)	46 / 18
Tobacco smoke (secondhand)	n/a	A (Y), M^C (Y), M^V (Y), M^F (Y)	46
Tobacco (biri) processing	n/a	UA^L (Y).	13

*   Agents in IARC Group 1 have been evaluated as being carcinogenic to humans, having sufficient evidence of carcinogenicity in humans or (exceptionally) strong evidence in humans of a mechanism of carcinogenicity for which sufficient evidence exists of carcinogenicity in experimental animals[42]

†   Estimates from NOES, NOHS, and other sources.   Estimates do not include agricultural workers.

N   Considered a potential occupational carcinogen by NIOSH

n/a   NOES data not available in RTECS for this chemical

O   Considered a potential occupational carcinogen by OSHA

Q   Effect inconsistent: seen in some studies and not in others and/or seen in some categories of exposed workers and not in others

For mutagenicity test codes, see Key for Tables 1–5

TABLE 3. IARC Group 2A* Industrial and Agricultural Chemicals, with Any Evidence of Mutagenicity

Chemical Name or Industry	Est. Minimum No. of Workers†	Cytological Test [agent or job title tested] (Effect Sent in Exposed?)	Reference
Formaldehyde[N,O]	1,500,000	PL^C (Q), PL^{SCE} (Q), M^V (Y), M^C (Y), M^F (Y), M^B (Y)	46
Diesel engine exhaust	1,300,000	UA^L (Y) FA^L (N), UA^L (N)	82 102
Silica, crystalline[N]	900,000	M^V (N), M^C (Y), M^B (N) PL^C (Y), PL^{SCE} (Y)	46 89
Perchloroethylene (Tetrachloroethylene)[N]	680,000	PL^C (N), PL^{SCE} (N), DNA^B (Y), M^C (Q), M^V (Y), M^F (N), M^B (N)	46
Acrylonitrile[N,O]	80,000	PL^C (N), M^V (N), M^C (Y), M^F (Y), M^B (Y)	46
Epichlorohydrin[N]	80,000	DNA^{AK} (Y), PL^C (Q), M^C (Q), M^F (Y), M^B (Y) PL^C (Y)	46 54
1,3-Butadiene[N]	50,000	M^V (Q), M^B (Y) PL^C (Y), PL^T (Y) PL^C (N), PI$^\mu$ (N), PL^{SCE} (N) PL^{HPRT} (Y) PL^{SCE} [diepoxybutane] (Y)	46 10 90 57 65
Creosotes	30,000	U^A (N), M^C (Y), A^L (Y) A^L (Y), UA (N)	46 16
Benzidine-based dyes[N]	25,000	M^B (Y), DNA^A (Y), A^L (Y)	46
Acrylamide[N]	10,000	Hb^A (Y), M^C (Y), DNA^A (Y), M^V (Y)	42
Dimethyl sulphate[N]	10,000	DNA^{AK} (Y), M^C (Y), M^V (Y), M^F (Y), M^B (Y)	46
Ethylene dibromide[N]	8,000	PL^C (N), PL^{SCE} (N), M^V (N), M^C (Y), A (Y)	46
Benz[a]anthracene	2,000		
Diethyl sulphate	2,000	DNA^{AK} (Y), M^C (Y), M^V (Y), M^F (Y), M^B (Y)	46
Benzo[a]pyrene	800	WDNA^A [foundry wrkrs,coke production] (Y)	46

TABLE 3. IARC Group 2A* Industrial and Agricultural Chemicals, with Any Evidence of Mutagenicity *(Cont.)*

Chemical Name or Industry	Est. Minimum No. of Workers†	Cytological Test [agent or job title tested] (Effect Sent in Exposed?)	Reference
N-nitrosodimethyl-amine[N,O]	700		
N-Methyl-N'-nitro-N-nitrosoguanidine (MNNG)	500	DNA^{AK} (Y), M^V (Y), M^C (Y), M^B (Y)	46
para-Chloro-ortho-toluidine and its strong acid salts	250		
Tris(2,3-dibromopropyl)phosphate	200	M^V (Y), M^C (Y), M^B (Y)	46
4,4-Methylene bis(2-chloroaniline) (MOCA)[N]	100	M^V (Y), M^C (Y), M^B (Y)	46
Dibenz[a,h]anthracene	n/a		
Dimethylcarbamoyl chloride[N]	n/a	M^V (Q), M^C (N), M^F (Y), M^B (Y)	46
IQ* (2-Amino-3-methylimidazo [4,5-f]quinoline)	n/a		
N-Methyl-N-nitrosourea (possible industrial use)	n/a		
N-Nitrosodiethylamine	n/a		
Petroleum refining	n/a		
Polychlorinated biphenyls[N]	n/a	M^V (Q), M^C (Y), M^B (N) PL^C (Y), PL^{SCE} (Y), PI$^\mu$ (Y)	46 47
Styrene oxide	n/a	M^C (Y), DNA^A (Y), M^V (Y)	42
Ultraviolet radiation A	n/a	M^C (Y), DNA^B (Y)	43
Ultraviolet radiation B	n/a	M^C (Y), DNA^B (Y)	43
Ultraviolet radiation C	n/a	M^C (Y), DNA^B (Y)	43

* Agents in IARC Group 2A are considered probably carcinogenic to humans. This category is used when there is limited evidence of carcinogenicity in humans and sufficient evidence of carcinogenicity in experimental animals[42]

† Estimates from NOES, NOHS, and other sources. Estimates do not include agricultural workers.

N Considered a potential occupational carcinogen by NIOSH

n/a NOES data not available in RTECS for this chemical

O Considered a potential occupational carcinogen by OSHA

Q Effect inconsistent: seen in some studies and not in others and/or seen in some categories of exposed workers and not in others

For mutagenicity test codes, see Key for Tables 1-5

TABLE 4. IARC 2B* Industrial and Agricultural Chemicals, with Any Evidence of Mutagenicity

Chemical Name or Industry	Est. Minimum No. of Workers†	Cytological Test [agent or job title tested] (Effect Seen in Exposed?)	Reference
Lead & inorganic lead compounds	1,650,000	PL^C (Q), PL^{SCE} (Y), M^V (Q), M^C (N), M^F (N), M^B (N), UA^L (N)	46, 7
Dichloromethane (methylene chloride)[N]	1,400,000	M^V (N), M^C (Q), M^F (Y), M^B (Y)	46
Gasoline[N]	740,000		
Carpentry and joinery	600,000		
Propylene oxide[N]	400,000	Hb^{AK} (Y), M^V (N), M^C (Y), M^F (Y), M^B (Y), DNA^A (Y)	46, 42
p-Dioxane[N]	400,000	DNA^B (Y), M^V (N), M^B (N)	46
Di-sec-octyl phthalate (pesticide)	300,000		
Styrene	300,000	PL^C (Y), $PI^{Iʰ}$ (Y), PL^{SCE} (Q); PL^C (Y), $PI^{Iʰ}$ (N); PL^{SCE} (N), $PI^{Iʰ}$ (N); DNA^A (Y), Hb^A (Y), $WDNA^B$ (Y); PL^C (Y), $PI^{Iʰ}$ (N); E^{GPA} (Q)	46, 6, 99, 42, 96, 22
Nitrilotriacetic acid salts	200,000		
Acetaldehyde[N]	200,000	M^V (Y), M^C (Y), A (Y), DNA^X (Y)	46
Antimony trioxide	200,000	A (N)	45
n,n-Dimethylformamide	100,000	PL^C (Q), M^F (Q), M^V (N), M^C (N), M^B (N)	45
Carbon tetrachloride[N]	100,000	M^V (Y), M^C (Q), M^F (Y), M^B (N)	46
Chloroform[N]	90,000	M^V (N), M^C (N), M^B (N)	46
Butylated hydroxyanisole (BHA)	80,000		
Calcium hypochlorite	80,000		
1,2-dichloroethane	80,000		
Hydrazine[N]	60,000	M^V (N), M^C (Q), M^F (Y), M^B (Y)	46

TABLE 4. IARC 2B* Industrial and Agricultural Chemicals, with Any Evidence of Mutagenicity *(Cont.)*

Chemical Name or Industry	Est. Minimum No. of Workers†	Cytological Test [agent or job title tested] (Effect Seen in Exposed?)	Reference
2-Biphenylol, sodium salt	50,000		
Acrylic acid, ethyl ester	40,000		
Disperse Blue 1	40,000		
Toluene diisocyanates[N]	30,000		
Thiourea	30,000		
p-Dichlorobenzene[N]	30,000		
o-Toluidine[N]	30,000	M^V (Q), M^C (Y), M^F (Q), A^L (Y)	46
Pentachlorophenol	25,000	PL^C (Q), PL^{SCE} (N), M^C (Q)	46
Potassium bromate	20,000		
Dichlorvos	20,000		
Phenytoin	20,000	M^V (Q), M^C (N), M^B (N)	46
Phenobarbital	20,000	M^V (N), M^C (Q), M^F (N), M^B (Q)	46
CI Acid Red 114	15,000		
Dacarbazine	15,000	M^C (Y)	46
4,4'-methylenedianiline[N]	15,000		
Magenta (with CI Basic Red 9)	10,000		
Chlordecone (Kepone)	10,000		
Ethylene thiourea[N]	10,000	M^V (N), M^C (N), M^F (Y), M^B (Q)	46
Propane, 1,2-epoxy-3-phenoxy- (phenyl glycidal ether)	10,000		
2,3,7,8-Tetrachlorodibenzo-p-dioxin (TCDD)[N]	n/a	PL^C (Q), M^V (N), M^C (N), M^B (N)	46
Ceramic fibers	n/a		
Chlorophenols	n/a	M^V [trichlorophenol] (Y), M^F (Y), M^B (N)	46

TABLE 4. IARC 2B* Industrial and Agricultural Chemicals, with Any Evidence of Mutagenicity *(Cont.)*

Chemical Name or Industry	Est. Minimum No. of Workers†	Cytological Test [agent or job title tested] (Effect Seen in Exposed?)	Reference
Chlorophenoxy herbicides	n/a	PL^C (N), PL^{SCE} (N), M^V (N), M^C (Y), M^F (Y), M^B (N)	46
Textile manufacturing industry	n/a	UA^{LB} [arylamines] (Y)	86
Welding fumes^N	n/a	PL^C (Y), PL^{SCE} (N), PL^{UDS} (N) DNA^X (Y), DNA^B (N)	50 74
1,2-Oxathiolane 2,2-dioxide (1,3-propane sultone)^N	n/a		
Chlordane^N	n/a	M^V (Q), M^C (N), M^B (N)	46
Anisole, 2,4-diamino-^{N}	n/a		
3,3'-dichlorobenzidine^N	n/a	M^C (Y), M^B (Y)	46
Toxaphene (chlorinated camphene)^N	n/a		
Ethyl methane sulphonate	n/a	SLE (Y), M^C (Y)	73
DDT	n/a		
Atrazine	n/a		
Heptachlor	n/a		
Amitrole	n/a		

*   Agents in IARC Group 2B are considered possible human carcinogens. This category is used when there is limited evidence of carcinogenicity in humans and less than sufficient evidence of carcinogenicity in experimental animals, or when there is inadequate evidence of carcinogenicity in humans but sufficient evidence of carcinogenicity in experimental animals[42]. The chemicals presented include those that have been studied by NIOSH, or are designated carcinogenic by NIOSH, or to which at least 10,000 workers are potentially exposed

†   Estimates from NOES, NOHS, and other sources. Estimates do not include agricultural workers.

N   Considered a potential occupational carcinogen by NIOSH

n/a   NOES data not available in RTECS for this chemical

O   Considered a potential occupational carcinogen by OSHA

Q   Effect inconsistent: seen in some studies and not in others and/or seen in some categories of exposed workers and not in others

For mutagenicity test codes, see Key for Tables 1–5

TABLE 5. IARC Group 3* Industrial and Agricultural Chemicals, with Any Evidence of Mutagenicity

Chemical Name or Industry	Est. Minimum No. of Workers†	Cytological Test [agent or job title tested] (Effect Seen in Exposed?)	Reference
Isopropyl alcohol	4,600,000		
Titanium oxide	2,700,000		
1,1,1-trichloroethane	2,500,000		
Xylene	2,100,000	PL^{SCE} (N), M^B (N)	45
Toluene	2,000,000	PL^{SCE} (Q), PL^C (Q)	45
Mineral oils, highly refined	2,000,000	UA^L (Y), A^L (N), M^C (Y) DNA^B (?)	46 30
Carbon black	1,700,000	A (Y), A^L (Y)	46
Talc (powder), no asbestos	1,300,000	M^C (N), M^V (N), M^F (N), M^B (N)	46
Hydrochloric acid	1,200,000		
Kerosene	1,000,000		
Hydrogen peroxide,30% or 90%	1,000,000		
Iron(III) oxide	950,000		
Polyethylene	850,000		
Mineral oil,white	600,000	A^L (N)	46
2-Biphenylol	600,000		
p-Cresol,2,6-di-tert-butyl-	550,000		
Phenol	550,000	M^C (Y), M^B (N)	45
Acrylic acid,polymers	550,000		
Chlorox	550,000		
Polyvinyl alcohol	500,000		
Ethylene,chloro-,polymer	450,000		
Asphalt (& bitumens)	450,000	A (Q) Ua^{BL} (Y)	46 69
Hydroquinone	400,000		
Cyclohexanone	400,000	A^L (N), M^V (Y)	45
Hexachlorophene	400,000		
Styrene polymer	400,000		
Chromium metal	350,000	PL^C (Q)	81
Phthalic acid,benzyl butyl ester	300,000		
Styrene polymer with 1,3-butadiene	300,000		

TABLE 5. IARC Group 3* Industrial and Agricultural Chemicals, with Any Evidence of Mutagenicity *(Cont.)*

Chemical Name or Industry	Est. Minimum No. of Workers†	Cytological Test [agent or job title tested] (Effect Seen in Exposed?)	Reference
Acetic acid,vinyl ester,polymer	300,000		
Sodium sulfite (2:1)	300,000		
Sodium bisulfite (1:1)	250,000		
Acetic acid,benzyl ester	250,000		
Propene polymers	250,000		
1,2-epoxybutane	250,000	A (Y), M^C (Y)	45
Tetrafluoroethylene,polymer	200,000		
Coumarin	200,000		
Morpholine	200,000	M^B (N), M^C (N), M^V (N)	45
C.I. Food Red 15	150,000		
C.I. Food Yellow 3	150,000		
Eugenol (pesticide)	150,000		
Rutile	150,000		
Dimethoxane (pesticide)	150,000		
Polymethylmethacrylate	150,000		
Methacrylic acid,methyl ester	150,000		
Polyethylene	150,000		
Silica,amorphous - diatomaceous earth	150,000	M^B (N), M^C (N)	46
Petroleum	150,000		
Poly(1-vinyl-2-pyrrolidinone)	150,000		
Chlorodifluoromethane	150,000		
1,3-Butadiene,2-chloro-,polymers	100,000		
Furfural	100,000		
Limonene	100,000		
Cosmetic Pigment Yellow Red DVR	100,000		
Acrylonitrile-butadiene-styrene copolymer	100,000		
Diesel fuels	100,000		
Resorcinol	100,000		
Nitrous oxide (anesthetic)	100,000	PL^{SCE} (Y), PL^C (Y), UA^L [NO & halothane] (N)	48
Acrylic acid	95,000		
Fuel oil,No.2	95,000		

TABLE 5. IARC Group 3* Industrial and Agricultural Chemicals, with Any Evidence of Mutagenicity *(Cont.)*

Chemical Name or Industry	Est. Minimum No. of Workers†	Cytological Test [agent or job title tested] (Effect Seen in Exposed?)	Reference
Halothane (anesthetic)	90,000	PL^{SCE} (Y), PL^{C} (Y), UA^{L} [halothane & NO] (N)	48
o-dichlorobenzene (pesticide)	90,000	M^{B} (N), M^{F} (N)	46
Piperonyl butoxide (pesticide)	85,000		
Chromium(III) oxide (2:3)	85,000		
Pyrosulfurous acid,diNa salt	85,000		
Benzoyl peroxide	85,000		
Poly(iminocarbonylpentamethylene)	85,000		
Sodium fluoride	85,000	DNA^{B} (N), M^{V} (N), M^{C} (Q), M^{F} (N), M^{B} (N)	46
Hypochlorous acid,calcium salt	80,000		
C.I. Acid Blue 1	80,000		
Sodium fluorosilicate (pesticide)	75,000		
Mercury	70,000		
Wollasonite	70,000		
Acetanilide,4'-hydroxy-	65,000		
Cyclohexylamine	60,000		
Isophthalonitrile,tetrachloro- (pesticide)	60,000		
Food blue dye 1	55,000		
Sulfur dioxide	55,000		
C.I. Solvent Red 19	50,000		
Disulfide,bis(diethylthiocarbamoyl)	50,000		
Diphenylmethane-4,4'-diisocyanate	50,000		
C.I. Pigment Red 3	50,000		
p-Phenylenediamine	45,000		
Chloroethane	45,000		
Thiram (pesticide)	45,000		
Polymethylenepolyphenyl isocyanate	45,000		
Mercury(II) chloride	45,000		
C.I. Solvent Yellow 14	40,000		
2(3H)-Furanone,dihydro-	40,000		
Melamine	40,000		
Carrageen	40,000		
Ethanol,2-(4-amino-2-nitroanilino)-	40,000		

TABLE 5. IARC Group 3* Industrial and Agricultural Chemicals, with Any Evidence of Mutagenicity *(Cont.)*

Chemical Name or Industry	Est. Minimum No. of Workers†	Cytological Test [agent or job title tested] (Effect Seen in Exposed?)	Reference
Ampicillin	40,000		
Aniline	40,000	M^V (Y), M^C (Q), M^F (N), M^B (N)	46
Tannic acid	40,000		
C.I. Basic Red 1	40,000		
Cholesterol	40,000	M^C (N), M^B (N)	46
m-Phenylenediamine	40,000		
2-Propenoic acid,butyl ester	35,000		
C.I. Acid Red 2	35,000		
C.I. Food Red 4	35,000		
Tetraethylplumbane	35,000		
Trichloroacetic acid	35,000		
Zinc dimethyldithiocarmate (pesticide)	30,000		
Potassium pyrosulfite	30,000		
Ether,bis(pentabromophenyl)	30,000		
N,N-dimethyl-aniline	30,000		
Theophylline	25,000		
p-Phenylenediamine,2-nitro-	25,000		
Hematite	25,000		
C.I. Acid Orange 10	25,000		
Selenium	25,000		
Antimony trisulfide	25,000		
Anatase	25,000		
Methylstyrene	25,000		
Bisphenol A diglycidyl ether	25,000		
2H-Azepin-2-one,hexahydro-	25,000		
5-Fluorouracil	20,000	PL^C (N), PL^{SCE} (N), M^V (Q), M^C (Y), M^F (Y)	46
Ampicillin sodium	20,000		
Propene polymers	20,000		
C.I. Acid Orange 3	20,000		
Polyurethane foam	20,000		
Fluoranthene	20,000		
Acrylamide,N-(hydroxymethyl)-	20,000		

TABLE 5. IARC Group 3* Industrial and Agricultural Chemicals, with Any Evidence of Mutagenicity *(Cont.)*

Chemical Name or Industry	Est. Minimum No. of Workers†	Cytological Test [agent or job title tested] (Effect Seen in Exposed?)	Reference
Valium	20,000		
C.I. Solvent Yellow 77	20,000		
Phenol,2-amino-4-nitro-	20,000		
C.I. Solvent Red 24	20,000		
Caffeine	15,000		
Malathion (pesticide)	15,000		
Leurocristine sulfate (1:1)	15,000		
Chromium (III) sulfate (2:3)	15,000	M^V (N), M^C (Q), M^B (N)	46
Sodium chlorite	15,000		
C.I. Acid Green 5	15,000		
Potassium hypochlorite	15,000		
1,3-Butadiene,2-chloro-	15,000		
o-Phenylenediamine,4-nitro-	15,000		
Methotrexate	15,000		
Bactrim	15,000		
Phosphorofluoridic acid,diNa salt	15,000		
Sevin (pesticide)	15,000		
Furoxone	15,000		
Lindane	15,000		
Lithium hypochlorite (pesticide)	15,000		
Acrylonitrile,polymer with styrene	15,000		
Adipic acid,bis(2-ethylhexyl) ester	15,000		
p-Benzoquinone	15,000		
Tetrafluoroethylene	10,000		
Actinomycin D	10,000	PL^{SCE} (N), M^C (Y)	46
Phenol,2-amino-5-nitro-	10,000		
Lasix (pesticide)	10,000		
Vincaleukoblastine,sulfate(1:1)(salt)	10,000		
C.I. Acid Red 27	10,000		
o-Toluidine,5-nitro-	10,000		
8-Quinolinol	10,000		
C.I. Food Red 1	10,000		

TABLE 5. IARC Group 3* Industrial and Agricultural Chemicals, with Any Evidence of Mutagenicity *(Cont.)*

Chemical Name or Industry	Est. Minimum No. of Workers†	Cytological Test [agent or job title tested] (Effect Seen in Exposed?)	Reference
Pyrocatechol	10,000		
Ampicillin trihydrate	10,000		
C.I. Basic Violet 14	10,000		
Ethyl bromide	10,000		
Ethylene	10,000	Hb^A (Y), M^V (N), M^B (N)	42
Phenol,4-amino-2-nitro-	10,000		
Chloral hydrate	10,000		
Acrylic acid,2-ethylhexyl ester	10,000		
Tagamet	10,000		
Selenious acid,disodium salt	10,000		
Chromium phosphate	10,000		
p-Amino-benzoic acid (PABA)	10,000		
Chloromethane	10,000		
volatile anesthetics	n/a	PL^C (Y), PL^{SCE} (N), M^V (N), M^C (Q), M^F (Q)	46
leather goods manufacture	n/a		
leather tanning & processing	n/a	PL^C (Q), Pl^u (N)	80 63
lumber & sawmill industries	n/a		
pulp & paper manufacture	n/a	M^C (Y)	46
organolead compounds	n/a		
Methyl bromide	n/a		
Acrolein	n/a		
Parathion	n/a		
Methyl parathion	n/a		
Kelthane	n/a		
Maneb	n/a		

*   Agents in IARC Group 3 are not classifiable as to their carcinogenicity to humans. This category is used for chemicals for which there is (inadequate evidence of human carcinogenicity and inadequate or limited evidence in experimental animals[42].   The chemicals presented include those that have been studied by NIOSH or to which at least 10,000 workers are potentially exposed.

†   Estimates from NOES, NOHS, and other sources.   Estimates do not include agricultural workers.

N   Considered a potential occupational carcinogen by NIOSH

n/a   NOES data not available in RTECS for this chemical

O   Considered a potential occupational carcinogen by OSHA

Q   Effect inconsistent: seen in some studies and not in others and/or seen in some categories of exposed workers and not in others

For mutagenicity test codes, see Key for Tables 1-5

MARTIN G. CHERNIACK, MD, MPH

EPIDEMIOLOGY OF OCCUPATIONAL DISORDERS OF THE UPPER EXTREMITY

From the Section of Occupational and Environmental Medicine
University of Connecticut Health Center
Farmington, Connecticut

Reprint requests to:
Martin G. Cherniack, MD, MPH
Section of Occupational and Environmental Medicine
University of Connecticut Health Center
Dowling North, MC6210
Farmington, CT 06030-6210

Occupational disorders of the upper extremity (ODUE) have been variously categorized as repetition strain injuries, cumulative trauma disorders, and cervicobrachial diseases. They have sometimes earned the sensational epithet of "new industrial epidemic" or "occupational disease of the 1990s." To an extent, even such provocative hyperbole does not seem out of place, given the real conflicts that complicate the most basic case definitions of ODUEs. While there are many impediments to a representative descriptive epidemiologic review, there are still quite solid reasons for establishing disease prevalence in both the general population and in selected work settings, even if the population numerators reflect different points of view on what constitutes a case. These reasons are based in the established facts of increased case reporting of ODUEs, usually as repetitive strain or cumulative trauma disorders, to workers' compensation commissions and other surveillance vehicles and in a rapidly evolving interest among clinicians in categorizing types of chronic soft tissue disorders through the application of more sophisticated analytic tools.

The meteoric rise in reports of ODUE in less than two decades is familiar to professionals associated with the arenas of occupational medicine, workers' compensation, and industrial case management. In Wisconsin, workers' compensation claims for carpal tunnel syndrome (CTS) rose from 432 to 2,429 (462%) from 1983–1988.[31] In California for the same years, doctors' first reports of CTS to the state's physician surveillance system rose from 329 to 2,775 (743%) cases.[47] In Connecticut, all repetitive trauma cases reported to the Department of Labor's Bureau of Labor Statistics rose more than tenfold from 1979–1983, from 471 to 5,526 (1073%) reported cases.[54] These trends have not been invisible to academic professionals. The frequency of articles in prominent occupational medicine journals addressing work-related upper extremity disorders has followed the general pattern of increased disease reporting; the once occasional piece on musculoskeletal injury has been supplanted by a regular stream of publication.

While the numbers speak to a substantial burden of disease and morbidity, an ongoing debate on the significance of these increases remains unsettled. The term *significance* can be applied with both its common biomedical usages—as a measure of mathematical recognition and as a qualitative estimation of the severity of a disease. Comparing annual incidence in the highest-risk plant populations (meat packing) to estimated population norms, some observers have described an age- and gender-specific risk ratio for CTS on the order of 100-fold. A similar order of risk was reported in the state of Washington from 1984–88 among employed workers, where the incidence of CTS based on workers' compensation claims was almost 15 times higher in meat packing and shellfish packing than in the average industry.[19] In Oregon, however, an opposite conclusion was reached: that impaired nerve conduction across the carpal tunnel, the benchmark of CTS, was unrelated either to type or duration of employment or to hand activity at work.[58] The disparities between passive case reporting and prevalence estimations based in clinical surveys involve differences in methodology and principles of population selection. Nevertheless, differing conclusions of such magnitude, in excess of an order of magnitude, can only partly be accounted for by divergent methods or investigator predilections. They most likely reflect inherent qualities or variable presentations in diseases themselves. Stated another way, the wide separation in work-related case rates of ODUE, recorded by active and passive systems, may not indicate a difference in case definitions directed to a common set of symptoms and pathology. Instead, the diseases being described may be different, segregated by the selected method of measurement.

Some reasons for ambiguity in both clinical and public health characterizations of ODUE are readily apparent. There are distinct reporting biases. For example, during the first three years of mandatory physician reporting of occupational diseases in Connecticut, diagnoses of CTS grew by 277%, and diagnoses of the totality of upper extremity repetitive trauma disorders increased by almost 100%.[54] In a state with static employment and demography, this must reflect the evolving process of physician familiarization with a new reporting system. Moreover, consternation over apparent epidemic increases in repetition strain injury (RSI) cases—in particular, the recognition that they make now up more than half of reported occupational diseases[1]—is perhaps less astonishing and ominous when placed in a somewhat different context. The occurrence of ODUEs must be weighed against the larger pool of lost-time occupational injuries to which RSI cases contribute not more than 3%. A growing sophistication on the part of practitioners also has resulted in the location of acute and singular injuries within a spectrum of chronic musculoskeletal disease. Moreover, regional mechanical problems of the lower back, which are usually counted as injuries rather than cumulative traumatic diseases, continue to dominate over ODUEs in terms of cost and lost work time.

Some problems of definition arise from the vagueness that occurs when clinically divisible upper extremity disorders are grouped as repetitive strain or cumulative trauma.

This springs legitimately from the fact that RSI is not singly a disease classification but conventionally has had at least three separate usages. As a clinical definition, RSI or cumulative trauma disorder (CTD) serves as a diagnostic umbrella for various upper extremity pathologies, including nerve entrapments, tendonitides, arthritides, and muscle injuries. In the terminology of administrative medicine and disease surveillance, RSI serves as a descriptive catalogue for the rising number of nonacute arm injuries which have been recorded by public health and workers compensation surveillance systems. In popular terminology, RSI identifies a troubling complex of symptoms associated with the technology of electronic keyboarding and implies an etiology that may combine individual emotional or group psychological dimensions.[38,73]

FREQUENCY AND PREVALENCE OF UPPER EXTREMITY DISORDERS

Frequency in the General Population

In cataloguing ODUEs, several observers have attempted to differentiate between anatomically definable disorders and vaguer symptom complexes.[8,13] There is a countervailing argument that the predominant portion of recorded upper extremity disorders, and therefore the source of the apparent recent increase, arises from poorly defined repetitive strain injuries. These, in turn, purportedly belong to medical neologism and are not an indicator of significant physical pathology.[25,33,41,42] Miller and Topliss reviewed 229 cases of diagnosed repetitive trauma and found anatomic diagnoses in only 29 cases.[51] Ireland, in dismissing the Australian RSI epidemic of the early 1980s as nonphysiologic disease, developed a partial list of true occupational upper extremity disorders related to overuse and distinguished them from the more amorphous RSI[34] (Table 1). However, physician inventiveness may not entirely explain the phenomenon of rising RSI cases, at least in Connecticut (see Table 1). Ireland's list of true upper extremity occupational diseases, which he contrasts to the vaguer presumably psychosocial entity of RSI, is quite similar to the

TABLE 1. Presumed and Observed Diagnoses of Occupational Disorders of the Upper Extremity

NonRSI Disorders of the Upper Extremity*	Observed Repetitive Trauma Injuries Connecticut 1992–1995**	Cases Observed in Connecticut (%)†
Rotator cuff tendinitis	Carpal tunnel syndrome	34%
Bicipital tendinitis	Tendinitis/Rotator cuff	26
Tennis elbow	Lateral epicondylitis/Tennis elbow	9
Golfer's elbow	Hand-arm vibration syndrome	6
Ulnar neuritis	Vibration white finger	4
Olecranon bursitis	Tenosynovitis	3
Radial tunnel syndrome	Repetitive strain, pain, overuse	3
DeQuervain's stenosing-tenosynovitis	DeQuervain's syndrome	3
Flexor tendinitis/carpal tunnel syndrome	Ulnar neuritis/neuropathy	3
Digital flexor tendinitis	Pain syndromes	3
	Ganglion/cyst	3
	Bursitis	3
	Trigger finger	1
	Myositis	1
	Other	1

* Partial list of nonRSI type upper extremity disorders as reported by Ireland, 1995.
** List of actual diagnoses classified as repetitive trauma disorders in Connecticut, 1996.
† Total percentage is 103% due to rounding.

upper extremity diagnoses actually made by physicians reporting to Connecticut's occupational disease reporting system. Moreover, vague symptom complexes, including the formal diagnosis of RSI, made up more than 10% of the ODUE diagnoses. Most diagnoses involved familiar pathologic classifications, even though the grouped result suggested an increase in CTD or RSI. At least in this example, the surveillance diagnosis coincides with well-defined rather than ill-defined clinical entities. While this comparison cannot determine if RSI has been included in standard diagnoses in other locales, it does suggest that these physicians attempted to be diagnostically specific.

Several practical problems also limit a descriptive assessment of ODUEs. Because many upper extremity disorders have not been well characterized in the general population, an appreciation of their frequencies in the overall adult population is not really possible and must also come from surveys of reported symptoms in identified workplaces that have been the object of focused studies. Carpal tunnel syndrome is the exception because of its greater notoriety and presumably distinctive features. It can be characterized both in terms of its workplace point prevalence and its prevalence in the general population.

In a community study in Rochester, Minnesota, Stevens described a CTS incidence rate of 149 cases in women and 47 cases in men per 100,000 person-years.[80] These were physician-reported results to the Rochester Epidemiology Project, based on various criteria but with a characteristic symptom pattern being the necessary baseline. A conversion of period prevalence into prevalence produces a rate of 4.2% among women and 1.3% among men. Dutch investigators used a combination of questionnaires, nerve conduction tests, and historical case review to determine prevalence of CTS based on a sample of 715 randomly selected residents of Maastricht.[17] Among women, 6.8% had occult symptoms of CTS and 3.8% had been previously diagnosed; 1.2% of men had been either previously diagnosed or had occult symptoms. These prevalences would need to be adjusted downward by about 15% to equal the age distribution of a comparable American community.

The largest population-based study of carpal tunnel syndrome and symptomatic hand pain in the United States was conducted in 1988 as part of the National Health and Nutrition Survey.[68,83,84] Survey results were entirely anamnestic, the positive choices being self reports of carpal tunnel syndrome in the previous 6 months or medical confirmation in the same interval. Thus, the results are an indicator of period prevalence rather than yearly incidence. The questionnaire was directed to 177,300 adults, subdivided into ever worked (170,200) and never worked (7,100) subpopulations. While dispensing with the objective criteria of the above two studies and relying on self-report, the case definition in fact required knowledge of a formal diagnosis rather than report of a symptom pattern. The period prevalence of self-reported CTS was 1.83% of women and 1.17% of men with a history of having recently worked, with slightly higher percentages of reported disease in participants without a history of recent work. Tanaka et al. reported that 0.53% of the recently working population who had self-reported CTS had also seen a physician for the condition in the prior year.[84]

Tanaka and McGlothlin's report also provides insight into the extent pool of patients with chronic hand symptoms.[82] Among their group of "recent workers," 21.6% reported significant hand symptoms in the preceding year; of these, 24.5% attributed their symptoms to injury and 42.4% could be classified as strain or pain. Only 3% of the chronic hand symptom group (0.2% of the "recent workers" cohort) were counted among the self-reported CTS cases. Even with this small degree of overlap, it seems probable that chronic distal upper extremity symptoms are common in the American workforce and that cumulative trauma and injury reporting categories established by BLS/OSHA have failed to capture this broader expression of symptoms.

Frequency of Carpal Tunnel Syndrome in the Working Population

The National Health Interview Survey, while offering some provision for the impact of employment, is broad in its representation and lacks a sufficient case definition. A more refined perspective on the relationship between CTS and the employed workforce can be deduced from workplace studies sufficiently inclusive to create a representative sample of job categories. More selective sector-specific comparisons provide another perspective by identifying specialized populations with specific risks.

In one of the earlier estimates of symptoms prevalence, Silverstein et al. determined the presence of CTS in automobile manufacturing based on a combination of symptoms (median nerve symptomatology) and signs (Phelan's or Tinel's) and identified CTS in 0.6% of the overall workforce and in 5.6% with the highest observed risk among four exposure groups.[78] Symptoms prevalence in groups 1 and 2, whose employment involved considerably more hand use than the general workforce, was 0.9%. The same population also was assessed for prevalence of upper extremity cumulative trauma disorders based on physician examination.[77] Case prevalence in the lowest and highest risk groups was 1.5% and 25.6%, and for the comparable groups 1 and 2 it was 4.5%.

Using similar clinical symptom criteria and a more rigorous electrophysiologic diagnostic standard, Nathan et al. diagnosed probable CTS in 20% of a diverse workforce divided into 5 employment groups.[55,56,58] An astonishing 39% had nerve conduction studies consistent with a diagnosis of carpal tunnel syndrome based on well-accepted criteria. In groups 1 and 2, where exposures were characterized as light or very light, 27.8% of the population had abnormal studies. The Oregon cohort study, while longitudinal in its original design, also underlines the instability and difficulties in follow-up and retention of a clinically affected population. Fully 33% of the original cohort was lost between its 1984 initial evaluation and 1989 follow-up.[55,57] Thus, there is no easy way to determine whether the homogeneity in symptom prevalence in 1984 and 1989 reflects absence of progression or drop-out and replacement among survivors. The authors believe the former explanation is correct.

A similarly designed cross-sectional study of Japanese factory workers demonstrated abnormal nerve conduction in 17.2% of the examined industrial population but a diagnostic symptom complex consistent with CTS in only 2.5%.[59] There was no stratification by job or exposure category. While the implication exists that cultural factors influence the description of pain and symptoms, there is also a suggestion in both the Japanese and American study populations that the link between characteristic symptoms and a confirmatory pathology may not be very well defined.

Table 2 summarizes the frequency of CTS in the general and working populations based on the above studies. While allotting for differences in test populations and testing methods, one surprising pattern is that the "gold standard," nerve conduction studies, appears to bolster the case rate, which remains lower when subjective criteria and clinical signs alone are relied upon. Customarily, symptom-based case definitions are thought to be broader and more inclusive than defining "gold standard" objective tests.

TABLE 2. Period Prevalence of Carpal Tunnel Syndrome

Population Cohort	Source	Method	Years	Female Cases/1000	Male Cases/1000	Age at Peak Occurrence
		Population-Based Studies				
US general	NHIS[68]	Self-report	1988	18	12	45–54
Netherlands	DeKrom et al.[17]	Self-report and testing	1983–1985	68	12	45–54
Rochester, MN	Stevens et al.[80]	MD diagnosed	1976–1980	9	3	45–54 55–64

Population	Source	Method		Years	% Diagnosed
		General Working Populations			
Oregon	Nathan et al.[55]	Nerve conduction studies (NCS) NCS (and symptoms)		1984–1985	39% 20%
Michigan	Silverstein[78]	Questionnaire		1987	0.6%
US (Employed)	NHIS[68]	MD diagnosed and Examination		1988	0.5%

Prevalence of Upper Extremity Disorders in Selected Industries

Both carpal tunnel syndrome and other cumulative trauma disorders of the upper extremity have been more extensively characterized in specific workforces and industries than in the general population. While selective, industry-to-industry comparisons can at least clarify whether these conditions are disorders of general living whose expression is unrelated to the workplace[24] or whether specific workplaces may heighten risk, even if the understanding of etiology remains hypothetical.[45,74,76] Industry-specific analyses fall into two basic types: (1) active surveys of working populations and (2) passive analyses of frequency differences from surveillance data. Both are presented below.

ACTIVE SURVEYS OF UPPER EXTREMITY DISORDERS

Newspaper and Office Work

Upper extremity disorders associated with the electronic keyboard have occupied a significant place in the repetitive strain and carpal tunnel literature, both as the source for etiological description of the diseases[69] and as the subject of several well-publicized generic investigations.[60,61] A principal theme in this medical literature has been the apparent contradiction between an elevated frequency of pain syndromes affecting the neck, shoulder, and wrist in occupations involving dedicated keyboarding[28,63] and a relatively low number of quantifiable entrapment disorders.[26]

Investigators from the National Institute for Occupational Safety and Health studying Newsday employees found work-related musculoskeletal disorders in 41% of this white collar workforce.[7,61] Body part symptom prevalence was distributed as follows: 26% to the neck, 17% to the shoulder, 10% to the elbow, 22% to the hand or wrist, and 25% to other or unclear regions. In 20% of the instances of positive symptom reporting, the pain occurred daily. One interesting piece of potentially validating evidence involved the elbow. The degree of chronicity was significantly higher at the elbow than at other anatomic sites, which supports the general medical view of epicondylitis as a more clinically intractable condition than most other soft tissue upper extremity disorders.[16,87] In a similar anamnestic study of 1,150 newspaper employees, CTS was estimated in 1.5% of the workforce[75a]. In a small cohort of office workers, including graphic artists, Franzblau et al. described an even higher prevalence of neck and shoulder symptoms, in excess of 70% of the most physically stressed workforce, but electrophysiologically confirmed carpal tunnel syndrome was more unusual (4.6%).[20]

The presence of nerve entrapment-like symptomatology with normal electrical studies has been characteristic of the keyboarding population, and it runs counter to case series in clinical practice where CTS clinical presentations have been accompanied by confirmatory nerve conduction studies in 80–90% of cases.[22,50,58,79] Two responses to this inconsistency have been the appropriate caveat against the presumptive value of surgical relief in all symptomatic cases[24] and the more contentious supposition that the reports of pain and paresthesias associated with keyboarding are institutional translations of normality into disease and lack underlying physical pathology.[25,41] A different and potentially more fruitful direction may come from the electrophysiologic and neurophysiologic laboratories, where there is evidence that small discrete or remote neurologic injury can produce a pattern of compression symptomatology at a variety of anatomic locales.[6,40,44,45]

Grocery Store Clerks

In a study of 56 grocery store workers, 17 (23%) met a case definition of CTS based on symptoms only.[67] In 5 (9%) of the cases, there was an abnormal motor nerve velocity at the median nerve. Selection was an important consideration because there were no abnormal tests in the subgroup whose jobs involved low repetition-force tasks, but 4 of 12 workers with high-exposure jobs had positive nerve conduction tests. In a questionnaire survey of 1,345 female grocery store workers, Morgenstern et al. found that 12.0% of the workforce met CTS case criteria based on the presence of 4 out of 4 symptom categories and 23.5% responded positively to 3 out of 4 symptoms categories.[53] Based on several models, the authors estimated that the attributable risk fraction of CTS due to work was about 60%.

Meat, Fish, and Poultry Workers

In an often quoted paper representing the extreme of workplace risk, Masear et al. described a 15% annual prevalence of CTS in the meat processing industry.[48] In a longitudinal study of Scandinavian meat processors, the case rates of tenosynovitis and peritendinitis were 11.0 cases per 100 person-years for men and 21.4 cases per 100 person-years for women in strenuous jobs. The rate was more than 1.0 case per 100 person-years for either gender in nonstrenuous jobs.[39] An analysis of the incidence of epicondylitis produced a somewhat narrower range of risk between men and women with strenuous and nonstrenuous jobs. The case rate in strenuous jobs was 5.2 per 100 person-years for men and 8.9 per 100 person-years for women. Baseline risk was 0.9 cases and 0.1 cases per 100 person-years for men and women, respectively. A cross-sectional validation study performed on the same workforce, underlined the inherent difficulties in making comparative case definitions for soft tissue disorders of the upper extremity.[86] Among women in strenuous and nonstrenuous jobs, 21.9% (strenuous) and 12.2% (nonstrenuous) reported symptoms in the preceding week. On examination by a physiatrist, 13.0% of women with strenuous jobs and 8.3% with nonstrenuous jobs had palpable epicondylar tenderness. Actual epicondylitis was diagnosed in 1% of each group. One question is whether strenuous work produces more profound symptom expression against a stable background prevalence of regional symptoms, which normally have a more moderate symptoms presentation. It is also striking that actual lost work-time was relatively infrequent in these northern European populations, whereas surgical intervention and morbidity were higher in the above-mentioned American carpal tunnel cohort.[48]

In a study of 157 poultry workers, a variety of quantitative measures were taken, including strength, vibration threshold, median nerve motor velocity, and the presence of Tinel's and Phelan's signs.[90] Clinical symptoms were also recorded. About 60% of the workforce had significantly abnormal upper extremity signs and symptoms, 31% had abnormal nerve conduction studies, and more than half had either grip weakness or symptoms of numbness. In a case review of 112 consecutive poultry workers evaluated for hand symptoms, 35% had either CTS symptoms or characteristically abnormal nerve conduction studies.[37] The authors underscored the points that most hand and wrist symptoms, even in a high-risk population, do not qualify as CTS based on nerve conduction and other clinical criteria. Significantly, where there were classic CTS symptoms, nerve conduction studies were positive 80–90% of the time, but as has been seen in other studies, abnormal tests appear to be over-represented in the nonsymptomatic population. One third of nerve conduction studies were positive in the absence of supporting clinical signs. This curious finding is discussed below.

Fish processing is another reportedly high-risk industry.[19] In a group of Scandinavian female processing workers, neck/shoulder and hand/wrist symptoms were three times more common than in controls.[65] Odds ratios were reduced in workers older than 44, however, compared to the immediately preceding cohort. The latter observation, in the author's estimation, was partly the result of a survivor/drop-out effect because musculoskeletal pain was cited as the principal reason for terminating work by a quarter of the nonincumbent workforce.

Other Sources of Employment

Recent studies have identified several other occupations that pose particular risks for upper extremity disorders. In a study of workers in ski manufacturing, adopting a case definition of positive nerve conduction studies (ulnar to median differential) and either signs or symptoms of CTS, 32.5% of workers with highly repetitive jobs and 18.2% of workers with nonrepetitive jobs met the case definition.[5] This was reduced to 15.4% and 3.1% with substitution of a tighter case definition. Using the NIOSH CTD questionnaire and case definitions,[30] a group of 308 electricians were surveyed for the prevalence of CTDs.[32] The group was young (median age 26 years), and noninjury-related chronic hand symptoms were present in 24% of the population. In a clinical examination of 82 sewing machine workers, 42% were disease free; there were no cases of carpal tunnel syndrome; and lateral epicondylitis was present in 5% of the population.[2] On the other hand, cervicobrachial myalgia was diagnosed in 47% of the population and cervical syndrome in another 17%. The important relationship between neck/shoulder and distal syndromes is discussed later in this chapter. In a questionnaire study of 101 cardiac ultrasonographers, 63% had some evidence of median nerve distributed complaints, while 6% met a rigid symptom profile for CTS and 3% had been previously diagnosed with CTS.[85]

SURVEILLANCE DATA REGARDING CTS AND OTHER UPPER EXTREMITY DISORDERS

Current surveillance systems for upper extremity disorders that rely solely on existing data reporting have several obvious limitations: either total absence or very limited capacity for validation of a surveillance case definition; an absence of quantitative inputs to the case definition; and a relationship between reported and actual cases that is difficult to quantify. On the other hand, there is a plausible basis for qualitatively translating incidence and prevalence data from specific sectors into disease comparisons between industries. OSHA's National Labor Survey in 1993 uncovered a case rate of CTS of 10.4 cases 10,000 and 7.4 cases of tendinitis per 10,000 in manufacturing, the sector with the highest incidence.[10] This is considerably less than the number of cases reported to the NHIS for the United States "recently worked" population. In Connecticut, workers' compensation first reports suggested a level of injury that was similar to OSHA's: 25.5 cases of RSI per 10,000 in manufacturing, 34% of which were CTS.[54]

In general, a limited level of overlap exists between various surveillance systems. In Connecticut, one of the greatest divergences existed between a physician's first reports to workers' compensation and reports of occupational disease to the health department.[54] In 1992, workers' compensation reports of CTS exceeded physicians' surveillance reports by 355%, and there was overlap in fewer than 10% of instances. A lack of correspondence between actual and probable cases was observed in Santa Clara County in California, where physicians' case reports uncovered only 13% of probable cases of CTS, determined by more specific subpopulation analyses.[47] Even with mandatory surveillance, CTS and RSI case rates were seriously underreported. Moreover, the wide discrepancy between cases reported to workers' compensation are fewer by a factor of almost ten than probable cases among the employed reported to the National Health Interview Survey. While many of the interview-established cases may not have been work-related, the fraction appears much too low, if the work-related fractions cited by Morgenstern et al. are applicable.[53]

Despite the many problems with determining a natural case rate from workers' compensation data, interindustry relative risks can be appreciated. Washington State is unique in its capacity to couple medical diagnosis with employment through its Labor and Industries Insurance System.[19] Overall, the CTS incidence rate of 17.4/10,000 full-time employees (FTEs) was higher than in the less centralized surveillance systems in place in California and Connecticut. Sector-specific studies were corroborative of the active studies presented above. Seafood and meat processing and packing case rates were the highest of all, ranging from 18.2–25.7 cases/1000 FTE. On the other hand, case rates in service and retail industries were less than 1.0 case/1000 FTE. There was more than a 100-fold differential between the highest and lowest exposure industries.

It is perhaps significant that the two surveillance studies of CTS based on medical record linkage had similar case rates: 1.19/1000 (age-adjusted case rate) in Rochester, Minnesota,[80] and 1.74/1000 in Washington.[19] Age-specific frequencies vary substantially depending on whether there is work-related selection. In the Rochester community-based cohort, the case rate peaked in the 45–54 year-old cohort and remained elevated well into the seventh decade.[80] In the Washington cohort, the case rate peaked for ages 35–44.[17] The age-specific case rates in Maastricht was similar to that observed in Minnesota,[17] where there was also no selection by working status. The similarities between case rates in Minnesota and Washington disguise different contributions of gender in working and general populations. For example, in the Rochester cohort from 1976–80, cases were 2.54 times more prevalent in females than in males. In Washington, the female-to-male ratio was 1.24. In the NHIS survey, self reported cases in the "recently worked" had a female-to-male ratio of 1.56, which appears to be closer to the proportion seen in working cohorts rather than in the general population.

TABLE 3.   Upper Extremity Clinical Diagnoses Associated with Overuse

Nerve Entrapment Disorders	Tendinitides	Orthopedic Disorders	Other Diagnoses
Radial tunnel syndrome	Flexor tendinitis	Rotator cuff	Trigger-point fasciitis
Posterior interosseous syndrome	Extensor tendinitis	Traumatic arthritis	Hand-arm vibration syndrome
Wartenburg's syndrome	Epicondylitis	Bone callous	Thoracic outlet syndrome
Cubital tunnel syndrome	Biceps tendinitis		Myofasciitis
Canal of Guyon syndrome	Tenosynotivitis crepitans		
Anterior interosseous syndrome	Trigger digit		
Carpal tunnel syndrome	DeQuervain's		
Pronator syndrome	EIP syndrome		

CASE DEFINITIONS

Incidence data on case frequency has been dependent on the method of investigation, whether through active study or surveillance. Another problematic area involves case definition. When survey data and clinical findings correspond poorly, the distinction is sometimes raised between surveillance definition and clinical definition, but this may only serve to obscure the fact that even subtle alterations or variations in case definition can profoundly affect case rates.

Table 3 lists common clinical diagnostic entities associated with overuse or injury to the upper extremity. As was evident in Table 1, CTS is the dominant diagnosis, but medically initiated surveillance tends to produce clinicopathologic categories like those listed in Table 3. These relatively specific anatomic diagnoses are limited in their ability to characterize diffuse pain syndromes or syndromes characterized by increasing acquired dysfunction. An alternative approach has relied on a more generic a priori case definition. Two such models of inclusive case definition are provided in Table 4.

The first, a symptoms dependent definition, is amenable to questionnaire evaluation and has been used with adaptation in studies performed by NIOSH.[77] The emphasis is on pain and symptoms rather than on measures of physical performance, such as those used in Definition 2.[90] A comparison of the two approaches produces a somewhat counterintuitive result—that the more objective measure detects a higher proportion of abnormality than inquiry driven by questionnaire dichotomies. For example, using their case definition, Silverstein et al. found an 8.9% plantwide prevalence for CTDs, with an adjusted odds ratio of 29.1 in the most highly exposed group compared to the nonexposed group.[77] In Young's study of poultry process workers, fully 62% had signs and symptoms of CTD.[90]

A similar discordance between the extent of positive cases and evaluation criteria applies to the diagnosis of CTS. In some respects, uncertainties affecting case definition are even more acutely drawn around carpal tunnel syndrome, since criteria may include relatively well recognized signs, such as Phelan's and Tinel's sign, and a median nerve dermatomal distribution; characteristic motor and sensory delays on nerve conduction studies; and a generic history and physical examination. The controversy over the superiority of experience-driven clinical diagnosis or consensual case definition is richly expressed in the case of carpal tunnel syndrome. The NIOSH case definition follows an a priori line of common sense and synthesis, taking an inclusionary approach to diagnosis (Table 5). By NIOSH's criteria, a

TABLE 4.   Inclusive Criteria for RSI

Definition 1*
Interview:
Symptoms of pain, numbness, or tingling
Symptoms lasting more than 1 week or more than 20 times in the previous year, or both
No evidence of acute traumatic onset
No related systemic diseases
Onset since working on current job
Physical examination:
Characteristic signs of muscle, tendon, peripheral nerve lesions
Rule out other conditions with referred symptoms
Definition 2**
Signs and quantitative tests:
Grip strength
Pinch strength
Cutaneous pressure
Vibration threshold
Terminal motor latency of median nerve
Tinel's sign
Phalen's test
Symptoms: (summed to a cumulative score)
Pain
Numbness
Swelling
Weakness

 * From Silverstein BA, Fine LJ, Armstrong TJ: Hand wrist cumulative trauma disorders in industry. Br J Ind Med 43:779–784, 1986.
** From Young LV, Seaton MK, Feely CA, et al: Detecting cumulative trauma disorders in workers performing repetitive tasks. Am J Ind Med 27:419–431, 1995.

work-related case is defined by the presence of three conditions and, complementarily, a nonwork-related case of CTS would need to meet the first two criteria.[49] As noted, in most of the categories of employment evaluated cross-sectionally by Silverstein et al., the prevalence of CTS was less than 1.0%.[78]

One way of eliciting the effectiveness of the case definition is to assess validity by applying these criteria to diagnosed cases; another way is to compare this surveillance case definition with more quantitative and restrictive criteria. By way of comparison with both of these measures, the NIOSH case definition falls far short of generic utility.

Katz et al. specifically applied the NIOSH surveillance case definition to a clinical population, absent electrodiagnostic studies.[36] The electrophysiologic case definition was quite loose: a median motor latency of > 4.0 m/sec, a median sensory latency of > 3.7 m/sec, or median sensory velocity of < 50 m/sec. Using the nerve conduction

TABLE 5.   NIOSH Surveillance Case Definition
of Work-related Carpal Tunnel Syndrome

Symptoms suggestive of CTS: Paresthesia, hypesthesia, pain or numbness affecting at least part of the median nerve distribution of the hand(s).
Objective findings consistent with CTS: Tinel's sign, and/or Phelan's sign, and/or decreased or absent sense of pinprick in a median nerve distribution.
Evidence of work relatedness: Frequent, repetitive use of the affected hand or wrist; and/or regular tasks requiring the generation or high force on the affected side; and/or regular or sustained tasks requiring awkward hand position, such as pinch grip or extreme, flexion, extension, or finger use in flexion; and/or regular use of vibrating hand tools, and/or frequent or prolonged pressure over the palm or wrist.

"gold standard," the NIOSH case definition had a sensitivity of 0.67, a specificity of 0.58, positive and negative predictive values of 0.50, and a 38% rate of misclassification. Using an even more discriminating approach to sensitivity testing, based on multiple case definitions, Cherniack et al. demonstrated that small variations in clinical certitude or nerve conduction criteria—well within the ranges included in the various criteria listed in the previously cited studies that relied on nerve conduction alone—could affect case rates and intertest correlations by more than 40%.[12]

A further consideration is the apparent anomaly that the inclusivity of broad clinical case definition may fail in its primary purpose, through a high level of unanticipated case exclusion. It has been suggested that in the natural history of median nerve mononeuropathy, Tinel's sign tends to be a late finding, coinciding with significant and presumably advanced sensory dysfunction.[62] Moreover, while the balance of attention to the sensitivity and specificity of nerve conduction studies has been directed to the approximately 10% of clinical patients with characteristic symptoms and signs and negative electrodiagnostic studies,[22,55] the more provocative problem involves the apparently asymptomatic individual with positive nerve conduction studies, whose existence seems to exceed the expected 5%. Redmond and Rivner found electrodiagnostic CTS in almost 50% of an asymptomatic clinical population.[75] This is uncomfortably similar to the Oregon workforce surveyed by Nathan et al., who described electrodiagnostic abnormalities in nearly 40% of their industrial cohort. What can be said about so high a prevalence of electrical abnormality, relatively unlinked to the symptom complex that has been the presumed concomitant of that abnormality?[55,58]

In this context, the seemingly benign and noncontroversial call for a better best test[36,62] may miss the point or at least produce unproductive choices. Given the complexity of compartment syndromes, with resultant discordances between measurable altered physiology, quantitative sensory dysfunction, and anamnestic symptom patterns, a unifactorial best test is likely to increase the detection of cases while failing to strengthen correlations with other expressions of signs and symptoms. In a population sense, the frequency of CTS could not be articulated independent of a specific statement on test definition.

REPETITIVE STRAIN INJURIES

The Australian Experience

Many of the controversies that surround the frequency and importance of occupational disorders of the upper extremity involve the Australian experience of the late 1970s and early 1980s, during which the term RSI was coined as a workplace malady. Between 1978–1982 in New South Wales, the diagnosis of repetitive strain injuries of the upper extremity rose by 300%, chiefly among female office workers using electronic keyboards.[4,9,18] The mercurial increase in cases followed by a precipitous decline in the face of institutional skepticism and diminished compensation has resulted in the characterization of RSI as a psychological or sociological disease, distinct from more uncommon, anatomically consistent, and conceptually concise overuse injuries.[3,14,41,42,88] More sympathetically, RSI among keyboard operators has been described as an adaptive group psychological response to the trauma of technological innovation, much like the "nystagmus" that affected miners with the introduction of the incandescent helmet.[33]

There is more to the story. Cohen et al. have argued that loose criteria and a too liberal acceptance of RSI was followed by an equally nonrigorous dismissal of the clinical condition.[15] They argue that nociceptive abnormalities and hyperalgesia may be a consequence of biomechanical exertions in the contemporary workplace. While there is argument on the relevance of diffuse neurologic symptoms caused by proximal postural distortions or aberrant peripheral neurologic stimuli,[11,44] the model of hyperalgesic response to proximal nerve injury has considerable physiologic plausibility.[6,40] In this model, torsion or transient compartmental pressure at specific points of large nerve vulnerability (the brachial plexus, the cubital tunnel, the carpal tunnel) may generate diffuse symptoms at multiple loci.

There is still another piece of this story. Remarking on the incidence of RSI in South Australia, Gun has shown that repetitive movement disorders of the upper extremity in blue collar workers were always more prevalent than in keyboardists and have persisted, gradually rising without a pattern of mercurial recognition and dismissal.[23] The reported compensable incidence rate of approximately 2 cases per 1,000 person-years, compare with those observed in Connecticut. From this perspective, the RSI "epidemic" in keyboardists concealed a more broadly based rise in incidence that has not abated.

In summary, the Australian experience was not quite so chimerical as the common view holds. Discomfort in keyboardists, regardless of its severity and quantification, has not disappeared, and the general prevalence of underlying upper extremity disorders in the working population seems consistent with the experience of North America.

RSI, Cervicobrachial Disorders, and Shoulder Pain

This chapter has emphasized the epidemiology of ODUE rather than their causes. However, there are disturbing problems of case definition, particularly the inference that the multiplicity of pathologies and symptom discordance are likely to be grouped in a manner shaped by the choice of survey or test instruments. The formative notion of clinical carpal tunnel syndrome advanced by Phelan[70,71,72] grew out of the treatment of a relatively well-defined middle-aged female population, whose pathology did appear to be restricted to the wrist and hand. Similarly, Yamaguchi's case series from the Mayo Clinic, which was referral based, was focused on hand and wrist problems, although there was a more broadly noted association with peritendinitis affecting a broader region of the upper extremity.[89] On the other hand, more recent observations on CTS have cited the concomitance of neck and shoulder symptoms with the more familiar distal disorders such as "cervicobrachial syndrome."[15] In Japan and Sweden, unlike the United States and Australia, the apparent outbreak of overuse syndromes has been reported as shoulder-neck disorders more often than CTS.[29,46,64,66] Several observers have attempted to integrate these observations through a dynamic model, emphasizing dysfunctional work postures, compensatory overuse of smaller muscle groups, and proximal and distal compartment syndromes, producing nerve entrapment.[35,43,45,69] While there is insufficient space to properly address these important lines of work, it is possible to address workplace epidemiologic issues around shoulder/neck disorders as they relate to the more familiar type affecting the distal upper extremity.

In a major review of odds ratios of shoulder-neck diseases for different occupations, Hagberg and Wegman found the highest prevalence of symptoms and diagnosed disease in meat carriers and slaughterhouse workers, as has been the case with CTS in the United States.[27] Miners and dentists were two other occupational groups having high prevalence rates. A recent study of neck and upper limb disorders in female workers reported associated risks with neck flexion, insufficient proximal strength, and repetition.[63] Although these factors are often associated with more distal abnormalities, there was no association in this cohort with coincident elbow and wrist symptoms. Shoulder symptoms were frequent among women engaged in light sedentary work, but there was considerably more seasonal variation than usually cited for more distal diseases of the hand and wrist.[81] While based on limited samples involving very different types of work, and despite apparently overlapping risk factors, there appear to be differences in the epidemiology of proximal and distal disorders of the upper extremity.

CONCLUSION

In a review of carpal tunnel syndrome cases for the State of Wisconsin Workers Compensation Commission, Moore describes his rejection of 35% of cases, principally because of nonconfirmatory nerve conduction studies.[52] He cites concordance with Katz et al.,[36] who found a 38% misclassification rate on a nondiagnosed population comparing nerve conduction criteria with the NIOSH SENSOR (sentinel event notification system for occupational risks) clinical case definition.[49] However, as already noted, the findings by Katz et al. took quite a different direction, suggesting that electrodiagnostic studies would uncover more positive cases than criteria based on signs and symptoms in a previously undiagnosed population. Most likely, the differences in these two results can be explained by the structure of the two studies, the first being a medicolegal review of reported (established cases), the second being a comparison of the application of two different case definitions to a previously undiagnosed clinical population. These distinctions merely emphasize the point that much of the debate over work-relatedness is misplaced, hinging on discordances between testing strategies, case definitions, and underlying purposes rather than the strength of associations in a relatively controlled context. Of course, control of context is especially difficult for industrial studies, where variations in work exposure, selective survival of existing cohorts, and small size all undercut quantitative comparison. This has curious implications for professional review. In the case of CTS, where there is a definitive test with the capacity of case definition, specialized evaluation seems to increase case detection. On the other hand, where a diagnosis must rest on signs and symptoms, such as cervical strain, professional review, usually based on physical examination, has tended to reduce the number of cases compared to the self-report of symptoms.

The available data support several tentative conclusions. For one thing, there are considerable sector differences in reported prevalence of ODUE, with physically intensive jobs involving stereotypic activity, such as slaughterhouse and packing work, having the highest rates of reported cases. There also is limited evidence that physicians are using cumulative trauma or repetitive strain as surrogates for diffuse and unfocused, or even spurious, upper extremity pain and discomfort. Whether correctly classified, most cases of ODUE are given a tissue-specific diagnosis. While perhaps attributable to limited information, it appears that the epidemiology of ODUE does not support a single unitary hypothesis of origins and symptom expression that extends from the neck to the distal finger.

The attention that is sometimes paid to differentiating surveillance from clinical definitions also appears to be of limited use. While significant upper extremity pathology seems to exist in several industrial sectors, there is a good deal of arbitrariness and selection inherent in its characterization. While there are complicating factors of age and gender, as the NHIS survey demonstrated, most adults work, and the bulk of their physical activity is extended in the workplace, regardless of the physical demands of the job.[84] Thus, there is no suitable nonworking adult comparison population. Because there are a multiplicity of work sites and potential injury sites, the likelihood of developing a consistent measure for determining ODUE is also problematic. This is more acutely a problem if symptoms are loosely correlated with pathophysiology and detectable wear and tear changes are common. The availability of portable electrical tests for screening, such as skin surface EMG machines, and simplified neurodiagnostic devices may further complicate rather than circumscribe this picture. A recent comparison of results obtained on industrial workers using a current threshold perception device, compared with symptoms and nerve conduction, revealed a high level of abnormality but with poor overlap both for symptoms and abnormal nerve conduction studies.[21]

The recommendation that testing strategies and case definition should be industry specific, anatomically specific, and test specific obviates a relatively universal diagnostic standard, such as the use of pulmonary function testing in occupational chest disease. While this poses less of a problem for diagnostics and therapeutics, it complicates concerns driven by assigning liability and compensation. The latter set of considerations are not medical and epidemiologic and when faced by occupational medicine practitioners, as in the case of "black lung," a different approach has been required, one that has been more administrative than biomedical. The same distinction may be useful for the medicolegal management of ODUEs.

REFERENCES

1. Adams FG, Tianti BL: Occupational Disease in Connecticut. Hartford, CT, Occupational Health Working Group, 1990.
2. Andersen JH, Gaardboe O: Musculoskeletal disorders of the neck and upper limb among sewing machine operators. Am J Ind Med 24:689–700, 1993.
3. Awerback M: RSI, or "kangaroo paw" [letter]. Med J Aust 142:237–238, 1985.
4. Bammer G, Martin B: The arguments about RSI: An examination. Comm Health Stud 12:322–558, 1988.
5. Barnhard S, Deers PA, Miller M, et al: Carpal tunnel syndrome among ski manufacturing workers. Scand J Work Environ Health 17:46–52, 1991.
6. Baumann TK, Simone DA, Shain CN, LaMotte RH: Neurogenic hyperalgesia: The search for the primary cutaneous afferent fibers that contribute to capsaicin-induced pain and hyperalgesia. J Neurophys 66:212–227, 1991.
7. Bernard B, Sauter S, Fine L, et al: Job task and psychosocial risk factors for work-related musculoskeletal disorders among newspaper employees. Scand J Work Environ Health 20:417–426, 1994.
8. Bird HA, Hill J: Repetitive strain disorder: Towards diagnostic criteria. Ann Rheum Dis 51:974–977, 1992.
9. Browne CD, Nolan BM, Faithfull DK: Occupational repetition strain injuries: Guidelines for diagnosis and management. Med J Aust 140:329–332, 1984.
10. Bureau of Labor Statistics: Occupational Injuries and Illnesses in the United States by Industry. Washington, DC, U.S. Dept. of Labor, 1992, pp 42–46, bulletin 2399.
11. Butler D, Gifford L: The concept of adverse mechanical tension in the nervous system. Physiotherapy 75:622–636, 1989.
12. Cherniack M, Moalli D, Viscoli K: A comparison of traditional electrodiagnostic studies, electroneurometry and vibrometry in the diagnosis of carpal tunnel syndrome. J Hand Surg 21A:122–131, 1996.
13. Cherniack M: Upper extremity disorders. In Rosenstock L, Cullen MR (eds): Textbook of Clinical Occupational and Environmental Medicine. Philadelphia, WB Saunders, 1994, pp 376–388.
14. Cleland LG: RSI: A model of social iatrogenesis. Med J Aust 147:236–239, 1987.
15. Cohen MI, Arroyo JF, Champion GD, Browne CG: In search of the pathogenesis of refractory cervicobrachial pain syndrome: A deconstruction of the RSI phenomenon. Med J Aust 156:432–436, 1992.
16. Coonrad WRW, Hooper R: Tennis elbow: Its course, natural history, conservative and surgical management. J Bone Joint Surg 55A:1177–1182, 1973.
17. DeKrom MCTGM, Knipschild PG, Kester ADM, et al: Carpal tunnel syndrome prevalence in the general population. J Clin Epidemiol 45:373–376, 1992.

18. Ferguson D: The "new" industrial epidemic. Med J Aust 140:318–319, 1984.
19. Franklin GM, Haug JH, Heyer N, et al: Occupational carpal tunnel syndrome in Washington state, 1984–1988. Am J Public Health 81:741–746, 1991.
20. Franzblau A, Flaschner D, Albers J, et al: Medical screening of office workers for upper extremity cumulative trauma disorders. Arch Environ Health 48:164–170, 1993.
21. Franzblau A, Werner RA, Johnston E, Torrey S: Evaluation of current perception threshold testing as a screening procedure for carpal tunnel syndrome among industrial workers. J Occup Med 36:1015–1021, 1994.
22. Goldring DN, Rose DM, Selvarajan K: Clinical tests for carpal tunnel syndrome: An evaluation. Br J Rheumatol 26:388–390, 1988.
23. Gun RT: The incidence and distribution of RSI in South Australia 1980–81 to 1986–87. Med J Aust 153:376–380, 1990.
24. Hadler NM: Arm pain in the workplace. J Occup Med 34:113–119, 1992.
25. Hadler NM: Cumulative trauma disorders: An iatrogenic concept. J Occup Med 18:117–126, 1990.
26. Hadler NM: The role of work and of working in disorders of the upper extremity. Clin Rheumatol 3:121–141, 1989.
27. Hagberg M, Wegman DH: Prevalence rates and odds ratios of shoulder neck diseases in different occupational groups. Br J Ind Med 44:602–610, 1987.
28. Hagberg M: Occupational musculoskeletal stress and disorders of the neck and shoulder: A review of possible pathophysiology. Int Arch Occup Environ Health 53:269–278, 1984.
29. Hagberg M, Sundelin G: Discomfort and load on the upper trapezius muscle when operating a word-processor. Ergonomics 29:1637–1645, 1986.
30. Hales TR, Kertsche PK: Management of upper extremity cumulative trauma disorders. AAOHN J 40:118–128, 1992.
31. Hanrahan LP, Higgins D, Anderson H, et al: Project SENSOR. Wisconsin surveillance of occupational carpal tunnel syndrome. Wis Med J 990:80–83, 1991.
32. Hunting KL, Welch LS, Cuccherini BA, Seiger LA: Musculoskeletal symptoms among electricians. Am J Ind Med 25:149–163, 1994.
33. Ireland DCR: Psychological and physical aspects of occupational arm pain. J Hand Surg 13B:5–10, 1988.
34. Ireland DCR: Repetition strain injury: The Australian experience—1992 update. J Hand Surg 20A:S53–S56, 1995.
35. Janda V: Muscles and cervicogenic pain syndromes. In Grant R (ed): Clinics in Physical Therapy: Physical Therapy of the Cervical and Thoracic Spine. New York, Churchill Livingstone, 1988, pp 153–166.
36. Katz JN, Larson MG, Fossel AH, Liang MH: Validation of a surveillance case definition of carpal tunnel syndrome. Am J Public Health 81:189–193, 1991.
37. Kirschberg GJ, Fillingim R, Davis VP, Hogg R: Carpal tunnel syndrome: Classic clinical symptoms and electrodiagnostic studies in poultry workers with hand, wrist, and forearm pain. S Med J 87:328–331, 1994.
38. Kissler S, Finholt T: The mystery of RSI. Am Psychol 43:1004–1015, 1988.
39. Kurppa K, Viikari-Juntura E, Kuosma E, et al: Incidence of tenosynovitis or peritendinitis and epicondylitis in a meat-processing factory. Scand J Work Environ Health 17:32–37, 1991.
40. Lamotte RH, Shain CN, Simone DA, Tsai E-F P: Neurogenic hyperalgesia: Psychophysical studies of underlying mechanisms. J Neurophysiol 66:190–211, 1991.
41. Lucire Y; Neurosis in the workplace. Med J Aust 145:323–326, 1986.
42. Lucire Y: Social iatrogenesis of the Australian disease 'RSI.' Comm Health Stud 12:147–150, 1986.
43. Machleder HI, Moll F, Verity A: The anterior scalene muscle in thoracic compression syndrome: Histochemical and morphometric studies. Arch Surg 121:1141–1144, 1986.
44. Mackinnon SE, Dellon AL, Hudson AR, et al: Chronic nerve compression: An experimental model in the rat. Ann Plast Surg 13:112; 120, 1984.
45. Mackinnon SE, Novak CB: Clinical commentary: Pathogenesis of cumulative trauma disorder. J Hand Surg 19A:875–883, 1994.
46. Maeda K, Horiguchi S, Hosokawa M: History of the studies on occupational cervichobrachial disorders in Japan and remaining problems. J Hum Ergol 11:17–29, 1982.
47. Maizlish, et al: Surveillance and prevention of work-related carpal tunnel syndrome: An application of the Sentinel Events Notification System for occupational risks. Am J Ind Med 27:715–729, 1995.
48. Masear VR, Hayes JM, Hyde AG: An industrial cause of carpal tunnel syndrome. J Hand Surg 11A:222–227, 1986.
49. Matte TD, Baker ET, Honchar PA: The selection and definition of targeted work-related conditions for surveillance under SENSOR. Am J Public Health 79:21–25, 1989.

50. Melvin JL, Schuchmann JA, Lanese RR: Diagnostic specificity of motor and sensory nerve conduction variables in the carpal tunnel syndrome. Arch Phys Med Rehabil 54:69–74, 1973.

51. Miller MH, Topliss DJ: Chronic upper limb pain syndrome (repetitive strain injury) in the Australian workforce: A systematic cross-sectional rheumatological study of 229 patients. J Rheumatol 15:1705–1712, 1988.

52. Moore SJ: Clinical determination of work-relatedness in carpal tunnel syndrome. J Occup Rehabil 1:145–158, 1991.

53. Morgenstern H, Kelsh M, Kraus J, Margolis W: A cross-sectional study of hand/wrist symptoms in female grocery checkers. Am J Ind Med 20:209–218, 1991.

54. Morse T: Ergonomics and repetitive strain injuries of the arms and hands at work: A Connecticut report. Connecticut Department of Labor Annual Report (in press).

55. Nathan PA, Keniston RC, Myers LD, Meadows KD: Longitudinal study of median nerve sensory conduction in industry: Relationship to age, gender, hand dominance, occupational hand use, and clinical diagnosis. J Hand Surg 17A:850–857, 1992.

56. Nathan PA, Keniston RC, Myers LD, Meadows KD: Obesity as a risk factor for slowing of sensory conduction of the median nerve in industry: A cross-sectional and longitudinal study involving 429 workers. J Occup Med 34:379–383, 1992.

57. Nathan PA, Keniston RC: Carpal tunnel syndrome and its relation to general physical condition. Hand Clin 9:252–263, 1993.

58. Nathan PA, Meadows KD, Doyle LS: Occupation as a risk factor for impaired sensory conduction of the median nerve at the carpal tunnel. J Hand Surg 13B:167–170, 1988.

59. Nathan PA, Takigawa R, Keniston RC, et al: Slowing of sensory conduction of the median nerve and carpal tunnel syndrome in Japanese and American industrial workers. J Hand Surg 19B:30–34, 1994.

60. National Institute for Occupational Safety and Health: NIOSH Health Hazard Evaluation Report: US WEST Communications, Phoenix, AZ, Minneapolis, MN, Denver, CO. Cincinnati, NIOSH, 1992, HETA 89-299-2230.

61. National Institute for Occupational Safety and Health: NIOSH Health Hazard Evaluation Report: Newsday, Inc., Melville, NY. Cincinnati, NIOSH, 1990. HETA 89-250-2046.

62. Novak CB, Mackinnon SE, Brownlee R, Kelly L: Provocative sensory testing in carpal tunnel syndrome. J Hand Surg 17B:204–208, 1992.

63. Ohlsson K, Attelwell RG, Pålsson B, et al: Repetitive industrial work and neck and upper limb disorders in females. Am J Ind Med 27:731–747, 1995.

64. Ohlsson K, Attewell R, Skerfving S: Self-reported symptoms in the neck and upper limbs of female assembly workers: Impact of length of employment, work pace, and selection. Scand J Work Environ Health 15:75–80, 1979.

65. Ohlsson K, Hansson, G-Å, Balogh I, et al: Disorders of the neck and upper limbs in women in the fish processing industry. Occup Environ Med 51:826–832, 1994.

66. Onishi N, Nomura H, Sakai K, et al: Shoulder muscle tenderness and physical features of female industrial workers. J Hum Ergol 5:87–102, 1976.

67. Osorio AM, Ames RG, Jones J, et al: Carpal tunnel syndrome among grocery store workers. Am J Ind Med 25:239–245, 1994.

68. Park C, Wagner DK, Pierce J: Health conditions among the currently employed, United States 1988. Hyattsville, MD, National Center for Health Statistics, 1993. DHHS publication 93-1514.

69. Pascarelli EF, Kella JJ: Soft-tissue injuries related to use of the computer keyboard: A clinical study of 53 severely injured persons. J Occup Med 35:523–532, 1993.

70. Phalen GS: Spontaneous compression of the median nerve at the wrist. JAMA 145:128–1133, 1951.

71. Phalen GS: The carpal-tunnel syndrome. J Bone Joint Surg 48A:211–228, 1966.

72. Phelan GS: The carpal-tunnel syndrome: Clinical evaluation of 598 hands. Clin Orthop 83:229–240, 1972.

73. Pickett CW, Lees RE: A cross-sectional study of health complaints among 79 data entry operators using video display terminals. J Soc Occup Med 41:113–116, 1991.

74. Putz-Anderson, Doyle GT, Hales TR: Ergonomic analysis to characterize task constraint and repetitiveness as risk factors for musculoskeletal disorders in telecommunication office work. Scand J Work Environ Health 2:123–126, 1992.

75. Redmond MD, Rivne MH: False positive electrodiagnostic tests in carpal tunnel syndrome. Muscle Nerve 11:511–517, 1988.

75a. Rosencrance JC, Cook JM, Zimmerman CL: Active surveillance of cumulative trauma disorders. J Orthop Rehab Ther 19:267–276, 1994.

76. Schoenmarklin RW, Marras WS: Effects of handle angle and work orientation on hammering: Part I—Wrist motion and hammering performance. Hum Factors 31:397–411, 1989.

77. Silverstein BA, Fine LJ, Armstrong TJ: Hand wrist cumulative trauma disorders in industry. Br J Ind
    Med 43:779–784, 1986.
78. Silverstein BA, Fine LJ, Armstrong TJ: Occupational factors and carpal tunnel syndrome. Am J Ind
    Med 11:343–358, 1987.
79. Spindler HA, Dellon AL: Nerve conduction studies and sensibility testing in carpal tunnel syndrome.
    J Hand Surg 3:260–263, 1982.
80. Stevens JC, Sun S, Beard CM, et al: Carpal tunnel syndrome in Rochester, Minnesota, 1961 to 1980.
    Neurology 38:134–138, 1988.
81. Takala E-P, Viikari-Juntura E, Moneta GB, et al: Seasonal variation in neck and shoulder symptoms.
    Scand J Work Environ Health 18:257–261, 1991.
82. Tanaka S, McGlothlin JD: A conceptual quantitative model for prevention of work-related carpal
    tunnel syndrome (CTS). Int J Ind Ergonom 11:181–193, 1993.
83. Tanaka S, Wild DK, Seligman PJ, et al: The U.S. prevalence of self-reported carpal tunnel syndrome:
    1988 National Health Interview Survey Data. Am J Public Health 84:1846–1848, 1994.
84. Tanaka S, Wild MS, Seligman PJ, Halperin WE, et al: Prevalence and work relatedness of self-re-
    ported carpal tunnel syndrome among US workers: Analysis of the occupational health supple-
    ment data of 1988 National Health Interview Survey. Am J Ind Med 27:451–478, 1995.
85. Vanderpool HE, Friis EA, Smith BS, Harms KL: Prevalence of carpal tunnel syndrome and other
    work-related musculoskeletal problems in cardiac sonographers. J Occup Med 35:604–610, 1993.
86. Viikari-Untura E, Kurppa K, Kuosma E, et al: Prevalence of epicondylitis and elbow pain in the
    meat-processing industry. Scand J Work Environ Health 17:38–45, 1991.
87. Watrous BG, Ho G: Elbow pain. Prim Care 15:732–735, 1988.
88. Weintraub MI: Regional pain is usually hysterical. Arch Neurol 45:914–915, 1988.
89. Yamaguchi DM, Lipscomb PR, Soule EH: Carpal tunnel syndrome. Minn Med 48:22–33, 1965.
90. Young LV, Seaton MK, Feely CA, et al: Detecting cumulative trauma disorders in workers perform-
    ing repetitive tasks. Am J Ind Med 27:419–431, 1995.

TERRENCE J. STOBBE, PhD

OCCUPATIONAL ERGONOMICS AND INJURY PREVENTION

From the Industrial & Management
Systems Engineering
Department
College of Engineering and Mineral
Resources
West Virginia University
Morgantown, West Virginia

Reprint requests to:
Dr. Terrence Stobbe
Industrial & Management Systems
Engineering Department
P.O. Box 6107
West Virginia University
Morgantown, WV 26506

The American workplace is facing a crisis: the cost of work-related injuries and illnesses is overwhelming the workers' compensation system. Too many workers are getting injured, they cost too much to compensate, employers feel they cannot spend any more on compensation, and workplace injuries and illnesses continue to occur. In addition, the American workforce is suffering the loss of many skilled people who are no longer able to contribute because they are injured or ill. The most rapidly increasing type of injury/ illness is cumulative trauma disorders. Almost all CTDs are musculoskeletal injuries brought on by a mismatch between the worker and the workplace. These disorders usually affect the back and the upper extremities.

Most CTDs are preventable by eliminating the worker/workplace mismatch. There are two ways to approach this. Historically, the approach has been to design a workplace and then try to fit workers into the workplace through training, worker selection, and other administrative schemes. It has not worked. The reason is simple: you cannot train workers to do something that exceeds their physical capability without placing them at risk of injury. Similarly, you cannot simply tell them to do the task safely or carefully and expect the mismatch problem to be solved. The failure of the "fitting worker to workplace" approach is borne out by the current rapid increase in musculoskeletal injury rates. Instead, we need to understand the range of workers' capabilities and then design the workplace to match them. This involves applying ergonomic principles to workplace design.

WHAT IS ERGONOMICS?

What is ergonomics, and how does it relate to the prevention of musculoskeletal injury in the workplace? Ergonomics is the science of matching workers and workplaces in a manner that improves worker productivity while lowering the worker's risk of injury and discomfort. More specifically, ergonomics is the study of human abilities and limitations and the application of this information to the design of the man-made environment.

Let us consider a simple example using a familiar workplace: the computer workstation. Has anyone who has worked at a computer never experienced one or more of the following symptoms: sore neck, sore shoulders, sore wrists, sore forearms, eyestrain, sore back, sore hands. Probably not. All of these complaints have their root in the mismatch discussed above. They continue to occur despite the fact that ergonomic guidelines that address computer workstation design have existed for at least 15 years. The guidelines describe the ways in which the workplace designer can match the worker to the workstation. For example, the guidelines suggest the proper location of the visual display terminal and copy material to avoid neck and shoulder problems, the proper chair design to avoid back problems, and the proper locations of the keyboard and arm support to avoid hand, wrist, and forearm problems. When these guidelines are followed and the mismatch is eliminated, worker complaints about a workstation are minimized or eliminated.

Although this chapter focuses on ergonomics and musculoskeletal injuries, the field is somewhat broader. Before addressing musculoskeletal injury, an overview of the field and a brief history of ergonomics are in order. The history of ergonomics, or human factors engineering as it was originally known in the United States, is the history of trying to improve human performance. Attempts to improve performance date back to the beginning of recorded history (mostly tool and weapon changes to improve hunting and warfare performance). Modern ergonomics developed out of military necessity during World War II. This period of development was oriented toward "fixing" design problems that prevented efficient performance with aircraft, warships, tanks, and other weapons.[6] At the beginning of the war, it was standard practice to blame the pilot/operator for crashed aircraft and ships, but by the end of the war it was clear that when a mismatch occurred between the operator's abilities and equipment's operational characteristics, the result was a failure that was beyond the operator's control. Operators must be able to see, read, reach, move, interpret, and hear the controls and displays used to operate the equipment; if they cannot, poor performance or failure will likely occur.

The consequences of mismatches during this so-called "knobs and dials" era was highlighted by the magnitude of the losses created by the mismatches. The pilot who misreads the altimeter and lands at a location other than an airport creates tremendous monetary and humanitarian costs; the operator who cannot use a weapon effectively has a fighting efficiency that is below the expected and, as a result, other equipment can be damaged or even a battle lost. The insights of this era were based on an expanded knowledge of human physiologic and psychophysical capabilities, but the fixes were based on man-machine performance rather than operator protection.

Beginning in the 1970s, a shift started to occur. The Occupational Safety and Health Administration was created, workers' compensation costs were rising, and basic research was being done on the physiologic and psychophysical causes of workplace injuries and illnesses. Most of the initial work focused on work-related low back pain because of its cost significance,[5,13,14,29] but work-related research on carpal tunnel syndrome also began to be published.[4,34] In 1981, the National Institute for Occupational Safety and Health published its Work Practices Guide to Manual Lifting, which provided guidelines for preventing low back injury during lifting.[23,24] The basis for the guidelines was matching workers and selected lifting tasks based on the expected physiologic, psychophysical, and biomechanical capabilities of workers (including their muscular strength). Unlike the "knobs and dials" era, where the purpose was man-machine performance enhancement, the main purpose had become avoidance of musculoskeletal injury. Since that time, the injury prevention side of the ergonomics field has grown dramatically, and in 1994, a national program was implemented by the Board of Certified Professional Ergonomists to test and certify practicing ergonomists.

A number of textbooks describe the field of ergonomics.[9,16,21,27] In short, ergonomics includes the study of functional and structural anthropometry; vision and visual performance; noise, hearing, and auditory performance; psychomotor skills and performance; psychophysical abilities such as lifting strength; the effects of vibration; the effects of repetitive work, awkward postures, and the development of cumulative trauma disorders; seating and workstation design; tool design; work physiology; the effects of thermal stress; and memory, human information processing, and decision making. To some degree, all of these topics are related to injury prevention in the workplace. However, the primary workplace issue of the 1990s is musculoskeletal injury and illness prevention; which means the control and prevention of low back injuries and cumulative trauma disorders, especially of the upper extremities.

MUSCULOSKELETAL INJURIES AND ILLNESSES

The terminology musculoskeletal injuries and illnesses is used for two reasons. First, musculoskeletal problems can be the result of an acute injury (lifting and twisting something heavy and causing immediate low back pain, or receiving a blow on the wrist, which causes tissue swelling that may lead to carpal tunnel syndrome), or they can result from chronic exposure to physically stressful conditions (lifting moderate weights hundreds of times per day for many years or operating a vibrating tool with a forceful grasp in a flexed wrist position for eight hours per day for an extended time). The second reason is that the 50 states have differing workers' compensation laws governing the compensability of these musculoskeletal injuries and illnesses (in some states it must be an injury and in some it is an illness or disease). This chapter uses the term musculoskeletal incident to include both injuries and illnesses.

Musculoskeletal incidents may affect muscles, tendons, ligaments, fasciae, bones, nerves, or any combination of these tissues. The incidents manifest in a variety of medical symptoms, including any, some, or all of the following: sharp pains, dull aches, tingling or numbness associated with compressed nerves, burning sensations, swelling, redness, tenderness to the touch, and pain on movement of the affected body part.

In many, if not most, cases, the exact mechanism of injury and the precise tissues that have been injured are unknown and, hence, the specific proper treatment cannot easily be identified. Rather, the medical condition's cause is presumed based on the combination of the immediate history of acute trauma, the person's work activity history, and the physician's personal experience with musculoskeletal incidents. The medical diagnosis is based on the symptoms and the presumed cause. The medical treatment often appears to be the same regardless of the cause and diagnosis. That is, treatment may include any combination of the following:

TABLE 1. Distribution of Body Parts Injured (% by Year), as Estimated by the
Bureau of Labor Statistics

Body Part	1992	1993
Back	28.0	27.3
Upper extremity	22.8	23.0
Lower extremity	19.2	19.5
Trunk (not back)	11.1	11.3
Head/neck	8.5	8.7
Other	10.3	9.8
Total	99.9	99.6

rest, exercise, and stretching; heat and cold; pain killers, muscle relaxants, and anti-inflammatory drugs; splinting and complete immobilization; and physical therapy and surgery. The combination in a specific case will depend on the treating physician's preference.

This chapter addresses two types of musculoskeletal incidents of particular interest to ergonomists: back pain (especially low back pain) and cumulative trauma disorders (especially those of the upper extremities). These incidents usually can be eliminated or minimized by the proper application of ergonomic principles.

Low Back Pain

Low back pain is one of the most universal medical conditions known to humans. It dates roughly to the time that humans began walking on two legs and appears to have become more of a problem with the passing of time. Statistics estimate that low back pain will affect 60–90% of the population at some time in their lives. In the United States, it accounts for 40% of the lost workdays and 33% of workers' compensation costs, and it is the most frequent cause of lost workdays.[8,20]

Data from the Bureau of Labor Statistics are presented in Table 1.[10,11] Table 1 shows the distribution of injuries by body part in 1992 and 1993; back incidents accounted for more than a fourth of all incidents. Table 2 summarizes the data by the event that provoked the incident; lifting incidents account for less than 20% of the back injuries. In both tables, the data remained consistent from 1992 to 1993.

Good comparison data can be found in a number of sources.[12,17,30–32] Stobbe's data, collected in the coal mining, health care, and tire manufacturing industries,

TABLE 2. Causative Events for Back Injuries (% of All Injuries), as Estimated by the
Bureau of Labor Statistics

Event	1992	1993
Contact with object or equipment	27.4	27.3
Overexertion (lifting)	17.1	16.9
Falls	15.3	15.7
Overexertion (not lifting)	11.2	11.3
Harmful substance exp	4.8	5.0
Repetitive motion	3.9	4.2
Slip/trip (with or without fall)	3.5	3.7
Other	16.9	15.9
Total	90.1	100.0

shows that across industries there was considerable variation in the causative event. The all-industry average for lifting was 29% and ranged from 18–39%.[31] Khalil reported that 41.5% of back incidents involved slips and falls and 24.9% involved lifting.[20] Snook used workers' compensation data to estimate the contribution of various events.[29]

How does ergonomics help reduce the occurrence of back injury? It can help in three ways. It helps (1) to understand what the event was, (2) to understand why the event occurred, and (3) using that information along with human capacity data, to modify event scenarios such that they fall within published workplace/work task design guidelines.

Traditionally, injury preventionists have determined the what of back injury— whether an event was caused by lifting, walking, slipping or tripping, falling, or another cause. In most cases, the investigation stops here, and we end up learning the percentage of injuries that were due to lifting, falling, and or chemical exposure. However, this information does not help to stop back injuries. It lends itself to solutions such as "lift more carefully," which is a functionally meaningless comment. To solve the problem, we must understand the event. Table 3 lists the minimal information that should be obtained about an event if we hope to prevent similar events. With this more detailed information, we can begin to understand the scenarios in which an event occurred and develop system-based control strategies that consider all aspects of the event as candidates for intervention strategies (as opposed to the modification of lifting behavior—a control strategy that offers little hope of success in a poorly designed workplace). These system-based control strategies may include employee screening, task elimination, changes in packaging, changes in package weight, changes in package or lifter location before or after the lift, changes in lifting posture, use of mechanical lifting aids, removal of the person from the task, and changes in package-lifter coupling (for example, adding handles).

The control strategy discussion is appropriate for responding to back injury events, but it does little to identify situations that contribute to a back injury or to prevent back injuries. Prevention must be based on an understanding of the types of situations that are known to cause back injuries, coupled with routine workplace assessments to determine where these situations exist. There are three situations that

TABLE 3. Partial List of Questions to Ask When Investigating a Back Injury

Describe the overall event.

Describe the specific event.

What was being handled/lifted/lowered?

What happened physically, including coupling between lifter and object?

How heavy was the object?

How was it grasped, regrasped?

Describe the injured person's actions at the time of the injury.

Where were the object and lifter located?

Why was the injured person doing that work?

Why was the injured person doing that work that way?

What alternative methods existed?

Was the injured person aware of them?

Why didn't the injured person use an alternate method?

Was the injured person aware of the risk associated with lifting?

are known to cause back injuries: overloading, sudden movement or unexpected loading, and asymmetric loading.

The human body is a relatively complex mechanical system that, like all mechanical systems, fails when the load exceeds its mechanical capacity. Overloading occurs when the load is excessive. Traditionally, the question of at what point the load becomes excessive was approached by the setting of arbitrary limits on the weight of loads to be lifted. However, this approach was unsuccessful for a number of reasons, including the fact that the real issue is biomechanical: the critical factor is the torque about the low back, not the weight lifted.[15] The torque is a function of the load weight, the load's position relative to the low back, and the lifter's posture (which determines the torque created by the body's own weight). The risk factor also is a function of both the torque associated with an individual lift and the cumulative torque due to repeated lifts over a work shift and perhaps a working lifetime.[23,24]

Overloading can be created by a number of situations, including excessive torque due to the following:

1. An objects' weight, e.g., trying to lift 150 or 200 pounds;

2. An object's location, e.g. lifting a light or moderate weight object at arm's length;

3. An object's bulkiness, which causes the center of gravity to be far from the lifter and makes the object hard to control, e.g., a large or irregularly shaped object;

4. A worker's choice of lifting method, which combines the effects of posture and location to create excessive torque, e.g., a worker who chooses to lift from a stooped posture with an arm that is fully extended;

5. Repeated lifting that has caused muscle fatigue and decreased lifting capacity, e.g., a person who lifts 40,000 or 50,000 pounds over the course of a workshift;

6. Extended work periods in a static forward flexed posture.

Sudden movement or unexpected loading is also a frequent contributing cause of back injury—and probably a variety of other musculoskeletal incident events. Sudden movement or unexpected loading occurs when a person experiences a quickly applied external load that must be resisted or compensated for by the neuromuscular system. The situation is highly dynamic, and injury may occur when the neuromuscular system cannot adjust quickly enough to the external load. The system does not know the magnitude and direction of the external force; neither is it fast enough to react appropriately in the few milliseconds that the external force is being applied. The injury may be the result of an external force creating an eccentric contraction in which the external force is much greater than the muscular strength and, therefore, a soft tissue strain or sprain occurs. The injury also may result from the external force moving a body part outside its normal range of motion, perhaps coupled with an eccentric contraction—again producing a soft tissue injury.

Examples of sudden movement situations include the following:

1. A sudden stop when pushing or pulling an object, e.g., pulling a cart whose wheels get stuck in a floor rut, which results in a sudden stop that jerks the person doing the pulling back toward the cart;

2. A sudden start when pushing or pulling an object, e.g., pulling on a hose or cable that is stuck or hung up which suddenly breaks loose, causing the high pulling/pushing force that is being applied by the puller to be unresisted;

3. Jolts of large and unpredictable magnitude and direction that are experienced by mobile equipment operators, e.g., being tossed from side to side and up and down while operating a front end loader or a forklift;

4. Sudden shifts in the load a person is lifting or carrying, e.g., a container of liquid that tilts and causes all of the liquid to flow to one side;

5. The loss of control of a lifted/carried object, which causes the lifter to reposition his or her hands suddenly and unpredictably, changing the biomechanical loading;

6. Lifting or catching moderate to heavy loads that are in motion at the time the worker attempts to establish control over them, e.g., catching and stacking boxes or bags at the end of a conveyor.

Studies by Stobbe et al. in the mining, health care, and tire manufacturing industries have shown that sudden movements were a contributing cause of injury in about half of all low back injuries.[31-33] Lifting was a contributing cause in only 29% of the incidents.

Asymmetric lifting has long been recognized as a contributing cause in many low back incidents. Asymmetric lifting occurs when the load is lifted, held, or carried to the right or left of the center line of the body. This results in torsional and shear loads on the spine, which significantly increase the risk of injury. In addition, asymmetric lifting requires a complicated neuromuscular response, which means there must be considerable coordination of active muscles. Any discoordination due to inattention, load shift, loss of balance, or other external factors may lead to a soft tissue strain or sprain.

Asymmetric lifting is a normal human behavior. It occurs despite all training to the contrary because it usually takes less energy to lift by bending and reaching to the side than it does to shift the feet, bend and lift, and then shift the feet again. In addition, workplace design can unconsciously encourage asymmetric lifting by locating a lift's origin and destination such that a person can stand and access both with a bend and reach followed by a lift and twist followed by a reach and release. When the workplace design makes it easiest to work in the wrong way, the work will be done the wrong way.

This section has discussed low back injuries and three work situations most likely to produce them. Prevention is most effectively carried out by conducting workplace assessments to identify places where the three situations exist. Once identified, the situations can be modified or eliminated through the application of ergonomic design principles, lifting guidelines established by NIOSH, and attentiveness to situations in which sudden or unexpected loading may occur. A number of sources provide an excellent basis for ergonomics-based workplace-design changes.[15,16,20-24,36] The following general suggestions also might prove helpful:

• Despite the best training efforts, Murphy's Law will prevail. Therefore, prevent the injury by fixing the workplace rather than trying to change the worker.

• The incidence of lifting injuries on jobs where people work in an erect posture is extremely low. If people keep all lifted loads between the knees and shoulders, they will not need to bend the torso or reach overhead, and back injuries will become a rare event.

• When a high-risk situation exists, ask the workers for the "easiest" way to work and then include "easiest" in your redesign. They will do "easiest" anyway, so make the lowest risk method the "easiest" method.

• Explain the sudden movement concept to workers, and ask them to help identify the sudden movement risks on their job. Then redesign the task or workplace to minimize or remove the risks.

• Evaluate work stations to identify asymmetric lifting and lift-and-twist situations. Redesign to minimize or eliminate them.

TABLE 4.   Common Work-Related Cumulative Trauma Disorders

Carpal tunnel syndrome	Peritendinitis
Tendinitis	Trigger finger
Tenosynovitis	Trigger points
Ulnar nerve entrapment	Cubital tunnel syndrome
deQuervain's disease	Ganglionic cyst
Ulnar arterial thrombosis	Thoracic outlet syndrome
Rotator cuff tears	Tension neck syndrome
Pronator teres syndrome	Epicondylitis
Perineural fibrosis of the digital nerves	Degenerative joint disease

Cumulative Trauma Disorders

Force, frequency, posture, duration, insufficient recovery time, localized pressure, thermal stress, vibration, and acute trauma and microtrauma are the causal terms most frequently associated with cumulative trauma disorders.[1,26,28] Cumulative trauma disorders are defined as disorders of the bones, tendons, ligaments, joints, muscles, and nerves that result from the repeated use of the affected body part. By definition, CTDs develop cumulatively over a relatively long time. Each repetition of an activity causes mechanical wear and tear or trauma to one or more body parts. A similar result can occur when an incident causes a local microtrauma that would normally heal without incident. Instead, the job's required movements further irritate the area of microtrauma and prevent normal healing. These are the typical mechanisms that can lead to a CTD.

Table 4 lists some of the common CTDs that have work-related causes. While CTD-type injuries have existed for years, only during the 1980s and 1990s have they become industrially significant. Like back injuries, CTDs are painful, hard to diagnose, resistant to treatment, and their specific causative characteristics are difficult to determine. Unlike back injuries, the frequency of CTDs is increasing rapidly. Table 5 shows that during a recent 5-year period, the reported incidence of CTDs more than doubled, with the annual increase ranging from 7–28%.

The cause of this dramatic increase in CTDs is unknown. It is not due to a sudden increase in the repetitiveness or difficulty of industrial work. It is more likely due to an increased awareness on the part of the medical profession, workers and unions, and occupational health and safety professionals. In addition, research conducted by ergonomists over the past 20 years has linked the listed workplace risk factors with the occurrence of specific CTDs.

The four primary risk factors are the muscular force applied, the frequency and duration of application, and the use of awkward (non-neutral) postures while working.

TABLE 5.   Number of Cumulative Trauma Disorders Reported in the United States, as Estimated by the Bureau of Labor Statistics

Year	Number of Reported Cases	Percentage Increase from the Previous Year
1989	147,000	28
1990	185,000	26
1991	224,000	21
1992	282,000	26
1993	302,000	1

Considering these four risk factors, along with individual susceptibility, it is probably true that on any given job where the risk factors are present, there is some combination of force, frequency, duration, and posture that will initiate a CTD. Unfortunately, we cannot yet specify what this combination is; nor can we determine the contribution of nonwork activities—golf, fishing, gardening, sewing—to the development of a CTD.

Many more epidemiologic studies need to be conducted before the critical risk factor exposure levels can be defined. These studies will be challenging, because both the typical job and the typical life have many risk factors (made up of a variety of tasks, each with a number of body motions). The complexity of this problem will render these studies ineffective, and perhaps misleading, if they are conducted at the macro level. Rather, detailed job analyses that describe individual work behaviors and practices will be needed to identify individual specific risk factor exposures, which can then be correlated with disease incidence.

Since we cannot adequately explain the origin or the diagnosis of these disorders, proper and effective individual treatment is difficult. The best solution is prevention, but given the nonspecific nature of CTD causation, we are usually left with reducing exposure to the risk factors rather than removing the causal factors.

The widely recognized risk factors for CTDs listed at the beginning of this section are discussed below.

FORCE

The amount of effort that is used while performing a task is a risk factor because it determines the amount of force (tension, compression, shear) on the affected parts of the body. The greater the relative force, the greater the risk of tissue damage. The term relative force is used because the closer a loaded muscle is to its strength capacity, the greater the risk of tissue damage. For example, a 50-pound load supported by the legs is a relatively small load, but a 5-pound load on a finger is relatively large.

The first step in reducing the force used while performing a job is to understand its cause. Common causes of high relative force are the handled object's weight, shape, and size, the object's location, and worker misperception. Depending on the task and object, it may be possible to modify the object to lower the strength required to use it. A little creativity will almost always allow a health and safety professional to change the object's location or orientation to make it easier to work with, thus reducing the force requirement. Worker misperception can be addressed by training that is based on an understanding of the reason for the misperception.

POSTURE

In the context of CTDs, posture means the working position of each joint in the body relative to the range of the joint's motion. Joint positions near the center of the range of motion have low risk for CTDs, while joint positions at the extremes of the range of motion have high risk. These low-risk joint positions are sometimes referred to as neutral postures. For example, a neutral wrist posture is best understood by considering the normal handshake; there is no bending to the left or right (flexion/extension), there is no movement toward the thumb or little finger (ulnar/radial deviation), and the palm is not twisted up or down (supination or pronation).

As a joint moves away from the central part of its range of motion, the functional strength of the associated muscles will decrease. This causes the applied force to be a greater percentage of that muscle's or muscle group's strength capacity. In addition, as the muscles and connective tissues move away from the central part of the range of motion, they are stretched and vulnerable to injury. Finally, as the tissues approach the end of the range of motion, they are fully stretched, and further motion due to sudden movements or unexpected loads may cause tissue injury. In some cases, these non-neutral postures may cause nerve compression, which can lead to a variety of CTD-related symptoms. The key to improving work postures is to understand why they are being used. Common reasons include object location and orientation, tool design, product design, unnecessary work content, and poor work habits resulting from inadequate training. Creativity mixed with ergonomic principles can assist in locating and orienting the objects for neutral posture access. The same approach will be helpful for improving tool and product design.[2,19] In some cases, specific work elements cause the "risky" postures, and these elements can be engineered out of the work. Workers should know the symptoms and causes of CTDs, and they should be trained to avoid work activities known to cause them.

FREQUENCY

One result of modern industrial efficiency is repetitious work with limited content. On some jobs the repetition occurs thousands of times per shift. Each repetition involves the application of force and movements toward and away from central part of the range of motion. These movements cause the tendons to move in their sheaths. Although this movement is normal, too much motion may cause inflammation within the sheath. There are a number of ways this inflammation of the tendon or its sheath can occur: a breakdown in the lubricating system of the synovial fluid, an inability of the lubricating system to offset the friction created by the force and posture, or an irritation of the swelling that resulted from a microtrauma to the tissue. An example is a minor impact injury to a tendon or sheath that causes a tiny swelling. Under normal use, the swelling would heal without incident, but with repetitive movement of the tendon across the affected area, the swollen tissue is further irritated, which prevents healing and causes additional swelling. This eventually may manifest as a CTD.

Frequency is usually defined in terms of the number of times a movement occurs in a job cycle and the number of job cycles per shift. The "too frequent" rate is dependent on the person and the force and posture involved.

The first step in reducing frequency is understanding what must be done. Unnecessary motions can be eliminated. Posture and force changes can be implemented to reduce the effect of frequency. Finally, frequency can be reduced through job rotation and by lowering the production rate.

DURATION

Another critical job component is duration of exposure. In this context, duration has two meanings, the length of time a given force and posture are held and the length of the exposure during the shift. Both the frequency of adopting a posture and the length of time the posture is held are risk factors for CTDs. For example, on some tasks, a motion may be repeated three times per cycle with two cycles per minute, with each motion lasting a second or less. On others, there may be one high-risk motion per cycle and one cycle per minute, but the motion may last for 20 seconds. This prolonged static hold will lead to muscle fatigue, a decrease in strength, and increased risk of CTDs. If the motion involves a nerve compression, the prolonged compression increases the risk of nerve damage. The longer a worker is exposed to the risk factors during a shift, the greater the risk of developing a CTD.

VIBRATION

Vibration is a risk factor that enhances the effect of other risk factors. By itself, vibration will cause Raynaud's syndrome but will not cause a CTD. When the other main risk factors occur in the presence of vibration, they can cause a CTD at reduced exposure levels. The main effect of vibration is to inhibit vascular circulation. Another significant effect is that vibration typically results in a worker's increasing the grip force they apply to operate a tool. The most common sources of vibration are hand tools (pneumatic and electric) and large pieces of equipment and vehicles. The control of vibration is highly situation-specific, and the reader is referred to other sources for additional information.[18,36]

THERMAL (COLD) STRESS

Cold stress, like vibration, will not cause a CTD, but it can enhance the effects of the main risk factors and promote the development of CTDs at reduced risk factor exposure levels. This enhancing effect is probably the result of the vascular modifications caused by the cold. Common causes of cold stress are working outside, working in refrigerated areas, and working with pneumatic tools whose air exhausts directly onto the hand or arm. Cold stress can be controlled with appropriately selected gloves and clothing. Tool exhausts can be redirected or moved to a location where the exhaust does not affect the user.

PRESSURE

Grasping a tool or leaning on a counter creates localized pressure on tissue. This pressure modifies or interrupts the blood flow and may directly injure tendons, nerves, and muscles. When combined with force, posture, and repetition, localized pressure may enhance the effects of the other risk factors. The most common sources of localized pressure are objects such as tools, tables, and counters with sharp edges; and triggers on power tools. Localized pressure is generally the result of poor design of the tool or object. Additional information is provided by other sources.[2,19]

CONTROL OF CUMULATIVE TRAUMA DISORDERS

Control and prevention of CTDs is "simple:" minimize exposure to the risk factors. This is a key point—we control or prevent CTDs by removing the source of the activity or by reducing exposure to as many of the risk factors as possible. As exposure to risk factors is reduced, so is the risk of developing a CTD. In most cases, ergonomic interventions can be used to reduce exposure to risk factors.

At first glance, this approach may appear too indirect. Any specific causative exposures should be removed. However, this is true only if the exposures can be identified. With cumulative trauma disorders, the injury is the accumulated result of many exposures to a combination of the risk factors.

In practice, therefore, CTDs are prevented by studying the tasks that make up the job. The study is carried out through a combination of employee and supervisor interviews, onsite observations, review of videotapes, and, when possible, personal experience performing the task. The study should focus on the components of the task that involve risk factor exposure, and, wherever possible, the exposure should be quantified. The information is analyzed, and modifications of the tasks are developed. The modifications are evaluated by a team of individuals familiar with the job to determine their effect on the overall production system. The best overall solutions are implemented, and the modified task is reevaluated as described above. If necessary, additional modifications can be developed and implemented. This iterative process may go through a number of cycles before a task redesign is satisfactory.

There is no one best way to evaluate job tasks. Two good sources are OSHA's Draft Ergonomic Protection Standard and ANSI Z-365, which is expected to be published in 1997 (a draft version of the ANSI standard is available and provides excellent job evaluation guidance).[3,35] In practice, most professional ergonomists use their training and experience to develop their own approach to job evaluation. Health and safety professionals who are interested in using ergonomics are encouraged to read the literature, to attend short courses from at least two sources, and to spend time working directly with a professional ergonomist before embarking on their own program. A roster of certified professional ergonomists is available from the Board of Certified Professional Ergonomists in Bellingham, Washington.

SUMMARY

Ergonomics is the study of people at work. The current focus is on the prevention of work-induced musculoskeletal injuries through the application of sound ergonomic principles. This chapter has briefly outlined ergonomics and its history, has described low back pain and upper extremity cumulative trauma disorders from an ergonomic perspective, and has discussed control and prevention approaches for a few scenarios.

Ergonomic principles are based on a combination of science and engineering and a thorough understanding of human capabilities and limitations. When these principles are applied to the design of a job, task, process, or procedure, the incidence and severity of musculoskeletal injuries decrease. In many cases productivity and morale also improve. Workers are spared suffering, and employers are spared costs.

It is hoped that this discussion will encourage more health, safety, and business professionals to learn about and apply ergonomics in their workplaces for the improvement of the worker, product, and business.

Finally, many additional epidemiologic studies on the individual and joint effects of the CTD risk factors are needed. The knowledge gained from these studies will promote the more effective application of ergonomic principles to reduce worker suffering, improve products, and reduce costs.

ACKNOWLEDGMENT

The author wishes to thank Tom Bobick for his thorough and insightful review of this chapter. Mr. Bobick is a safety engineer with NIOSH and a doctoral candidate in industrial and management systems engineering at West Virginia University, Morgantown, West Virginia.

REFERENCES

1. American Industrial Hygiene Association: Ergonomics Guide to Cumulative Trauma Disorders of the Hand and Wrist. Fairfax, VA, AIHA, 1994.
2. American Industrial Hygiene Association: Ergonomics Guide to Hand Tool Design. Fairfax, VA, AIHA, 1996.
3. American National Standards Institute: ANSI Z-365, Draft Standard for the Control of Cumulative Trauma Disorders. New York, ANSI, 1996.
4. Armstrong TJ, Chaffin DB: Carpal tunnel syndrome and selected personal attributes. J Occup Med 21:481–486, 1979.
5. Ayoub MM, Dryden R, McDaniel J, et al: Predicting lifting capacity. Am Ind Hyg Assoc J 40:1075–1084, 1979.
6. Bailey RW: Human Performance Engineering. 2nd ed. Englewood Cliffs, NJ, Prentice Hall, 1989.

7. Bobick TG, Stobbe TJ, Plummer RW: An analysis of selected back injuries occurring in underground coal mining, IC9145. US Bureau of Mines, 1987.
8. Bobick TG, Pizatella TJ, Hsiao H, Amendola AA: Job-design characteristics that contribute to workplace-related musculoskeletal injuries. Orthop Phys Ther Clin North Am 4:375–385, 1995.
9. Bridger RS: Introduction to Ergonomics. New York, McGraw-Hill, 1995.
10. Bureau of Labor Statistics: Occupational injuries and illnesses: Counts, Rates, and Characteristics, 1992. Washington, DC, US Dept. of Labor, 1995.
11. Bureau of Labor Statistics: Occupational injuries and illnesses: Counts, Rates, and Characteristics, 1993. U.S. Washington, DC, US Dept. of Labor, 1996.
12. Carbines ME, Schwartz, GE: Strategies for Managing Disability Costs. Washington, DC, Washington Business Group on Health/Institute for Rehabilitation and Disability Management, 1987.
13. Chaffin DB: Human strength capability and low back pain. J Occup Med 16:248–254, 1974.
14. Chaffin DB, Herrin G, Keyserling WM: Pre-employment strength testing—An updated position. J Occup Med 20:403–408, 1978.
15. Chaffin DB, Andersson GBJ: Occupational Biomechanics. 2nd ed. New York, Wiley & Sons, 1991.
16. Eastman Kodak: Ergonomic Design for People at Work. New York, Van Nostrand Reinhold, 1983.
17. Frymoyer JW, Pope MH, Clements J: Risk factors in low back pain. J Bone Joint Surg 65A(2): 213–218, 1983.
18. Griffin MJ: Handbook of Human Vibration. San Diego, Academic Press, 1990.
19. Greenberg L, Chaffin DB: Workers and Their Tools. Midland, MI, Pendell, 1977.
20. Khalil TM, Abdel-Moty EM, Rosomoff RS, Rosomoff HL: Ergonomics in Back Pain. New York, Van Nostrand Reinhold, 1993.
21. Konz S: Work Design: Industrial Ergonomics. 3rd ed. Worthington, OH, Publishing Horizons, 1990.
22. Kroemer K, Kroemer H, Kroemer-Elbert K: Ergonomics. Englewood Cliffs, NJ, Prentice Hall, 1994.
23. National Institute for Occupational Safety and Health: Work practices guide for manual lifting. Washington, DC, NIOSH, 1981, publication 81-122.
24. National Institute for Occupational Safety and Health: Applications manual for the revised NIOSH lifting equation.Washington, DC, NIOSH, 1994, publication 94-110.
25. Pope MH, Frymoyer JW, Andersson GBJ: Occupational Low Back Pain. New York, Praeger, 1983.
26. Putz-Anderson V: Cumulative Trauma Disorders: A Manual for Musculoskeletal Diseases of the Upper Limbs. London, Taylor & Francis, 1988.
27. Sanders MS, McCormick EJ: Human Factors in Engineering and Design. 7th ed. New York, McGraw-Hill, 1993.
28. Silverstein BA, Fine LJ, Armstrong TJ: Hand wrist cumulative trauma disorders in industry. Br J Ind Med 43:779–784, 1986.
29. Snook SH, Campanelli A, Hart JW: A study of three preventive approaches to low-back injury. J Occup Med 20:478–481, 1978.
30. Snook SH, Jensen RC: Cost of occupational low back pain. In Pope MH (ed): Occupational Low Back Pain. New York, Praeger, 1984.
31. Stobbe TJ, Plummer RW: Sudden-movement/unexpected loading as a factor in back injuries. In Trends in Ergonomics/Human Factors V. Amsterdam, Elsevier Science Publishers, 1988.
32. Stobbe TJ, Plummer RW: Back Injuries in underground coal mining [research report]. Pittsburgh, US Bureau of Mines, 1989.
33. Stobbe TJ, Plummer RW: A study of back injuries in underground coal mining. In Advances in Industrial Ergonomics and Safety VI. Bristol, PA, Taylor & Francis, 1994.
34. Tichauer ER, Gage H: Ergonomic principles basic to hand tool design. Am Ind Hyg Assoc J 38:622–634, 1977.
35. United States Department of Labor, Occupational Safety and Health Administration: Draft ergonomic protection standard, Washington, DC, OSHA, 1995.
36. Wasserman DE: Human Aspects of Occupational Vibrations. Amsterdam, Elsevier, 1987.
37. Woodson WE, Tillman B, Tillman P: Human Factors Design Handbook. 2nd ed. New York, McGraw-Hill, 1991.

GRACE KAWAS LEMASTERS, PhD

EPIDEMIOLOGY OF REPRODUCTIVE HAZARDS IN THE WORKPLACE

From the Department of
Environmental Health
University of Cincinnati College
of Medicine
Cincinnati, Ohio

Reprint requests to:
Grace K. Lemasters, PhD
Department of Environmental
Health
University of Cincinnati College
of Medicine
231 Bethesda Avenue
Cincinnati, OH 45267-0182

In 1960 the percentages of women and men in the United States civilian labor force younger than 35 were 32.7% and 37%; today these values have risen to 42.6%, and 44.9%, respectively.[75] However, since 1960 the percentage of married men in the labor force has decreased from 89.2% to 77.4% and has almost doubled for married women, from 31.9% to 60.7%. Further, the percentage of women younger than 44 having a child while in the labor force increased from 38% in 1980 to 54% in 1992. The fetal loss rate per 1,000 women increased one percentage point, from 14.1% to 15.1% during the same time, and the percentage of low birthweight (< 2,500 grams) infants increased from 6.8% to 7.1%.

Concerns exist as to whether the fertility potential of men is declining. This concern has been sparked by findings that testicular cancer has increased and that the average human sperm count has declined by half since the 1930s.[15] Others, however, state that these perceived changes are related to methodologic and technical procedures and differences in study subjects. Based on a meta-analysis of 60 historical studies[15] and analysis of data from sperm banks, there may be some reason for alarm.[5] A study of 1,351 healthy men has shown a decrease of 2.1% in sperm concentrations per year, a decrease in sperm motility, and an increase in abnormal spermatozoa.[5] What associations the above findings have with exposures in the workplace can only be speculated.

REPRODUCTIVE AND DEVELOPMENTAL TOXICOLOGY

Reproductive toxicity is defined as a condition causing deleterious responses in the postpubertal male or female, manifested by interference with normal physiologic processes or regulatory mechanisms, organ functioning, or the genetic integrity of the sperm or eggs. Exposure related to reproductive toxicity may occur at any time in the life of the individual from conception throughout sexual maturity. Developmental toxicity is defined as a condition producing adverse effects on the developing organism reflected in prenatal or early postnatal death, altered growth, structural abnormalities, and functional deficits.

Reproductive toxicity studies require consideration of gender differences in absorption, distribution, metabolism, storage, and excretion of xenobiotics. The maximum oxygen uptake for women is 57% that of men but more closely approximates 91% that of men when adjusted for lean body weight.[49] Changes during pregnancy in body weight, plasma proteins, plasma volume, body fat, cardiac output, extracellular fluid volume, and total body water generally increase xenobiotic uptake and distribution.[44–47] For example, during pregnancy minute ventilation capacity increases by nearly 50% over the nonpregnant state, potentially increasing exposure to air contaminants. While initial distribution of a toxicant is regulated by blood flow, tissue concentration is determined by affinity.[3] Because women have a higher fat-to-body mass ratio than men, lipophilic xenobiotics may show an increased body burden within the fat compartments. Adipose tissue metabolism differs from muscle tissue, contributing to women's generally slower metabolic rate.[42] Lipophilic compounds sequestered in adipose tissue later may be mobilized due to increased metabolic demand related to strenuous activity or by the physiologic demands of a pregnancy. Important determinants of the toxicokinetic action of xenobiotics include the residence time in tissue and metabolism, not only in the liver but also in the lung, kidney, intestinal tract, and skin, placenta, and fetal tissues. Lipid solubility, protein binding, dose, and route of exposure to the toxicant affect the rate of biotransformation. Most xenobiotics are eliminated by renal, hepatic, or pulmonary routes. Renal blood flow, glomerular filtration, tubular secretion, and reabsorption are greater in men than in women. Elimination may be further compromised during pregnancy.

After the union of the egg and sperm, the zygote may experience insult in a hostile uterine environment. The transport time of a fertilized ovum prior to implantation is 2–6 days. Initially, the zygote may be exposed to xenobiotics that penetrate into the uterine fluids. Absorption of these chemicals may be accompanied by degenerative changes that cause failure to implant. Although the preimplantation loss rate in humans is high, the embryo at this early stage—before cells have differentiated—may be resistant to teratogenic insult. Late embryogenesis and the early fetal period is characterized by differentiation, mobilization, and cellular and tissue organization. During this period of organogenesis, the embryo is at greatest risk for a teratogenic insult. The fetal period extends from embryogenesis to birth and begins around the 54th to 60th day of gestation. The fetus is capable of xenobiotic metabolism as early as 6 weeks' gestation, causing the fetus to act as a potential biological "sink." Some xenobiotics found in fetal blood at levels equivalent to those in maternal blood include lead, arsenic, benzene, trichloroethylene, vinyl chloride, manganese, and methyl mercury.[8] During the fetal period, toxic insult can lead to adverse outcomes related to growth, histogenesis, and functional immaturity.

Hence, a couple's reproductive success ultimately depends on a delicate physiochemical regulation within and between the paternal, maternal, and embryo/fetal systems, requiring the management of exogenous as well as endogenous exposure conditions. Detection of exposure-response associations may be further compromised by differences in individual susceptibility and maternal factors such as nutritional deficiency, health status, and lifestyle.

CHARACTERIZING EXPOSURE

Exposure Parameters

Varying patterns in route, level, and timing of exposure are factors related to the difficult identification of reproductive and developmental toxicants. The additive or synergistic effects associated with multiple exposures may alter the response of the adult or the developing conceptus. Individuals generally experience multiple exposures from several sources simultaneously, i.e., from air, water, and food either while at home or in the workplace.

Reproductive and developmental studies have an added precision requirement—needing to link exposure during a fairly narrow but critical time. A pregnancy lasts only 40 weeks and spermatogenesis about 10 weeks. Therefore, an acute exposure within these narrow time bands may have profound adverse effects. If, for example, fetal loss or birth defects are the effect of interest, exposures occurring just prior to conception or during early pregnancy constitute a critical period. Exposure markers for teratogens are generally targeted during the period of organogenesis, up to days 55–60 of gestation, but for some anomalies, e.g., of the central nervous system, eye and genitalia, exposures should be assessed throughout the pregnancy. If, however, birthweight is being investigated, second or third trimester exposures are critical periods for growth.

A measure of variability referred to as an overall time window ratio has been proposed to evaluate the extent of misclassification bias that can occur if there is a vulnerable period during which the xenobiotic exerts its effect.[26] The higher the overall time window, the greater the potential for misclassification. Characterizing an exposure variable as occurring "anytime during pregnancy" or "anytime during spermatogenesis" may be too gross a measure to detect an agent that exerts its effect during an even narrower time. Studies suggest that women can recall exposures during pregnancy, even those changing on a monthly basis, across the 9 months of gestation and especially those related to infections, medical treatments such as medications, x-rays, and ultrasound, and exposures associated with painting, lacquering, varnishing, and pesticides.[26] If a woman has had multiple jobs or has been laid off work during a critical time such as organogenesis, there is great opportunity for exposure misclassification. To minimize occupational exposure misclassification, information should be gathered concerning specific job duties, periods of time off, rotation patterns among jobs, the use of protective equipment including masks and clothing, and medical and other exposures, especially during critical periods. Questions such as "Were you pregnant while working at this job task?" and "Approximately during which month of your pregnancy did you perform these job activities?" may be good memory jogs to decrease errors in linking jobs to reproductive events.

Exposure Dosimetry

Figure 1 is a schematic diagram of the concepts of external, absorbed, internal, and the biologically effective dose underlining exposure characterization. One of the most common sources for characterizing a worker's exposure is external measures such as job title and work activities documented by questionnaire or company records. Work histories gathered from the employee have been shown to be a fairly

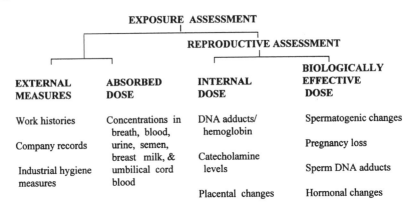

FIGURE 1. Exposure and reproductive health assessment. (Adapted from Lemasters GK, Schulte PA: Biologic markers in the epidemiology of reproduction. In Schulte P (ed): Molecular Epidemiology: Principles and Practices. San Diego, Academic Press, 1993.)

reliable and valid source of information, but they depend on several factors, including number of jobs held, length of time since employment, short tenure on the job, and level of education.[9,13,70] In one study, supervisors were asked to independently identify exposures by job tasks of women in the semiconductor industry, and the answers were compared to the women's reports.[56] The supervisors' reports compared favorably with the women's, suggesting good recall. Jobs may be linked with other surrogate measures of exposure, such as production records or chemical usage information, as was done with exposure to 1,2-dibromo-3-chloropropane (DBCP) in a pesticide manufacturing facility.[78] Based simply on the job tasks reported by the men, DBCP was initially identified as the primary agent causing male infertility even though the company used 100 chemicals to manufacture more than 200 compounds. The job tasks were then linked to the number of pounds produced of that particular chemical in a specific process area. Availability of industrial hygiene measurements and work histories will further augment confidence in categorized levels of exposure. Even with the addition of industrial hygiene measures, there still may be considerable error in exposure estimation, and exposures may not reflect the concentrations of the agent in actual biological fluids. If other routes of entry, such as absorption through the skin, are more relevant than inhalation or the worker is using personal protective equipment, the industrial hygiene measurements also may contribute to exposure misclassification.

Absorbed dose is defined as the concentration of a compound in biological fluids, including breath, blood, urine, saliva, breast milk, umbilical cord blood, and seminal fluids (Fig. 1). Although the most commonly used media to evaluate absorbed dose are blood and urine, they may not always be the most optimal, especially if exposures are low and quantities of fluid relatively sparse. In addition, blood and urine require the handling of body fluids; obtaining blood is invasive, and obtaining urine may require the bulky collection and storage of 24-hour samples.

In contrast, breath sampling for volatile organic compounds is a noninvasive alternative that can detect low levels of exposure, and concentrations in breath have correlated well with external industrial hygiene measurements and blood concentrations.[22,54,76] Pharmacokinetic modeling of absorbed dose requires consideration of residence time of the agent in tissues. To continue with the example of volatile organic compounds, a four-compartment model of absorbed dose may be considered when calculating the optimal time for breath collection. Because of a rapid exponential emptying of the blood, to evaluate the first compartment, breath samples must be collected within 1–13 minutes after exposure. This measurement captures the immediately preceding peak exposures. The second compartment is vessel rich tissue with a residence time of 1–2 hours. The hypothalamus-pituitary axis and reproductive organs can be considered vessel-rich tissues. Thus, hormonal changes or menstrual system disorders may better correlate with the samples collected 1–2 hours after exposure rather than immediately after exposure. The third compartment, representing vessel poor tissue, has a residence time in the upper limits of 4–8 hours. The fourth may be more representative of fat storage, with a residence time of 50–100 hours.[22,54,76] Measurements of compounds in other media, i.e., saliva or semen, require entirely different pharmacokinetic considerations. Thus, before determining the type and timing of biological sample collection for evaluating the absorbed dose, an understanding of the route of exposure and timing of sampling related to the tissue residence time is necessary.

As shown in Figure 1, the next levels of exposure characterization examine internal dose and the closely related concept of the biological effective dose. Internal dose is defined as the level of chemicals bound to the site of biological activity.[36] Examples of internal dosimetry are the evaluation of lead in the placenta or newborn tissue, or increased levels of catecholamines. The biological effective dose may be the most difficult "dose" measure to obtain because it refers to actual biological changes or the outcome of interest. An example of the efficacy and precision of combining several approaches was described by Everson et al.,[19] who evaluated the association between DNA damage in the human placenta (internal dose) and maternal smoking history (applied "dose"), with birthweight (biological effective dose). The association between maternal smoking and birthweight was assessed by using questionnaire data, biochemical measures for smoking exposure, and molecular methods. No association was found between birthweight and biochemical measures of smoking. A clearly significant association was uncovered between birthweight and the DNA adduct levels. This association served as a demonstration that DNA adduct levels were probably an accurate dosimeter, reflecting exposure to cigarette smoke. This study demonstrates the need to integrate various methodologies in order to assess how specific environmental agents might impair reproductive health.

Exposure Scales

The quality of the exposure data will determine the appropriate exposure scale available for statistical analysis.[40] The decision to use either a nominal, ordinal, or continuous exposure scale implies certain assumptions about expected underlying relationships. The nominal scale classifies each outcome as exposed or unexposed. The scale assumes that any level of exposure may be related to the adverse outcome. If a threshold exists at which the exposure affects the conceptus, a true risk may not be identified if most gestational exposures are below this threshold. The ordinal scale groups exposure into categories that can be analyzed without assuming a dose-response relationship. This scale assumes that the outcome of interest may be placed into a specific category during the critical period. The continuous scale measures actual level, generally using either the applied dose, industrial hygiene measurements, or an absorbed dose measurement. Use of this measure assumes a dose-response relationship and in reproductive studies can yield erroneous results.[62] A low-level in utero exposure, for example, might result in a teratogenic effect, whereas a high exposure may be associated with embryo death or infertility. If malformations were the only outcome of interest, a high exposure could appear protective because early embryonic death would preclude the observation of any malformation. Hence, exposure modeling is both a science and an art. When the goal is to uncover these sometimes subtle and elusive links, an understanding of the possible biological mechanisms, timing and level of exposure, appropriate sampling techniques, and pharmacokinetic models is required to evaluate and statistically define the optimal exposure model.

OUTCOMES

Although hormonal imbalance and menstrual disorders generally may be viewed as less serious than many health endpoints, the health and financial impact of these conditions is immense. Besides personal discomfort, day-to-day disruptions, and inconvenience due to chronic symptoms associated with menstrual pain and heavy flow, the presence of hormonal imbalances may be an indication of the rate and severity of other diseases, such as cardiovascular disease, endometrial and breast cancer, and osteoporosis. Severe menstrual symptoms also are associated with regular absences from work in 3–10% of all fertile women.[72] Accordingly, the national cost estimate for missed work days due to menstrual illness for women younger than 44 ranges from $94 million to $308 million per day missed.[74]

Female Hormonal Studies

A detailed description of the reproductive neuroendocrine system is provided elsewhere.[48,60] In brief, a woman's ability to maintain healthy reproductive functioning is controlled by complex components of the central nervous system, including the hypothalamus and pituitary functioning in synchrony with the reproductive organs of the vagina, uterus, fallopian tubes, and the ovaries. At birth, each ovary has 3 million to 4 million follicles. By puberty the number has decreased to fewer than 400,000. Early reproductive senescence can occur if xenobiotic agents block oogenesis in the fetus or destroy oocytes, causing premature ovarian failure. Damage to the ovulatory process also may be expressed in disorders of menstruation, subfecundity, or early fetal loss.

Xenobiotics have been shown to affect the female hormonal axis.[16] Bernstein et al.[10] examined the impact of cigarette smoking on human chorionic gonadotropins (hCG), estradiol, and sex-hormone globulin-binding capacity. Decreased levels of estradiol (p = 0.03), sex-hormone globulin-binding capacity (p = 0.18), and the hCG (p = 0.01) in smokers were evident over the 43–113 days of gestation. The difference between smokers and nonsmokers with regard to estradiol may be explained by the associated hCG effect, i.e., adjusting the estradiol outcome measures by the hCG levels almost completely accounted for the group differences in estradiol. The key to assessing such environmental/hormonal response is understanding whether the hormonal values are related to the exposure or are related secondarily to another response.[39]

Elevated follicular phase of luteinizing hormone (LH) levels are associated with increased spontaneous abortion rates and reduced conception rates, perhaps due to premature maturation of the oocyte.[57,66,68] Absence of the preovulatory LH surge precludes ovulation. LH surge amplitude, measured in urine, is lower in cycles with luteal phase deficiency.[6] Aberrations in the duration or quantity of progestin production (luteal phase deficiency) can lead to subfertility. Ovulation may appear normal, but if luteal function is abnormal, conception or pregnancy maintenance may be jeopardized.[50,69]

Urinary estrogen tends to be higher during the late follicular phase and mid-luteal phase during cycles of early pregnancy loss than for successful conception cycles.[7] Elevated early follicular phase levels of follicle stimulating hormone (FSH) are associated with low conception rates and infertility and with disruption of LH and progesterone secretion.[2,43,55,61] Elevated FSH secretion is also an early index of menopause onset.[31,65] Decreased FSH levels, accompanied by chronic anovulation and an elevated LH/FSH ratio, are characteristic of polycystic ovarian disease. Hormone stability studies conducted by the National Institute for Occupational Safety and Health outline the conditions under which hormones and glucuronides maintain their stability.[32] Few hormonal studies have been conducted in the occupational setting, and their potential has yet to be exploited.

Studies of Menstrual Disorders

According to a recent thorough review of the literature, although the characteristics of a normal cycle vary considerably between women, variations within an individual are small.[25] The average age of menarche is about 12.5 years (range 9–16 years). The average duration of menses is 2–7 days, and the average interval between menses is 28.1 days (range 23–35 days). Variation in the interval between menses for an individual should not exceed 5 days. During each menses the average blood loss is 30–100 ml. Menstrual abnormalities can be divided into three categories: cycle length, characteristics of bleeding patterns, and the presence of pain.[27] The most dramatic disruption of cycle rhythm is complete absence of menses. Primary amenorrhea is defined as the failure to menstruate by age 16, and secondary amenorrhea is the cessation of menses for 3 months or longer before age 40. An abnormal cycle pattern was defined in a survey of nurses by (1) the presence of secondary amenorrhea, (2) menstrual intervals of fewer than 25 days and greater than 31 days, and/or (3) duration of menstrual flow of fewer than 2 or greater than 7 days.[67] Prevalence of variability in cycle length was reported at about 25%.

One abnormal characteristic of bleeding pattern is excessive flow, referred to as hypermenorrhea. The prevalence of hypermenorrhea has been reported to vary between 8%[37] and nearly 30%.[63] In a Swedish population study, the mean volume of blood loss per episode was 43.4 ml, and an upper limit of normal was defined as about 80 ml.[24] This study showed that women have no criterion on which to grade the severity of their own blood loss in terms of "light" versus "heavy" flow. A more objective measure of the amount of flow may be the number of sanitary pads or tampons needed. If more than six pads or tampons are used each day or if clots are present, the flow can be defined as abnormally heavy and used as a measure of hypermenorrhea. Although some variability will exist due to variation in hygienic patterns, any bias between an exposed and unexposed group should be nondifferential.

Pain also is used to characterize the menstrual cycle. Dysmenorrhea or painful menstruation may include lower abdominal cramping, backache, aching thighs, nausea, diarrhea, headache, anorexia, irritability, and poor concentration. Severe dysmenorrhea may be defined by any one of the following: a combination of the above symptoms and/or need for bed rest, missing work as a result of the pain, or requiring medication for pain. Menstrual dysfunction, dysmenorrhea, and increased duration of cycle in workers exposed to toluene, benzene, and perchloroethylene were significantly increased in the rubber, leather shoemaking, and dry cleaning industries.[11,14,20,28,52,71,73,80] A study of workers exposed to styrene indicated no menstrual effects;[37] however, studies of women exposed to paint solvents and to formaldehyde showed significant effects.[23] Other studies of menstrual disorders and exposures include lead, active and passive cigarette smoke, vibration, exercise, and shift work (Table 1).[17,21,35,41,51] Hence, toxic exposures can alter hormonal and menstrual patterns by a number of mechanisms, including inhibition or damage to ovarian follicles, effects on the central nervous system involving the endocrine system, damage to hormone-secreting organs, or disruption of the hormone balance that regulates ovulation and the menstrual cycle.

Pregnancy Outcome Studies

The developmental stage of the zygote, defined in days from the last menstrual period, progresses from the blastocyst stage at days 15–20, with implantation occurring on day 20 or 21, to the embryonic period from days 21–62, and the fetal period from day 63 until the designated period of viability, ranging from 140–195 days. Estimates of the probability of pregnancy termination at one of these stages depends on both the definition of fetal loss and the method used to measure the event. Considerable variability in the definition of early versus late fetal loss exists, ranging from the end of week 20 to week 28. In the United States, the gestational age used to delineate a fetal loss from a stillborn is widely accepted to be 20 weeks. In a review of nine retrospective or cross-sectional studies, the fetal loss rates before 20 weeks' gestation ranged from 5.5–12.6%.[34] In prospective studies, the incidence rate of fetal loss among clinically recognized pregnancies has a relatively narrow range: 12–15% for the gestational period up to 28 weeks.[79]

When occult abortions or early "chemical" losses identified by an elevated hCG are included, the total spontaneous abortion rate jumps to 22%.[79] Limiting factors for using this approach in occupational field studies are cost and resources needed to coordinate collection, storage, and analysis of urine samples, and especially onerous is

TABLE 1. A Summary of Occupational Exposures and Risk Factors Associated with Menstrual Disorders

Risk Factors	Amenorrhea, Oligomenorrhea	Hypermenorrhea, Polymenorrhea	Irregular Cycles/ Metrorrhagia	Dysmenorrhea	Type Unspecified
Antineoplastics	X		X		
Fluorine					X
Weaving-industry compounds			X		
Cotton/textiles-industry compounds		X			X
Formaldehyde				X	X
Hormones	X		X		X
Carbon disulfide		X			
Benzol (benzene)					X
Vibration		X		X	
Croton aldehyde		X		X	
Petrol		X		X	
Jet air travel	X	X	X	X	
Trinitrotoluene	X	X	X		
Solvents	X	X	X	X	
Chloroprene					X
Cadmium					X
Shift work			X	X	
Superphosphates			X		
Perchloroethylene			X	X	

the need for a large population. In a study of women workers exposed to video display terminals and early pregnancy loss, about 7,000 women were screened to acquire a sufficient sample.[43] The requirement of needing 10 times the sample size to achieve an adequate population stems from reduction in the available number of women because of ineligibility due to age, sterility, and the enrollment of only women who use relatively ineffective forms of contraception or no contraception.

More conventional occupational studies use questionnaires to identify spontaneous abortions. Data are collected with mailed instruments or in personal or telephone interviews. Questions that are usually included in reproductive histories include all pregnancy outcomes, prenatal care, family history of adverse pregnancy outcomes, marital history, nutritional status, prepregnancy weight, height, weight gain, use of cigarettes and alcohol, use of prescription and nonprescription drugs, health status of the mother during and prior to a pregnancy, exposures at home and in the workplace to physical and chemical agents such as vibration, radiation, metals, solvents, and pesticides, and exposures of the father. Possible male-mediated effects associated with fetal loss were shown with paternal exposure to mercury and anesthetic gases and a suggestive but inconsistent finding related to exposures to lead, rubber manufacturing, selected solvents, and some pesticides.[59] Maternal employment may itself be a risk factor for adverse pregnancy outcome or may act as a confounder in the assessment of occupational exposure and spontaneous abortion.[38] Some investigators suggest that women who stay in the workforce are more likely to have had an adverse pregnancy history; others, however, believe this group is an inherently more fit subpopulation due to their having higher incomes and better prenatal care.

Among the many factors linked with infant survival, physical underdevelopment associated with low birthweight presents one of the greatest risks. Significant weight gain of the fetus does not begin until the second trimester. The conceptus weighs 1 g at 8 weeks, 14 g at 12 weeks, and reaches 1.1 kg at 28 weeks. An additional 1.1 kg is gained every 6 weeks until term. Normal newborns weigh about 3,200 g at term. The newborn's weight depends on its rate of growth and its gestational age at delivery. An infant that is growth-retarded is said to be small for gestational age. An infant delivered preterm will have a reduced weight but will not necessarily be growth-retarded. A low-birthweight infant is defined as an infant weighing less than 2,500 g, very-low-birthweight is defined as less than 1,500 g, and extremely low-birthweight is less than 1,000 g.[77]

When examining patients for reduced growth, it is important to distinguish between asymmetrical and symmetrical growth retardation. Asymmetrical growth retardation, i.e., when the weight is affected more than the skeletal structure, is primarily associated with a risk factor operating during late pregnancy. Symmetrical growth retardation may more likely be associated with an etiology that operates over the entire length of gestation.[34] Asymmetry of growth also has been observed in studies of environmental exposures. In a study of 202 expectant mothers residing in neighborhoods at high risk for lead exposures, prenatal maternal blood samples were collected between the sixth and 28th week of gestation.[12] Prenatal blood lead levels were associated with both a decreased birthweight and length but not head circumference after adjustment for other relevant risk factors. A significant confounding effect also was observed between prenatal blood lead and maternal age and birthweight. For 30-year-old mothers with an estimated blood lead level of about 20 μg/dL, the offspring weighed approximately 2,500 g; however, babies born to 20-year-old mothers with similar lead levels weighed about 3,000 g. The investigators speculated that the difference may indicate that older women are more sensitive to the additional insult of lead exposure or that older women may have had a higher total lead burden from having had more years of exposure or higher ambient lead levels when they were children.

Cigarette smoking is one of the primary exogenous agents most directly linked with lower-weight offspring. Maternal smoking during pregnancy has been shown to increase the risk of a low-birthweight offspring two to three times and to cause an overall weight deficit of 150–400 g. Nicotine and carbon monoxide are considered the most likely causative agents since both are rapidly and preferentially transferred across the placenta. Nicotine is a powerful vasoconstrictor, and significant differences in the size of the umbilical vessels of smoking mothers has been demonstrated. Carbon monoxide levels in cigarette smoke range from 20,000–60,000 ppm. Carbon monoxide has an affinity for hemoglobin 210 times that of oxygen. During pregnancy, the blood oxygen capacity decreases up to 30%, and the fetus has a low arterial oxygen tension and is therefore even less able than the adult to compensate. Occupations with a possible high risk for carbon monoxide exposure for pregnant employees include industries associated with fuel exhaust, pulp and paper manufacture, blast furnace operations, breweries, carbon black, coke oven, organic chemical synthesizers, and petroleum refineries.

Male Reproductive Studies

Spermatogenesis is a time-locked synchronous process wherein the germ cell proceeds through a series of mitotic and meiotic divisions. Differentiation steps occur, releasing spermatozoa from the testes for transport through the epididymis. During this later phase, sperm cells are undergoing maturation while acquiring full motility and the ability to fertilize. The number of sperm achieving successful transport through the vaginal canal and oviduct for possible union with the oocyte decreases from between 50 million to 100 million at ejaculation to only a few dozen. Redundancy in male sperm production seems essential, and agents interfering with this redundancy are threatening to the species.

Spermatogenesis requires an intact hypothalamic-pituitary-testicular axis, and hormonal alterations may provide a measure of the successful integration of this system. Schrader and Kesner[61] have published an informative overview related to the male neuroendocrine effects and the multiple routes that xenobiotics can act to disrupt normal functioning. To summarize, the hypothalamus integrates signals from the central nervous system regulating gonadotropin secretion by the anterior pituitary gland. The Leydig, Sertoli and germ cells are acted upon by the hormonal secretions of the anterior pituitary gland to regulate spermatogenesis and hormone production by the testes. The gonadotropin-releasing hormone stimulates the anterior pituitary to release luteinizing hormone, follicle-stimulating hormone, and prolactin. Synthesis and release of testosterone is controlled by LH acting on the Leydig cells, while FSH stimulates biosynthesis of testosterone to estradiol in the Sertoli cells. LH stimulates Leydig cells in the testis to secrete testosterone. Testosterone diffuses from the interstitial space in the testis into the spermatogenic tubules and affects spermatogenesis, either directly or indirectly through the Sertoli cells.[64] FSH also acts on the Sertoli cells to stimulate spermatogenesis. Repeated measurements of FSH, LH, and testosterone, both pre- and postexposure, may be useful for assessing the temporal effects of exposure that precede a more permanent effect on a couple's fecundity. Prolactin acts synergistically with LH and testosterone to ultimately increase the amount of androgen-receptor complex.

Lead has been shown to directly affect the neuroendocrine system and is associated with reduced testosterone and elevated concentrations of serum LH and sex-hormone binding-globulin, and decreased sperm count.[4,58] Other toxicants, such as organochlorine pesticides, polychlorinated biphenyls, and polybrominated biphenyls, also may exert estrogenic agonist/antagonist activity that interferes with male reproductive functions. The possible effects of tobacco smoke on sperm concentration, morphology, and motility provides an interesting case study. Although study results have been mixed, it has been suggested that the effects of smoking on these semen parameters may be caused by the presence of intermediary factors such as increased levels of choline acetyltransferase inhibitors, catecholamines, prolactin, serum estradiol, or testosterone.[33] Alterations in any of these measurements might be early indicators of susceptibility that precede direct effects on sperm values. The challenge in using hormonal markers is to detect alterations sufficiently early in the exposure-disease process, and the goal is to distinguish whether hormonal imbalances are a consequence of a primary effect on the hypothalamus or pituitary axis or are a secondary result of disruption of the testicular-hypothalamic feedback mechanism. The ability to distinguish the marker as preexisting—acquired prior to the exposure period of interest or inherited—also is crucial.

Traditional measures of male fertility such as sperm count, concentration, motility, morphology, and morphometrics historically have proved useful in detecting reproductive toxicants such as lead, ethyline dibromide, and DBCP. Other biochemical markers of sperm quality are needed to identify deficiencies in sperm function. Sperm creatine-kinase activity to predict sperm fertilizing potential may be one such assay.[30] One study compared 33 fertile oligospermic men and 66 infertile men, with identical mean sperm concentrations—11.9 million sperm/ml—and similar mean motility values of 23.7 and 23.0, respectively. Sperm creatine-kinase was significantly lower in the fertile oligospermic group. These findings also were supported in normospermic men.[29]

A promising assay used to assess genetic cell damage due to workplace exposures is the sperm chromatin structure assay.[18] Originally developed and validated in livestock, the assay uses flow cytometric analysis of acridine orange-stained sperm to prove structural integrity of the sperm chromatin. Native DNA fluoresces green, and denatured DNA fluoresces red. DNA probes to discern genetic mutation and sperm chromosome karyotyping also may have considerable future relevance. Although genetic damage is difficult to detect, the need for detection is indicated by animal studies using the dominant lethal assay and epidemiologic studies of adverse pregnancy outcomes of the wives of workers exposed to agents such as fuels, exhaust, and degreasing compounds and workers holding jobs as janitors, plywood millworkers, foresters and loggers, and painters.[53]

RISK COMMUNICATION

There is probably no greater anxiety connected with workplace risk communication than that associated with exposures and adverse reproductive or developmental outcomes. Ahlborg et al.[1] recently recommended that risk communications should be based on the following principles: (1) do not act as an expert if you are not, (2) answer all questions truthfully, and (3) be careful not to do harm. Risk communication to employees usually occurs when it is believed that an increased risk already exists based on data from laboratory or human studies or based on the physical or chemical property of the agent(s). Risk communication is often undertaken due to some expressed concern and the risk is, in principle, unavoidable. The following

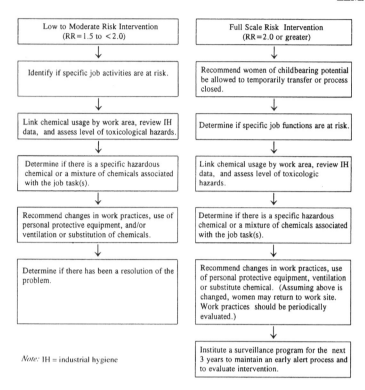

FIGURE 2.   Level of risk intervention.

illustration shows how the above principles were or were not applied in an actual case study.

A large U.S. manufacturer contacted the author regarding employees' concerns about a particular chemical exposure. Management understood that they had no internal resources to address questions from the workforce regarding possible exposures related to spontaneous abortions (principle 1). The female workers were concerned about a cluster of recent adverse pregnancy outcomes, particularly spontaneous abortions. The author was asked to visit the plant site, meet with the workers, evaluate the plant process and exposures, and make recommendations (principle 2). Based on the walk-through evaluation, discussions with employees, and a review of chemical usage pattern, a particular process was targeted for more in-depth evaluation due to possible hazardous exposures. Before air sampling could be performed, however, the equipment was suddenly removed and the particular manufacturing process permanently eliminated. The workers became upset that the company had seemingly interfered and possibly compromised the evaluation process (failure to adhere to principle 3).

The author had recommended that two key questions needed answering: "Was there a true elevation in adverse pregnancy outcomes?"and, if the answer is yes, "What changes were needed to rectify the situation?" To answer the first question, a systematic collection of pregnancy outcome information over the previous 3 years was suggested. This baseline information not only would have served to answer the first question but, with a reproductive surveillance program in place, it was considered key for future evaluations to determine if the recommended changes had improved the work environment. These recommendations were given both to management and the employees, and a cost-effective reproductive surveillance program was designed (principle 2).

Possible a priori intervention plans were outlined (Fig. 2). It was suggested that if the relative risk of an increase in spontaneous abortion from the baseline data collection was less than 1.5 (no difference to less than a 50% increase), the finding would be presumed to be most likely a chance occurrence and no major intervention would be needed. If, however, the relative risk was between 1.5 and 2.0 (50% to less than 100% increase in spontaneous abortions regardless of whether it was statistically significant), a moderate risk intervention program was proposed. The intervention plan was directed at determining if a particular group(s) was affected and determining if work policies or environmental changes were needed. A relative risk of 2 or greater in the spontaneous abortion rate in the exposed versus unexposed workforce—again, regardless of whether it was statistically significant—called for a full-scale risk-intervention strategy including removal from the workplace of women who were not using contraceptives.

The proposed recommendations were not carried out. The company withdrew its commitment, and the employees were informed of a sudden change in plans. The company informed the workers that its new plan was to conduct a toxicology literature review and a modified exposure assessment. At this point, the author terminated her relationship with the company. Was harm done to the employees (principle 3)? At the minimum, the company lost credibility with its workforce, fears may have increased, and, if a reproductive hazard exists, the company and workers will not know if implemented changes made any real difference. In other words, principle 3 was seriously compromised.

ACKNOWLEDGMENT

The author thanks Dr. James Lockey and Ms. Christina Lawson for their input and suggestions. The writing of this chapter was partially supported by NIH grant P30 ES06096.

REFERENCES

1. Ahlborg G Jr, Bonde JP, Hemminki K, et al: Communication concerning the risks of occupational exposures in pregnancy. Int J Occup Environ Health 2:64–69, 1996.
2. Ahmed Ebbiary NA, Lenton EA, Salt C, et al: The significance of elevated basal follicle stimulating hormone in regularly menstruating infertile women. Hum Reprod 9:245–252, 1994.
3. Amdur MO, Doull J, Klaasen CD, eds: Casarett & Doull's Toxicology: The Basic Science of Poisons. 4th ed. New York, Pergamon Press, 1991.
4. Assennato G, Paci C, Baser ME, et: Sperm count suppression without endocrine dysfunction in lead-exposed men. Arch Environ Health 41:387–390, 1986.
5. Auger J, Kunstmann JM, Czyglik F, Jouannet P: Decline in semen quality among fertile men in Paris during the past 20 years. N Engl J Med 332:281–285, 1995.
6. Ayabe T, Tsutsumi O, Momoeda M, et al: Impaired follicular growth and abnormal luteinizing hormone surge in luteal phase defect. Fertil Steril 61:652–56, 1994.
7. Baird DD, Weinberg CR, Wilcox AJ, et al: Hormonal profiles of natural conception cycles ending in early, unrecognized pregnancy loss. J Clin Endocrinol Metab 72:793–800, 1991.
8. Barlow SM, Sullivan FM: Reproductive Hazards of Industrial Chemicals. New York, Academic Press, 1982.
9. Baumgarten M, Siemiatycki J, Gibbs G: Validity of work histories obtained by interview for epidemiologic purposes. Am J Epidemiol 118:583–591, 1983.
10. Bernstein L, Pike ML, Lobo RA, et al: Cigarette smoking in pregnancy results in marked decrease in maternal hCG and oestradiol levels. Br J Obstet Gynaecol 9:92–96, 1989.
11. Beskrovnaia NJ: Gynecological morbidity among workers in rubber manufacture [translation]. Gig Tr Prof Zabol 8:36–38, 1979.
12. Bornschein RL, Grote J, Mitchell T, et al: Effects of prenatal lead exposure on infant size at birth. In Smith M, Grant L (eds): Lead Exposure and Child Development. Boston, Kluwer Academic Publishers, 1989.
13. Bourbannias R, Meyer F, Theriault G: Validity of self-reported work history. Br J Ind Med 45:29–32, 1988.
14. Butarewicz L, Gosk S, Gluszczopma M: Examination of the health of female workers in the leather industry, especially from the gynecological viewpoint [abstract]. Med Pr 20:137–140, 1969.
15. Carlsen E, Giwercman A, Keiding N, Skakkebaek N: Evidence of decreasing quality of semen during past 50 years. BMJ 305:609–613, 1992.

16. Cooper GS, Baird DD, Hulka BS, et al: Follicle-stimulating hormone concentrations in relation to active and passive smoking. Obstet Gynecol 85:407–411, 1995.

17. DeSouza MJ, Metzger DA: Reproductive dysfunction in amenorrheic athletes and anorexic patients: A review. Med Sci Sports Exerc 23:995–1007, 1991.

18. Evenson DP, Jost LK, Baer RK, et al: Individuality of DNA denaturation patterns in human sperm as measured by the sperm chromatin structure assay. Reprod Toxicol 5:115–125, 1991.

19. Everson RB, Randerath E, Santella RM, et al: Quantitative association between DNA damage in human placenta and maternal smoking and birth weight. J Natl Cancer Inst 80:567–576, 1988.

20. Ferroni C, Selis L, Mutti A, et al: Neurobehavioral and neuroendocrine effects of occupational exposure to perchlorethylene. Neurotoxicology 13:243–247, 1992.

21. Franks PA, Laughlin NK, Dierschke DJ, et al: Effects of lead on luteal function in rhesus monkeys. Biol Reprod 41:1055–1062, 1989.

22. Gordon SM, Kenny DV, Kelly TJ: Continuous real-time breath analysis for the measurement of half-lives of expired volatile organic compounds. J Exposure Anal Environ Epidemiol 3:75, 1993.

23. Griesemer RA, Ulsamer AG, Acos JC, et al: Report of the federal panel on formaldehyde. Environ Health Perspect 43:139–168, 1982.

24. Hallberg L, Hogdahl AM, Nillson C, et al: Menstrual loss—a population study: Variation at different ages and attempts to define normality. Acta Obstet Gynecol Scand 45:320–351, 1966.

25. Harlow SD, Ephross SA: Epidemiology of menstruation and its relevance to women's health. Epidemiol Rev 17:265–286, 1995.

26. Hertz-Picciotto I, Pastore L, Beaumont J: Timing and pattern of exposures during pregnancy and their implications for study methods. Am J Epidemiol 143:597–607, 1996.

27. Hibbard L, Judd H, Lamb E, et al: The Menstrual History. Steering Committee for Cooperative Teaching Association of Professors of Gynecology and Obstetrics. Atlanta, National Medical Audiovisual Center, 1973 (Revised 1977).

28. Huang XY: Influence on benzene and toluene to reproductive function of female workers in leather shoe making industry. Chin J Prev Med 25:89–91, 1991.

29. Huszar G, Corrales M, Vigue L: Correlation between sperm creatinine phosphokinase activity and sperm concentrations in normospermic and oligospermic men. Genet Res 19:67–75, 1988.

30. Huszar G, Vigue L, Corrales M: Sperm creatine kinase activity in fertile and infertile oligospermic men. J Androl 11:40–46, 1990.

31. Jaffe RB: The menopause and perimenopausal period. In Yen SSC, Jaffe RB (eds): Reproductive Endocrinology. Philadelphia, WB Saunders, 1986.

32. Kesner JS, Knecht EA, Krieg EJ Jr: Stability of urinary biomarkers of female reproductive hormones stored under various conditions. Reprod Toxicol 9(3):239–244, 1995.

33. Klaiber EL, Broverman DM: Dynamics of estradiol and testosterone and seminal fluid indexes in smokers and nonsmokers. Fertil Steril 50:630–634, 1988.

34. Kline J, Stein Z, Susser M: Conception to Birth—Epidemiology of Prenatal Development. Monograph in Epidemiology and Biostatistics. Vol 14. New York, Oxford University Press, 1989.

35. Laughlin NK, Bowman RE, Franks PA, Dierschke DJ: Altered menstrual cycles in rhesus monkeys induced by lead. Fund Appl Toxicol 9:722–729, 1987.

36. Lauwerys RR: Industrial Chemical Exposure: Guidelines for Biological Monitoring. Davis, CA, Biomedical Publications, 1983.

37. Lemasters GK, Hagen A, Samuels SJ: Reproductive outcomes in women exposed to solvents in 36 reinforced plastics companies. I. Menstrual dysfunction. J Occup Med 27:490–494, 1985.

38. Lemasters GK, Pinney S: Employment status as a confounder when assessing occupational exposures and spontaneous abortion. J Clin Epidemiol 42:975–981, 1989.

39. Lemasters GK, Schulte PA: Biologic markers in the epidemiology of reproduction. In Schulte P (ed): Molecular Epidemiology: Principles and Practices. San Diego, Academic Press, 1993, pp 385–406.

40. Lemasters GK, Selevan SG: The use of exposure data in occupational reproductive studies. Scand J Work Environ Health 10:1–6, 1984.

41. Lemasters GK: Occupational exposures and effects on male and female reproduction. In Rom WN (ed): Environmental and Occupational Medicine. 2nd ed. Boston, Little Brown & Co., 1992, pp 147–170.

42. Ljunggren H: Sex differences in body composition. In Brozek J (ed): Human Body Composition: Approaches and Applications. Oxford, Pergamon Press, 1963.

43. Marcus M, Gunfeld L, Berkowitz G, et al: Urinary follicle-stimulating hormone as a biological marker of ovarian toxicity. Fertil Steril 59:931–933, 1993.

44. Mattison DR: Physiological variations in pharmacokinetics during pregnancy. In Fabro S, Scialli AR, (eds): Drug and Chemical Dependency: Pharmacological and Toxicologic Principles. New York, Marcel Decker, 1986.

45. Mattison DR: Transdermal drug absorption during pregnancy. Clin Obstet Gynecol 33:718–727, 1990.
46. Mattison DR, Blann E, Malek A: Physiological alterations during pregnancy: Impact on toxicokinetics. Fundam Appl Toxicol 16:215–218, 1991.
47. Mattison DR, Malek A, Cistola C: Physiological adaptations to pregnancy: Impact on pharmacokinetics. In Aranda J, Yaffe S (eds): Pediatric Pharmacology: Therapeutic Principles in Practice. 2nd ed. Philadelphia, WB Saunders, 1992.
48. Mattison DR, Plowchalk DR, Meadows MJ, et al: Reproductive toxicity: Male and female reproductive systems as targets for chemical injury. Med Clin North Am 74:391–411, 1990.
49. McArdle WD, Williams D, Katch FI, et al: Exercise Physiology, Energy, Nutrition and Human Performance. Philadelphia, Lea & Febiger, 1981.
50. McNeely MJ, Soules MR: The diagnosis of luteal phase deficiency: A critical review. Fertil Steril 50:1–15, 1988.
51. Messing K, Saure-Cubizolles M-J, Bourgine M, Kaminski M: Menstrual-cycle characteristics and work conditions of workers in poultry slaughter houses and canneries. Scand J Work Environ Health 81:302–309, 1992.
52. Michon S: Connection between aromatic hydrocarbons and menstrual disorders analyzed [translation]. Pol Tyg Lek 20:1648–1649, 1965.
53. Olshan AF, Teschke K, Baird PA: Paternal occupation and congenital anomalies in offspring. Am J Ind Med 20:447–475, 1991.
54. Pellizzari ED, Wallace LA, Gordon SM: Elimination kinetics of volatile organics in humans using breath measurements. J Expo Anal Enviro Epidemiol 2:341–355, 1992.
55. Pearlstone AC, Fournet N, Gambone JC, et al: Ovulation induction in women age 40 and older: The importance of basal follicle-stimulating hormone level and chronological age. Fertil Steril 58:674–679, 1992.
56. Pinney SM, Lemasters GK: Spontaneous abortions and stillbirths in semiconductor employees. Occup Hyg 2:387–401, 1996.
57. Regan L, Owen EJ, Jacobs HS: Hypersecretion of luteinizing hormone, infertility, and miscarriage. Lancet 336:1141–1144, 1990.
58. Rodamilans M, Osaba MJ, To-Figueras J, et al: Lead toxicity on endocrine testicular function in an occupationally exposed population. Hum Toxicol 7:125–128, 1988.
59. Savitz DA, Sonnerfeld NL, Olshaw AF: Review of epidemiologic studies of paternal occupational exposure and spontaneous abortion. Am J Ind Med 25:361–383, 1994.
60. Schrader SM, Kesner JS: Male reproductive toxicology. In Paul M (ed): Occupational and Environmental Reproductive Hazards: A Guide for Clinicians. Baltimore, Williams & Wilkins, 1992.
61. Scott RT, Toner JP, Muasher SJ, et al: Follicle-stimulating hormone levels on cycle day 3 are predictive of in vitro fertilization outcome. Fertil Steril 51:651–654, 1989.
62. Selevan SG, Lemasters GK: The dose-response fallacy in human reproductive studies of toxic exposure. J Occup Med 29:451–454, 1987.
63. Shangold M, Rebar RW, Wentz AC, Schiff I: Evaluation and management of menstrual dysfunction in athletes. JAMA 263:1665–1669, 1990.
64. Sharpe RM: Follicle-stimulating hormone and spermatogenesis in the adult male. J Endocrinol 121:405–407, 1989.
65. Sherman BM, West JH, Korenman SG: The menopausal transition: Analysis of LH, FSH, estradiol, and progesterone concentrations during menstrual cycles of older women. J Clin Endocrinol Metabol 42:629–36, 1976.
66. Shoham Z, Jacobs HS, Insler V: Luteinizing hormone: Its role, mechanism of action, and detrimental effects when hyper secreted during the follicular phase. Fertil Steril. 59:1153–1161, 1993.
67. Shortridge LA: Assessment of menstrual variability in working populations. Reprod Toxicol 2:171–176, 1988.
68. Stanger JD, Yovich JL: Reduced in-vitro fertilization of human oocytes from patients with raised basal luteinizing hormone levels during the follicular phase. Br J Obstet Gynecol 92:385–393, 1985.
69. Stewart DR, Overstreet JW, Nakajima ST, Lasley BL: Enhanced ovarian steroid secretion before implantation in early human pregnancy. J Clin Endocrinol Metabol 76:1470–1476, 1993.
70. Stewart W, Tonascia J, Matanoski G: The validity of questionnaire-reported work history in live respondents. J Occup Med 29:795–800, 1987.
71. Syrovadko ON, Skormin VF, Pron'kova EN: Effect of working conditions on the health and some specific functions in female workers exposed to white spirit [translation]. Gig Tr Prof Zabol 16:5–8, 1975.
72. Tippy PK, Falvo DR, Smaga SA: Premenstrual symptoms and associated morbidity in a family practice setting. Fam Pract Res J 6:79–88, 1986.

73. Tp NG, Foo SC, Yoong T: Menstrual function in workers exposed to toluene. Br J Ind Med 49:799–803, 1992.
74. U.S. Department of Commerce: Statistical Abstract of the United States: The National Data Book. Washington, DC, Bureau of the Census, 1994.
75. U.S. Department of Commerce: Statistical Abstract of the United States: The National Data Book. 115th ed.Washington, DC, Bureau of the Census, 1995.
76. Wallace L, Pellizzari E, Gordon S: A linear model relating breath concentrations to experimental exposures: Application to a chamber study of four volunteers exposed to volatile organic chemicals. J Expo Anal Environ Epidemiol 3:75–102, 1993.
77. WHO Public Health Papers: Prevention of perinatal morbidity and mortality. Geneva, WHO, 1969, no. 42.
78. Whorton D, Krauss RM, Marshall S: Infertility in male pesticide workers. Lancet (17):1259–1261, 1977.
79. Wilcox AJ, Weinberg CR, O'Connor JF, et al: Incidence of early loss of pregnancy. N Engl J Med 319:189–194, 1988.
80. Zielhuis GA, Gijsen R, vander Gulden JWJ: Menstrual disorders among dry-cleaning workers. Scand J Work Environ Health 15:238, 1989 [letter].

PAUL HEWETT, PhD, CIH

INTERPRETATION AND USE OF OCCUPATIONAL EXPOSURE LIMITS FOR CHRONIC DISEASE AGENTS

From the National Institute for
   Occupational Safety and Health
Division of Respiratory Disease
   Studies
Environmental Investigations
   Branch
Morgantown, West Viriginia

Reprint requests to:
Paul Hewett, PhD, CIH
National Institute for Occupational
   Safety and Health
Division of Respiratory Disease
   Studies
Environmental Investigations
   Branch
1095 Willowdale Road
Morgantown, WV 26505-2888

Monson[1] recommended that the "role of the occupational epidemiologist must evolve into that of a person who assists in the setting of standards of exposure rather than that of a person who measures adverse effects of exposure." Burke[2] expressed similar concerns in discussing the role of epidemiology in developing federal, state, and local exposure limits: "[E]pidemiology is currently playing an increasing role in contemporary regulatory issues. . . . results of epidemiologic studies are being used by regulators to guide decisions. Shouldn't epidemiologists participate in determining how their data are applied?"

Monson and Burke suggest that occupational epidemiologists become active participants in the risk assessment process. After all, who knows the strengths and weaknesses of a study better than the occupational epidemiologist? Furthermore, exposure-response studies are rarely done out of mere scientific curiosity. Usually there is strong evidence that a substance causes one or more diseases, and it is desirable to quantify the risk or likelihood of developing such diseases in response to average or cumulative exposure or some other valid measure of exposure. The researcher knows and, in fact, expects that eventually a risk assessor will try to apply the study results in some practical, useful sense. Consequently, epidemiologists should be advocates of their research; that is, effective risk communicators who transmit their results and recommendations to risk assessors and risk managers, especially if their work reliably suggests that a current occupational exposure limit (OEL) is inadequate to the task of protecting exposed workers. But first, it is essential to understand how OELs are used by company-level risk managers—industrial hygienists[3]—to assess and control occupational exposures.

This chapter discusses occupational exposure limits (OELs) for chronic disease agents both as a product of occupational exposure risk assessment and as an essential component of occupational exposure risk management.[4] Topics include:

- the OEL concept as an essential link to occupational epidemiology
- how OELs are used as a tool in occupational exposure (risk) management
- the process of setting an OEL

Along the way several themes should emerge:

- An OEL minimally consists of three components: concentration, averaging time, and target (usually the individual worker). Changing any component results in a modified OEL, designated as OEL' (pronounced *OEL prime*). The OEL can be modified in many ways such that the resulting OEL' will not provide the same level of protection as the original OEL.
- An OEL for chronic disease agents is often based on a long-term, working-lifetime mean exposure that is perceived as acceptable for groups of workers. However, the OEL is defined as an upper limit for each single-shift TWA exposure. This is the only practical way of ensuring that the true long-term, working-lifetime mean exposure of each employee is maintained at protective levels and also provides a practical means of accounting for the uncertainty in the risk assessment that led to the OEL.
- Once an OEL is established, exposure (risk) management should be viewed as a quality control problem: the distribution of exposures for each worker should be controlled so that exposures rarely exceed the "upper control limit" (i.e., the OEL).
- The measurement and control of occupational exposures are similar in concept to the medical management of nonoccupational risk factors, such as elevated cholesterol. Consequently, those charged with risk assessment (i.e., occupational exposure management) responsibilities in each company should focus on ensuring that risk to each employee is continually controlled. This requires monitoring at regular intervals.

This chapter frequently refers to risk assessors and risk managers— terms that are sometimes used interchangeably or given widely different interpretations. To avoid confusion, the following conventions are adopted for this chapter: (1) because OELs are the end result of a risk assessment process, risk assessors are responsible for setting an OEL, and (2) risk managers are responsible for recognizing, evaluating, and controlling exposures.

OCCUPATIONAL EXPOSURE LIMITS
AND OCCUPATIONAL EPIDEMIOLOGY

Occupational exposure limits are the essential link between the process of risk assessment and the practice of risk management.[5] Although toxicology and animal studies are often reviewed and considered, for chronic disease agents it is often the exposure-response relationships from one or a handful of epidemiologic studies that form the basis for an OEL. In many cases the OEL represents a compact, distilled form of the relevant occupational epidemiology.

At its most basic, an OEL has three components: concentration, averaging time, and target.[6] For example, in 1987 the Occupational Safety and Health Administration[7] (OSHA) adopted a permissible exposure limit (PEL) for benzene of 1 ppm and specified the averaging time as a single shift (8 hours).[8] The target of all legal and most authoritative OELs is the individual worker. For example, legal OELs, such as OSHA's PELs, and authoritative OELs, such as the recommended exposure limits (RELs) of the National Institute for Occupational Safety and Health (NIOSH) and the threshold limit values (TLVs) of the American Conference of Governmental Industrial Hygienists (ACGIH), are intended in principle to be applied to the exposures experienced by each employee. It is conceivable, however, that a company will devise a corporate OEL that has another target, such as an exposure group, work area, task, or occupation.

The level of protection afforded the individual worker will change if any of the components of an OEL are modified from those originally defined or intended by the risk assessor. For example, the level of protection is increased when a company sets and meets an internal OEL that is less than the legal limit. On the other hand, the level of protection is reduced if a company has a policy of comparing the average of multiple time-weighted average (TWA, the average concentration across a single work shift) measurements to a legal or authoritative OEL in which the averaging time was originally defined as a single shift. (Other means of reducing the nominal level of protection are discussed later.)

The process of setting or revising an OEL, especially at the federal level, can be cumbersome. As a result, OSHA's PELs are approaching 30 years of age. Considering that Congress may require extensive federal risk assessments,[9] we may soon reach the point of near stagnation in regard to new or revised federal OELs. Consequently, industrial hygienists have come to rely increasingly on OELs developed by authoritative bodies, such as the ACGIH, American Industrial Hygiene Association (AIHA), and NIOSH. For substances without OELs or newly created substances (e.g., pharmaceuticals), companies often develop internal or corporate OELs.[5,10,11]

For purposes of discussion we can divide risk assessors into governmental and nongovernmental agents. Governmental risk assessors are generally required to implement a comprehensive process of risk assessment.[12] A reading of OSHA's preamble to the 1987 benzene standard gives insight into the extensive process that now precedes the issuance of new or revised PELs. NIOSH's 1995 criteria document for respirable coal mine dust[13] is also worth reviewing, because it conforms closely to the current federal risk assessment model. The REL was based on consideration of epidemiology, sampling and analytic feasibility,[14] and technologic feasibility.

Nongovernmental risk assessors, such as the ACGIH and the AIHA, often utilize a less rigorous risk assessment process that gives diminished weight to technologic feasibility and lacks the mandate to protect "all" workers. Companies producing or using chemicals for which there are no federal or authoritative OELs often devise interim, company-specific OELs.[11]

RISK ASSESSMENT, RISK MANAGEMENT, AND RISK COMMUNICATION

Risk assessment, risk management, and risk communication are known as the triad of risk science. The definition of each may differ, depending on one's viewpoint. For example, the National Research Council[12] defined the concepts of risk assessment and risk management as they pertain to the agencies of the federal government charged with regulating environmental and occupational contaminants, drugs, and toxic substances in foods. Corporate or plant-level risk assessors and risk managers, academicians, and consultants may have slightly different definitions.

Risk Assessment

The National Research Council (NRC)[12] defined risk assessment at the federal level as "the qualitative or quantitative characterization of the potential health effects of particular substances on individuals or populations". Governmental risk assessment can be broken down into four steps,[12,15]: (1) hazard identification, (2) dose-response assessment, (3) exposure assessment, and (4) risk characterization. According to the NRC, risk assessors assemble, analyze, and compare the health effects data. This information is then handed to the risk managers who are responsible for setting the air quality standard or occupational exposure limit after weighing the costs and examining feasibility issues. Others tend to view the recommendation of a reasonably "safe" level of exposure as the logical endpoint of the "risk assessment" process. Leung and Paustenbach[16] noted that

> A true risk assessment to *determine safe levels of occupational exposure* [emphasis added] actually requires exhaustive analysis of all the information obtained from studies of mutagenicity, acute toxicity, subchronic toxicity, chronic studies, pharmacokinetics, metabolism data, and epidemiology before a limit is recommended.

For Hallenbeck[17] the process of risk assessment involves identifying a potential hazard; characterizing its adverse effects in humans, animals, or cellular tests; determination of the relationship between dose or exposure and response; characterizing the exposures experienced by those employees in contact with the agent and the incidence or prevalence of disease; and, finally, the "recommendation of an acceptable concentration in air, food, or water." As stated before, this view is adopted in the present chapter.

Risk Management

The NRC[12] defined risk management as "the process of evaluating alternative regulatory options and selecting among them" and noted that a "risk assessment may be one of the bases of risk management." Risk management involves "value judgments" after considering the estimates of actual risk, the perceptions of risk in exposed populations and target industries, and the benefits and costs of control measures. In principle, a federal agency manages risk to the nation's workers in several ways: (1) by setting an OEL (concentration, averaging time, and target), (2) by requiring a minimal level of baseline monitoring and occasional resampling, (3) by requiring that exposures be adequately controlled, (4) by requiring a minimal level of medical monitoring, and (5) by occasionally auditing, through unannounced inspections, each company's ability to manage risk for its employees.

From the perspective of the plant manager or employer and the plant industrial hygienist, risk assessment is the process undertaken by the federal government or some authoritative organization to generate an OEL and related requirements. Risk management begins when the plant manager or employer hires the necessary staff or consultants and provides the resources for baseline evaluations, baseline exposure monitoring, periodic remonitoring, medical monitoring, and implementation and maintenance of controls, if necessary.

The first step in the process of risk management is the responsibility of the plant industrial hygienist: recognition that the hazardous substance is present in the plant. For the industrial hygienist the OEL is viewed as the output of a valid risk assessment process and functions as a practical tool for classifying work environments as either acceptable or unacceptable. The industrial hygienist accepts the concentration, averaging time, and target as specified, either explicitly or implicitly, by the OEL and seeks to maintain exposures at levels less than the OEL. The industrial hygienist utilizes the resources made available by upper management and determines whether the risk of disease is properly and effectively managed for each employee under the industrial hygienist's care. For the industrial hygienist, risk management— or, as some call it, occupational exposure management—consists simply of the traditional industrial hygiene triad of recognition, evaluation, and control. It can be safely said that the industrial hygienist is the ultimate occupational exposure (risk) manager.[18]

Risk Communication

At the federal level risk communication takes the form of OSHA and MSHA exposure standards and regulations, NIOSH-recommended exposure limits and publications, and the various OSHA, MSHA, and NIOSH training and educational programs. Risk communication to individual workers primarily falls to the industrial hygienist.[19]

CONSIDERATIONS WHEN SETTING OELS

In interpreting the occupational epidemiology and establishing an OEL, the risk assessor must address several issues. Three are considered here:
* Extrapolating from cohort to individual worker
* Selecting a level of "significant risk"
* Controlling lifetime risk with measurements of single-shift exposures

Extrapolating from Cohort to Individual Worker

In studies in which historical exposure data are available, the occupational epidemiologist constructs job-exposure matrices to determine the cumulative or average exposure of each member of the cohort for the period of the study. Consequently, the exposure experience of an exposure group is assigned to each worker in that group for each observation period, commonly each month or year of the study. Because individual workers move from group to group for differing amounts of time, the range of cumulative or average exposures may vary substantially, resulting in unique pairs of response measurements and cumulative or average exposures. The exposure-response analysis focuses on estimating the expected average response corresponding to specific levels of cumulative or average exposure. It is often possible, even desirable, to determine the cumulative or average exposure corresponding to a level of "significant risk." However, the level of response or risk at any average or cumulative exposure is an average level for a hypothetical group. Some individuals within the hypothetical group will experience a higher risk and others a lower risk.[20,21] The range of these differences reflects lack of knowledge about such factors as individual sensitivity and the fact that the estimates of exposure are usually crude and group-based and do not capture true individual exposure differences.

How then does one translate an acceptable average or cumulative exposure for a hypothetical exposed group to an individual worker? This question is relevant for two reasons:

1. Federal laws (and common sense) mandate that each worker or miner has a right to expect, to the extent possible, "safe and healthful working conditions" throughout his or her working life.[22,23] Thus risk managers at the corporate and plant level must control exposures and manage the risk of disease for each employee. It is not sufficient that the exposures are, on average, acceptable within an exposure group or across a plant or industry, because some individuals within the group will experience, on average, greater exposures.[20] In summary, the risk of disease should be properly managed for each employee.

2. Companies are increasingly aware that both OELs—federal, authoritative, or corporate—and effective risk management are necessary to minimize both employee

injury claims and "product liability suits" on the part of users of chemical products.[11] Again, it is necessary to set an OEL that is considered protective for each exposed individual and not just for some larger exposed population.

Selecting a Level of Significant Risk

The concept of "significant risk" has received a great deal of attention in regard to carcinogenic agents. OSHA now uses guidance provided by the U.S. Supreme Court and considers a risk of 1-in-1000, for a working lifetime, as significant (i.e., unacceptable) and necessitating some sort of regulatory action.[24] OSHA recently requested guidance in defining significant risk for noncarcinogenic disease endpoints.[25] NIOSH[13] referred to the significant risk concept of 1-in-1000 when recommending an exposure limit for respirable coal mine dust, a noncarcinogen that can produce irreversible disease.

The ACGIH has no stated policy regarding significant risk. TLVs are set at values that are "believed" to be protective of "nearly all workers." Many TLVs are based on concentrations with "no observed effect,"as reported in the literature, or levels at which the risk does not significantly exceed the risk in unexposed workers. Few, if any, TLVs are based on a rigorous risk assessment process with the goal of reducing risk to the 1-in-1000 guideline established during the OSHA benzene deliberations.[26] (This is not to say that TLVs are invalid, because they are often modified to reflect current health effects in the literature and may result in recommended control values more stringent that those of OSHA or NIOSH.)

Controlling Lifetime Risk with Single-Shift TWA Measurements

For purposes of risk assessment, it is desirable to estimate long-term cumulative or average exposures.[27] For purposes of risk management, it is usually not feasible to estimate the long-term average exposure of each employee.[28] The general practice is to set a single-shift OEL equal to the long-term average exposure that appears to be acceptable or suitably protective, based on exposure-response analyses. This practice recognizes (1) the need to devise OELs that can be used for purposes of day-to-day risk management, (2) the need to control the long-term, working-lifetime exposure of each individual worker to protective levels, and (3) the philosophical requirement that each OEL embody a safety factor.

Consequently, in a "controlled" work environment exposures rarely or infrequently exceed the OEL. The expectation is that by limiting the fraction of exposures exceeding an OEL, the true long-term mean exposure is indirectly controlled to an acceptable level for each individual. During its deliberations over revision of the benzene PEL, OSHA considered proposals for defining the PEL as either a 5-shift, 40-hour average or a long-term mean, calculated from n measurements collected over some defined period.[7] OSHA rejected these proposals as difficult to implement both by OSHA, when conducting inspections, and by most employers. Furthermore, OSHA observed that a long-term average exposure at the benzene PEL still contained significant residual risk. OSHA reasoned that only by defining the PEL as a limit for each single-shift TWA will individual workers be adequately protected. The NIOSH RELs are based on this philosophy, and it appears that the ACGIH TWA TLVs are also consistent with it.

In summary, occupational epidemiologists and risk assessors may think in terms of long-term, working-lifetime exposures when extracting protective exposure levels from exposure-response relationships; however, in suggesting acceptable levels of exposure for day-to-day risk management by industrial hygienists, the OEL should reflect the fact that exposures for chronic disease agents are measured across one shift at a time, and, given typical practices in industry, few measurements are available for any particular worker.

USING OCCUPATIONAL EXPOSURE LIMITS TO CONTROL EXPOSURES: CURRENT PRACTICE

A risk assessment of some sort is necessary to produce an OEL for a chronic disease agent. However, once an OEL is established, concern shifts from risk assessment to risk management. Risk management (also called occupational exposure management) has long been recognized as basically a problem of "quality control" or "statistical process control."[21,29–33] In terms of statistical process control, the OEL is an "upper specification limit" or "upper control limit." Consequently, the objective of an effective exposure monitoring program is periodically to obtain sufficient, valid, and representative exposure measurements so that the work environment for each individual worker is accurately classified as either acceptable or unacceptable for each "observation period."[34] Also, the objective of an effective exposure control program is to ensure that most, if not all, of the exposure measurements are less than the TWA OEL.[7,21,30,31,36,40] Exposure monitoring is a long-term responsibility that does not end until the substance in question is no longer used.[36] Processes change, controls deteriorate, and new workers are introduced. thus there is always a need for resampling and internal audits.[31]

Exposures need not be controlled to the extent that absolutely no random exposure ever exceeds a TWA TLV or TWA PEL. Even in a well-controlled work environment an occasional outlier may occur (interpretation of a single over-exposure is discussed later). Consequently, the practical goal of each employer or risk manager is to provide each employee a "controlled" work environment; that is, an environment in which exposures rarely or infrequently exceed the OEL. Such a goal does not lose sight of the fact that risk for chronic disease agents is usually best characterized by the average or mean exposure. By limiting single-shift excursions above the TWA OEL, the true long-term mean exposure for each employee is indirectly maintained at a level well below the TWA OEL.[7,35,36]

The primary goal of any exposure assessment strategy should be to determine whether the work environment is acceptable for each exposed worker. A common secondary goal is to determine whether the work environment is in compliance with the minimal requirements of a federal or state OEL.[37] Three basic approaches have evolved for determining the acceptability of a work environment:
- Individual-based exposure assessment strategies[38]
- Maximum risk employee-based exposure assessment strategies
- Group-based exposure assessment strategies

Individual-Based Exposure Assessment Strategy

Ideally, the exposures experienced by each employee should be regularly estimated, preferably by several exposure measurements collected either in campaign fashion (i.e., within a short period or during consecutive shifts) or across several months. The industrial hygienist then estimates various exposure parameters; for example, arithmetic and geometric means, 95th percentile exposure (and upper confidence limit for the 95th percentile, also called the upper tolerance limit), and the fraction of exposures expected to exceed the OEL. If the 95th percentile is less than the OEL, one can state that apparently the distribution of exposures is suitably controlled for the individual employee. If the 95% upper tolerance limit is less than the

OEL one can state, with 95% confidence, that exposures are controlled. However, regular monitoring of all exposed employees is, for practical reasons, not often implemented. For some occupations or work environments, in which there are only a few workers and exposures range from significant[39] to poorly controlled, periodic montioing of 100% of workers is entirely feasible and necessary.

Maximum Risk Employee-Based Exposure Assessment Strategies

Early in the 1970s NIOSH and OSHA recognized the need for sampling strategies and decision logics that would impose a "minimum burden to the employer (i.e., risk manager) while providing adequate protection to the exposed employees."[40] NIOSH devised an exposure assessment strategy designed around (1) selection of the "maximum risk employee" (MRE) or the "employee (per exposure group) presumed to have the highest exposure risk," and (2) collection of one or a few exposure measurements. NIOSH reasoned that if the exposures of the MRE are judged acceptable, based on the NIOSH logic,[41] then each individual worker in the exposure group represented by the MRE is adequately protected. Consequently, although the focus may be on one or more MREs per exposure group, the goal is to ensure that the exposures for each worker are adequately controlled.

The weaknesses of this strategy have been recognized.[40,42–44] The primary problem is that the strategy has poor power in regard to detecting truly unacceptable work environments.[42] However, even if NIOSH had recommended a statistically sound, rigorously designed strategy, it would have been roundly criticized as impractical for businesses of limited means. OSHA incorporated versions of this strategy in numerous 6(b) standards[45] but recognized that such a strategy represents a token commitment that does not accurately classify all work environments.[46] The ability of industrial hygienists to select reliably one or more MREs from an exposure group has also been questioned by several researchers. Nonetheless, for initial evaluations or when resources are limited or resampling intervals are broad, the MRE concept is both recommended and commonly used by industrial hygienists as a means of efficiently determining the acceptability of the work environment for members of an exposure group.[40,47–49,71,85]

Group-Based Exposure Assessment Strategies

Corn and Esmen[50] described an exposure assessment strategy based on the concept of an exposure group or, as they called it, an "exposure zone." Basically, workers are aggregated on the basis of work similarity, exposure agent(s), environment similarity, and identifiability. A single exposure measurement is collected from each of n randomly selected workers per exposure group and a standardized exposure parameter *phi* is calculated. The *phi* value (basically a Z-value) permits one to estimate the fraction or number of employees expected to have exposures in excess of the OEL.[50,51] If the expected number is one or greater, "a hygienic problem exists"[50] and should be addressed. This strategy was designed so that a decision is reached for each exposure group with a limited number of measurements. The measurements obtained from the group are believed to characterize the work performed by each group member and therefore can be extrapolated to all members of the exposure group, measured or not.

Similar strategies have been described by others.[31,36,52,53] Roach[31] described a "health risk surveillance" strategy in which the exposures for a reasonably homogeneous "job-exposure group" are acceptable if they are "consistently below one-third the exposure limit." Still and Wells[52] acknowledged the efficiencies of the "screening" sample approach (basically the MRE-based strategy discussed above) but leaned toward collecting sufficient measurements to estimate the 95th percentile exposure and its 95% upper confidence limit (the 95% upper tolerance limit), which would be compared with the TWA OEL. The AIHA Exposure Assessment Strategies Committee[36] added the concept of the "homogeneous exposure group" (HEG). An HEG is an exposure group in which the workers have "identical probabilities of exposure to a single environmental agent," although on any single day the exposures will vary. For an initial or baseline evaluation, the industrial hygienist should randomly select 6–10 workers per HEG and collect 6–10 measurements over a relatively short period. The industrial hygienist then analyzes the data and decides, using a combination of "statistical analysis and professional judgment," whether the "exposures demonstrate an acceptable work environment."[54] Exposures for an HEG are usually deemed acceptable if it is highly likely that 90 or 95% of the measurements are less than the OEL (determined by using upper tolerance limits). After the baseline data are collected, the adequacy of the "HEG assumption" can be determined by qualitatively examining the linearity of the log-probability plot of the exposure data. However, such a procedure primarily addresses the assumption that the data are lognormally distributed. The committee provided no criteria or objective procedures for determining whether a particular combination of workers and "process/agent/task" results in reasonably homogeneous exposures.

The European standard for exposure assessment adopted by the Comité Européen de Normalisation (CEN)[55] is also based on the HEG concept. CEN ackowledges that within an HEG exposures are subject to both "random and systematic" variation and provides a "rule of thumb" for assessing group homogeneity.[56] This standard contains simple decision rules for classifying each exposure measurement collected from an HEG. However, if six or more measurements are randomly collected, one can use statistics to estimate the probability of overexposure for individuals within the HEG. CEN suggests that if this probability is less than 0.1% and the work environment is reasonably stable, exposure monitoring can be reduced or eliminated until a significant change occurs. If this probability exceeds 5%, corrective action should take place. Otherwise, periodic monitoring should be used to confirm that the point estimate of the probability of overexposure remains less than 5%.

These strategies are obviously best suited to exposure groups that are reasonably homogeneous; that is, systematic differences among the individual exposure distributions of the group members are minor. If the exposure group is heterogeneous, with large systematic differences among individuals, such a strategy may miss group members who are routinely overexposed.[55] With the usual number of measurements collected per exposure group, one often has to accept on faith that the exposure groups are reasonably homogenous. Several researchers have shown that exposure groups often have a great deal of between-worker variability.[57,58] Consequently, this assumption may not be valid without an analysis of objective data.[59]

The overall goal remains the assessment of exposures for the individual worker, albeit in an indirect fashion. For the sake of efficiency,[60] it is assumed that exposures collected from the exposure group and inferences from the analysis of said exposures can be applied to any and all members of the exposure group.[36,48,50,52] This assumption is valid to the extent that the exposure group is reasonably homogeneous.

MODELS OF COMPLIANCE FOR CHRONIC DISEASE AGENTS

What does it mean to be "in compliance" with a TWA OEL? This question can be addressed by looking first at the distribution of shift average exposures (i.e., the distribution of TWAs) and next at the distribution of short-term exposures within a single shift.

Between-Shift Control Models

Figure 1 illustrates the between-shift variation expected in a minimally controlled work environment for an individual worker. Overexposures are infrequent, and the long-term mean is a fraction of the TWA OEL. There are basically two between-shift control models: the indirect and the direct. The commonly applied indirect control model holds that the distribution of exposures for an individual worker is controlled when overexposures occur infrequently. Several authors and authoritative sources recommend that the exceedance fraction (fraction of measurements above the OEL) should be no more than 0.05.[21,36,40,48,52,55,61] For example, NIOSH[40] stated the following goal for an effective exposure assessment program: "In statistical terms, the employer should try to attain 95% confidence that no more than 5% of employee days are over the standard."

Along similar lines OSHA[46] indicated that a well-designed exposure sampling strategy that results in "95% certainty" that employees are exposed below the PEL provides "compelling evidence that the exposure limits are being achieved." Although not stated with the rigor that a statistician would desire, OSHA's intent is clear: compelling evidence that compliance is routinely achieved can be developed by a statistical analysis of exposure measurements. For example, the often used one-sided upper tolerance limit test, in which one is 95% confident that 95% of the measurements are less than the OEL, is consistent with the NIOSH statement and may be considered "compelling evidence," as mentioned by OSHA.

Figure 2 shows several exposure distributions that may be considered minimally 'acceptable" according to the indirect control model. The range of GSDs (1.5–3.0) covers the range of most within-worker GSDs commonly observed in practice.

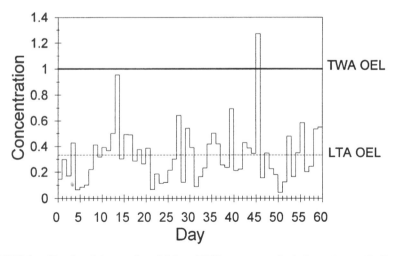

FIGURE 1. Simulated time series of 8-hour TWA exposures depicting a "controlled" work environment. Single shift excursions above the TWA OEL are "infrequent" and the long-term mean is approximately ⅓ (TWA OEL).

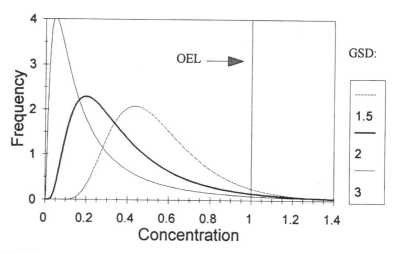

FIGURE 2. "Indirect control" model. Hypothetical single shift limit, or OEL, is set at 1. The exceedance fraction is fixed at 0.05 for each distribution.

GSD	Mean	% > OEL	% > OEL'	% > 1.5 • OEL	% > 2 • OEL
1.5	0.56	5%	2.3%	0.4%	< 0.1%
2.0	0.41	5%	3.2%	1.3%	0.4%
3.0	0.30	5%	3.8%	2.2%	1.1%

(The effective OEL, or OEL', is the critical value for issuing a citation (assuming $CV_T = 0.1$): OEL' = OEL • $(1 + 1.645 • CV_T) = 1.16 = 1(1 + 1.645 • CV_T) = 1.16$.)

The direct control model requires that the distribution of exposures for a worker be controlled to the point that the distribution mean is some fraction of the TWA OEL. For example, the AIHA[36] suggests that a "typical LTA (i.e., long-term average exposure limit) may be one-third of an 8-hr PEL."[62,63] Roach and Rappaport[64] suggest that exposures be controlled so that the long-term average exposure is one-tenth or one-fourth of the applicable ACGIH TLV, thus limiting the fraction of overexposures to 0.01–0.05. Figure 3 shows several exposure distributions that may be considered minimally acceptable according to the direct control model. The mean of each distribution is controlled to an LTA OEL set at $^1/_3$ • OEL, as suggested by the AIHA. The exceedance fraction varies from 0.002–0.061, depending on the underlying distribution.

Both models have limitations. The indirect control model has two chief limitations: (1) the long-term mean exposure is controlled to different levels, depending on the underlying GSD, and (2) the long-term mean exposures for distributions with GSDs less than 1.5 will exceed half of the TWA OEL and even approach the OEL for extremely low GSDs. Because this control model is commonly used, this lmitation points to the need for risk assessors to indicate clearly the long-term goal of a single-shift TWA OEL for a chronic disease agent. For example, routine compliance with a single-shift TWA OEL should result in a long-term, multiyear average exposure of each exposed employee that is no more than a specific fraction of the single-shift OEL, regardless of the underlying variability of exposures. The direct control method has several limitations: (1) single-shift exposures are occasionally expected to exceed greatly the TWA OEL for exposure distributions having GSDs greater than roughly three; (2) low variability distributions may be perceived as "overcontrolled;" and (3),

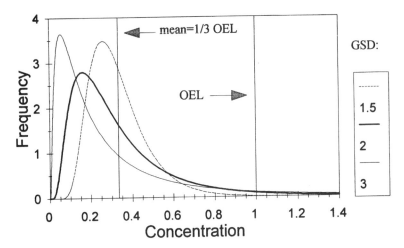

FIGURE 3. "Direct control" model. Hypothetical single shift limit, or OEL, is set at 1. The long term OEL is fixed at ⅓ the single shift OEL, per the recommendation of the AIHA.[36]

GSD	Mean	% > OEL	% > OEL'	% > 1.5 • OEL	% > 2 • OEL
1.5	0.333	0.2%	< 0.1%	< 0.1%	< 0.1%
2.0	0.333	2.7%	1.6%	0.6%	0.2%
3.0	0.333	6.1%	4.6%	2.7%	1.5%

(The effective OEL, or OEL', is the critical value for issuing a citation (assuming $CV_T = 0.1$): OEL' = $1(1 + 1.645 • CV_T) = 1.16$.)

in general, more measurements and time are necessary to determine whether exposures are controlled in relation to a long-term mean standard.

In reality, which model is adopted for an existing TWA OEL is largely academic. Convincing many employers to practice effective risk management by any model appears to be the major problem facing regulatory agencies. For the range of GSDs considered, either model, if effectively applied, will control an individual worker's long-term average exposure, i.e., the average TWA, to roughly half or less of the TWA OEL and limits single shift excursions above the OEL to a low percentage.[35] Either model also reduces the probability of a citation to less than 5% for an individual worker. For example, the legends of Figures 2 and 3 contain estimates of the fraction of exposures above the effective OEL, or the citation value.[65] These estimates range from less than 0.1% to 4.6% for the underlying GSDs considered. In summary, a minimally controlled distribution of exposures, using either model, controls to arguably acceptable values the long-term mean, single-shift excursions above the OEL and the probability of a citation.

A third compliance model, advanced in recent years, is mentioned only for the sake of completeness. This model focuses on characterizing the distribution of individual long-term mean exposures within an exposure group.[66,67] Implementation, as envisioned by Rappaport et al.,[67] requires repeat measurements from 10 or so workers per exposure group and uses a complex analysis procedure. Basically, the goal of this model is to control the probability that any single worker's long-term mean exceeds a LTA OEL to a low value (e.g., 0.10, as recommended by Rappaport et al.[67]) In principle, it is incorrect to apply this model to a TWA OEL; it is designed for determining compliance with an LTA OEL.

Within-Shift Control Model

The ACGIH recommends excursion limits for controlling within-shift exposures. The excursion limits and the supporting documentation readily permit the construction of a control model for the within-shift distribution of exposures. Basically, the ACGIH believes that within-shift excursions can be controlled in the majority of work environments so that short-term exposures, typically measured over 15-minute intervals, infrequently exceed three times the TWA TLV and rarely, if ever, exceed five times the TWA TLV. Figure 4 illustrates a minimally controlled distribution of within-shift exposures according to ACGIH recommendations. The ACGIH does not require routine assessment and control of TWA exposures with short-term measurements. The excursion limits appear to be directed at describing good practices and preventing abuse of the TWA TLV concept (discussed later). OSHA adopted a similar approach in the recently revised asbestos standard[68]: "Excursion limit. The employer shall ensure that no employee is exposed to an airborne concentration of asbestos in excess of [10 times the PEL] as averaged over a sampling period of thirty (30) minutes."

Interpretation of One or More Overexposures

The above models of compliance are useful for constructing a mental concept of what the distribution of exposures should look like for each employee. Sufficient exposure measurements for estimating, either by log-probability plotting or through a histogram, the distribution of exposures for any single exposure group are often unavailable, let alone sufficient measurements for characterizing the distribution of exposures for any single employee.[69] Figure 5 depicts a time series of 36 consecutive TWA measurements for a worker exposed to inorganic lead.[70] These measurements were collected as part of a research project. The single overexposure, when compared with the 1995–1996 ACGIH TLV for inorganic lead, is not likely to be a cause for great concern when considered in context with the other 35 measurements (the average measurement was 37% of the TLV). However, if only the measurement

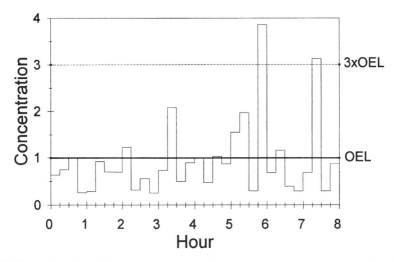

FIGURE 4. Simulated 15-minute short-term (average) exposures across a single 8-hour workshift where the within-shift exposures are minimally controlled (short-term excursions above 3 • OEL are infrequent and the TWA OEL is not exceeded).

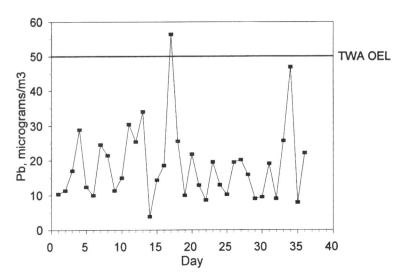

FIGURE 5. Consecutive measurements of airborne inorganic lead for "Worker A" of Cope et al.[47]

on day 17 were available, how would one or more overexposures be interpreted for purposes of effective risk management?

Authoritative sources recommend investigation of each overexposure.[31,40,47–49,52,55,71] The exceedance fraction calculations in the legends for Figures 2 and 3 suggest that in controlled work environments random exposures above the TWA OEL and, for example, 1.5 or 2 times the TWA OEL are infrequent to rare. Therefore, any over-exposure in which the number of measurements is small should be a cause for concern. Also, the work of Nicas et al.[72] suggests that overexposures should not be blamed on measurement error. Simply put, each overexposure should be investigated.[73] If compelling or convincing past exposure data[74] suggest that the overexposure is most likely an anomaly, it is reasonable to take no action beyond merely documenting the investigation. However, if no rational explanation can be found for the overexposures, one is compelled to conclude that a systematic change of some sort may have occurred; after all, in a controlled work environment overexposures should be rare to infrequent (for example, see Figs. 2 and 3). Follow-up actions may consist of fine tuning existing controls, installation or modification of controls, or evaluation of individual work practices. In any case, additional measurements are usually warranted to verify the need for additional controls or to evaluate the effectiveness of any intervention.

Criticisms and Defense of Occupational Exposure Levels

The ACGIH TLVs have been criticized for not being based on a rigorous risk assessment process and for being subject to industry influence.[26,64,75,76] The ACGIH[20,77] defended its policies, arguing that much of the criticism was either unwarranted or unsupported and that, in the absence of better documented or more rigorously developed standards, TLVs have long served to assist occupational health professionals in assessment and control of exposures.

Although many TLVs have since been revised downward and hundreds more added, OSHA continues to enforce the 1968 TLVs as permissible exposure limits (PELs). Despite the fact that the PELs are out of date and badly in need of revision, several researchers[43,44,78,79] have argued that in adopting the 1968 ACGIH TLVs, OSHA improperly defined the PELs for chronic disease agents as control limits on the average exposure across each shift rather than limits on the working-lifetime average exposure. However, such views appear to be in the minority. Stokinger,[80–84] Roach et al.,[85] and the many other authorities discussing the ACGIH TLVs provide abundant evidence that TWA TLVs, and by extension TWA PELs, were and are intended to be interpreted, for purposes of risk management, as upper limits for each TWA exposure.[86] Practicing industrial hygienists routinely interpret ACGIH TLVs and OSHA PELs as upper limits for the average exposure of each employee across each shift.[36,40,48,49,50,52] Furthermore, in the preface of the 1968 TLV booklet the ACGIH[87] clearly stated:

(1) Time-weighted averages permit excursions above the limit provided they are compensated by equivalent excursions below the limit *during the workday* [emphasis added].[88]

(2) Enlightened industrial hygiene practice inclines toward controlling exposures to below the limit rather than maintenance at the limit.

Nonetheless, the notion that OSHA "got it wrong" continues to be discussed.

Misinterpretation and Misuse of the Concept of Occupational Exposure Levels

There are numerous ways in which the OEL concept can be misinterpreted or misused:

• Interpreting OELs as "fine lines between safe and dangerous"
• Using an 8-hour TWA OEL to assess short-term exposures
• Using 8-hour TWA OELs to devise community air quality standards
• Applying 8-hour TWA OELs to "novel" work schedules
• Comparing an exposure group's average exposure to a TWA OEL
• Extending the averaging time from a single shift to multiple shifts
• Interpreting the TWA OEL as a long-term average (LTA) OEL

Stokinger[80,84,89] mentioned several ways in which the ACGIH TLVs were misinterpreted and misused. First, some interpreted the TLVs as "fine lines between safe and dangerous concentrations."[90] One or a few TWA measurements that are just under the TLV do not imply that exposures are adequately controlled during the remaining unmeasured shifts. Second, some were using 8-hour TWAs to assess short-term exposures. The TWA TLVs are not appropriate for high-exposure tasks that last only a fraction of the shift. For example, if a task lasts only 30 minutes, it is not permissible to permit up to 16 times the TWA TLV, even if the daily average is less than or equal to the TWA TLV. Beginning in the early 1970s, the TLV committee felt compelled to recommend specific within-shift excursion limits to prevent this type of abuse. For example: "Excursions in worker exposure levels may exceed 3 times the TLV-TWA for no more than a total of 30 minutes during a workday, and under no circumstances should they exceed 5 times the TLV-TWA, provided that the TLV-TWA is not exceeded."[91] Finally, TLVs were occasionally applied to community or environmental exposures. The TLVs were designed for healthy, working populations and should not be used for "limiting pollutants in urban community air" where exposures are 24 hours per day and susceptible subpopulations are affected.[92]

Brief and Scala[93] noted that the TLVs were designed for a traditional 8-hour work shift and 40-hour workweek. They proposed a conservative method for reducing the TLVs to reflect a "novel" work schedule. Extended workshifts and/or more than 40-hours of exposure per week reduce the recovery time for each worker and "stretch the reliability and even viability of the data base for the TLV."[94] The ACGIH[91] recommends that, among other models, the Brief and Scala model be used as guidance for reducing the TLV during a nontraditional work schedule. OSHA adopted a simpler scheme for the 1978 lead and the 1994 cadmium PELs.

Occasionally industrial hygienists compare the average exposure of an exposure group to a TWA OEL. This practice changs the OEL's target from the individual worker to the exposure group and is valid to the extent that the exposure group is homogeneous. For a group in which there are systematic and significant differences between worker exposures, a practice of routinely comparing the group average exposure to an OEL may permit some workers to be routinely overexposed.[21] Such a practice was considered and rejected by NIOSH[40] as a valid technique for determining compliance with legal OELs except under the extraordinary circumstance when the overall GSD for the exposure group is 1.15 or less (meaning that, for practical purposes, the exposure group is truly homogeneous).[95]

An OEL can be weakened by extending the averaging time for a single measurement from a single shift to multiple shifts.[49] For example, a practice of comparing the average of n TWAs to an OEL in effect creates an OEL$'$ defined as the average of n TWA measurements, which is contrary to the intended interpretation of the OSHA TWA PELs, NIOSH TWA RELs, and ACGIH TWA TLVs. Such a practice explicitly permits frequent single-shift overexposures and creates an OEL$'$ that does not provide the level of protection inherent in the original OEL. When issuing the 1978 final lead PEL, OSHA explicitly forbade multishift averaging:

> The proposed standard expressed the PEL as an 8-hour, time-weighted average "based on a 40-hour week." This [language] has been deleted [from the final standard] to avoid ambiguity since it was misconstrued by some commenters as a conversion of the PEL to a 40-hour average.[96]

The ACGIH[91,94] expressly forbids redefining the TLVs: "it is not appropriate for individuals or organizations to impose on the TLVs . . . their concepts of what the TLVs . . . should be or how they should be applied." Although it is abundantly clear to most practicing industrial hygienists that the TWA TLVs are defined as limits for each TWA exposure, a minority insist that the TWA TLVs represent long-term, even lifetime average exposures. Such a view basically redefines the TWA TLVs, extending the averaging time from a single shift to months or years or even the employee's working lifetime. Because the long-term average exposures permitted by this practice can be double or more over those that result when the TLV is properly interpreted as an upper control limit for each TWA, the level of protection provided by such a modified TLV cannot possibly equal the level of protection provided by the original TLV. Because OSHA's TWA PELs and NIOSH's TWA RELs are clearly defined as upper limits for each single-shift average exposure (TWA), it is clearly inappropriate to manage exposures as if they represented limits on long-term, average exposures.

SOURCES OF OCCUPATIONAL EXPOSURE LEVELS

The number of chemicals found in the nation's workplaces is literally in the tens of thousands.[11] However, OELs have been established for only 2000 or so substances. In general, plant industrial hygienists look to OSHA and MSHA for legal OELs and to the ACGIH, AIHA, and NIOSH for authoritative OELs. In the absence of a legal or authoritative OEL, many corporations devise internal or corporate OELs.[11]

American Conference of Governmental Industrial Hygienists

The history of the ACGIH and Tlvs has been well described elsewhere.[80,97] The ACGIH TLV list now contains over 700 recommended exposure limits for substances ranging from simple irritants to chronic disease agents and carcinogens. The ACGIH TLV committee consists primarily of professionals recruited from the ranks of government (federal and state) and academia. It is well known that for decades the TLVs represented the only available exposure guidelines and before the creation of OSHA, MSHA, and NIOSH served well the occupational health community. Given the lengthy process required to update each OSHA PEL, the current TLVs are considered by many to represent the best available information on acceptable exposures for the majority of the listed substances.

The ACGIH TLVs for airborne substances are defined as upper limits for the average concentration across the indicated averaging time. For substances with acute or short-term effects, the ACGIH recommends a short-term exposure limit (STEL).[98] The averaging time for this limit is 15 minutes. For slower-acting substances or substances that produce a chronic effect, the ACGIH recommends a TWA TLV. The averaging time for this limit is a single shift (8 hours). The ACGIH recommends that TWA TLVs be reduced when workshifts are longer than 8 hours and/or the work week consists of more than 40 hours.

ACGIH[91] introduces the TLVs with what is basically a risk assessment statement: "[TLVs] refer to airborne concentrations of substances and represent conditions under which it is believed that nearly all workers may be repeatedly exposed day after day without adverse effects." The ACGIH TLV committee believes that routine exposures at the level of the TLV will be protective but allows that a small percentage of workers may develop occupational illness. Consequently, one can be reasonably confident that this statement will hold true for an individual worker by ensuring that exposures are routinely maintained beneath the TLV. Thus, for risk management purposes, the ACGIH[91] defines the TWA TLVs as limits for the average exposure across each 8-hour shift. Stokinger[84] recommends that users consult the documentation for each TLV to determine the basis for the TLV and the "safety factor," if any, inherent in each TLV. For example, the 1971 documentation for the crystalline silica TWA TLV leaves no doubt about the TLV committee's intentions[99]: "The margin of safety of the quartz TLVs is not known. In the documented examples of virtual silicosis elimination, concentrations have averaged well below the TLV. It is suggested that quartz concentrations be maintained as far below the TLV as current practices will permit."

A nearly identical caution is given in the 1991 documentation.[94] The 1971 documentation for coal dust reveals that the TWA TLV was based on the interim results of a long-term study of British coal workers. The authors of the study estimated that 35 years of exposure at 2.2 mg/m^3 was correlated with a near zero probability of category 2 pneumoconiosis. The 1991 documentation[94] for benzene accepted a conclusion of the authors of a mortality study that 0.1 ppm as a working lifetime average would reduce the odds of "benzene-induced leukemic death" to near the odds for unexposed populations. These are examples of risk assessments looking at group average exposures and group average responses. For risk management purposes, the recommended TWA TLVs for silica, coal dust, and benzene are defined by the ACGIH as upper limits for single shift exposures in order to (1) adequately protect individual workers and (2) partially account for the uncertainty in the epidemiologic data. A review of the ACGIH 1991 documentation for OSHA's 6(b) substances, most of which are considered chronic disease agents, reveals that the ACGIH also advocates the use of within-shift excursion factors for nearly all of these substances[100] and in many cases states explicitly that TWA TLV is nearly equivalent to the corresponding OSHA PEL and NIOSH REL (which are defined as limits for single-shift exposures). The ACGIH TLV committee for chronic disease agents and carcinogens has several advantages over OSHA and NIOSH. For instance, the TLV committee can rapidly recommend new or revised TLVs in response to advances in the epidemiologic or toxicologic literature. The TLV committee is not required to examine closely issues of feasibility for all affected industries or to engage in lengthy cost-benefit debates. This happy state of affairs may be changing, because the ACGIH sometimes finds itself threatened with lawsuits upon recommending a reduction in a TLV, forcing the ACGIH to increase the level of documentation and to engage in lengthier risk assessment deliberations. Another advantage is that the ACGIH TLV committee is not required to recommend a TLV that protects the overwhelming majority of workers, but only one that is believed to be protective for "nearly all" workers.[91] Consequently, the ACGIH does not get mired in disputes with industry regarding definitions of significant risk. Others view this as a disadvantage, arguing that the TLVs do not provide adequate protection for enough workers[64] or for susceptible subgroups.[101] In summary, specific ACGIH TLVs may not be as protective as the more recent OELs of OSHA and NIOSH; taken as a whole, however, the TLVs reflect more accurately current changes in the understanding of the relationship between exposure and occupational disease.

American Industrial Hygiene Association

The AIHA issues guidelines for workplace environmental exposure levels (WEELs) for substances for which there are no authoritative or legal OELs.[102,103] The number of WEELs on the current list is less than 100. Candidate substances are solicited from the AIHA membership or suggested to the WEEL committee. Unlike the ACGIH, members of the AIHA WEEL committee can be currently employed by industry, but the procedures used by the WEEL committee are similar to those used by the ACGIH TLV committee. Like the TLV committee, the WEEL committee believes that each WEEL will "provide a level to which nearly all workers may be repeatedly exposed, for a working lifetime, without adverse health effects."[103] Also like the TLV committee, for risk management purposes the AIHA defines the WEELs as upper limits for each 8-hour work shift (assuming the typical 40-hour work week) or as ceiling values not to be exceeded during each shift.

Occupational Safety and Health Administration

OSHA[22] is permitted to "promulgate" occupational health standards that ensure "most adequately . . . to the extent feasible, on the basis of the best available evidence, that no employee will suffer material impairment of health or functional capacity even if such employee has regular exposure to the hazard dealt with by such standard for the period of his working life."

OSHA initially adopted existing consensus air quality standards and standards already in effect under the Walsh-Healy Public Contracts Act. These consisted of the 1968 ACGIH TLVs and various ANSI Z committee standards, which resulted in an initial list of PELs that numbered slightly more than 400. OSHA soon found that the promulgation process was cumbersome and slow because of the frequent demands for scientific certainty placed on government risk assessors and the fact that accurate exposure-response relationships are often difficult to obtain with the available exposure data, reflecting the general inability or unwillingness of industry to collect, maintain, and share quality exposure information. Although the Supreme Court, in the benzene decision, determined that "OSHA is not required to support its findings that a significant risk exists with anything approaching scientific certainty,"[104] the PEL revision process is sufficiently difficult and time-consuming that OSHA has managed to modify only eleven PELs.[105] Attempting to compensate for a lack of progress, in 1989 OSHA issued a comprehensive air contaminants standard that modified more than 400 PELs. Because of objections from both industry and labor, a court of appeals nullified the revised PELs.[106] As a result, the vast majority of the current PELs are based on criteria that are approaching 30 years of age. OSHA[18] recently announced its intention once again to start the PEL revision process and solicited comments about the selection of target chemicals, appropriate risk assessment methods for carcinogens and noncarcinogens, and determination of significant risk for carcinogens and noncarcinogens. OSHA listed 20 chemicals as candidates for revision and intends to revise the PELs for 20 or so substances at a time, thus avoiding the problems encountered during the earlier revision effort.

While OSHA contemplates revising the PELs, Congress is considering proposals to make risk assessment at the federal level more rigorous and thus presumably more defensible.[9] Because the PEL revision process is likely to be slow at best, resulting in significant delays before more protective PELs are adopted,[107] enlightened companies are likely to rely on the more current TLVs or to devise corporate OELs that use the latest epidemiologic and toxicologic data.

OSHA is compelled, for both practical and legal purposes, to define the PELs as values never to be exceeded. It is easy to envision the multitude of arguments that a company could make if OSHA attempted to issue a citation for violation of a TWA PEL defined as the upper limit for long-term or lifetime mean exposure. Similarly, if TWA PELs were defined as the 95th percentile exposure, many employers would be inclined to claim that any overexposure measured during an OSHA health inspection was one of the "allowed" overexposures.[108] However, because of the uncertainty in every exposure measurement, due to sampling and analytic error (variability), OSHA does not simply issue a citation whenever a measurement collected by a compliance officer exceeds the PEL. OSHA's policy is to calculate the lower confidence limit for each measurement and to issue a citation only when the lower confidence limit exceeds the PEL.[109] If the company has historical exposure data, the OSHA compliance officer is instructed[109] to "review the long-term pattern and compare it to the [OSHA] results. When OSHA's samples fit the long-term pattern, it helps to support the compliance determination. When OSHA's results differ substantially from the historical pattern, the [compliance officer] should investigate the cause of this difference and perhaps conduct additional sampling."

This practice underscores the importance of an employer's collecting and maintaining sufficient, recent exposure data to demonstrate convincingly that exposures are usually controlled (see previous discussion of models of compliance). However, the "outlier" excuse will not prevail if no historical exposure data exist or the data are dated or not comparable to OSHA's.[110] In such cases, the compliance officer will undoubtedly issue a citation and require the employer to evaluate the potential problem and to take corrective steps if necessary. OSHA's citation philosophy is entirely compatible with the previous discussion of the interpretation of one or more overexposures.

OSHA has considered and rejected as impractical industry proposals to define new TWA PELs as long-term values.[7] However, OSHA[7] noted in the preamble to the 1987 benzene standard:

[T]here is no requirement to control exposures so far below the PEL so as to ensure than absolutely no random exposures exceed the PEL. OSHA's longstanding enforcement policy, in recognition of the existence of the "occasional outlier," is designed to prevent citations being issued under such circumstances.

According to OSHA, excursions above the PEL may occasionally occur in a controlled work environment. In such an environment the true long-term mean exposure for each employee will be below the PEL. How far below is not specified, but in regard to the 1987 benzene standard, OSHA[7] stated:

(1) [V]irtually all employers keep long term average exposures under the PEL by a margin and where feasible under the action level with a margin." (p. 34508)

(2) Employers generally keep their exposures on average somewhat under the PEL so if the measurement is high on the day of inspection, the measured exposures will still be under the PEL. (p. 34535)

(3) In attempting to reduce the possibility of a random exposure exceeding the . . . PEL, employers will generally reduce average exposures to well below [the PEL]. (p. 34537)

Regarding the 1978 lead PEL, OSHA[96] stated:

OSHA recognizes that there will be day-to-day variability in airborne lead exposure experienced by a single employee. The permissible exposure limit is a maximum allowable value which is not to be exceeded: hence exposure must be controlled to an average value well below the permissible exposure limit in order to remain in compliance.

If one accepts the proposition that an "occasional outlier" implies that no more than 1 in 20 single-shift TWAs exceeds the PEL and assumes that exposures are lognormally distributed with characteristic GSDs in the range of 1.5–3, the true long-term mean for a "minimally controlled" work environment will be in range of $0.30 \cdot$ PEL to $0.56 \cdot$ PEL (for example, see Fig. 2.) Interested readers should review OSHA's well-conceived but hardly noticed "non-mandatory" appendix to the 1992 formaldehyde standard.[46] It provides considerable common-sense guidance for the design and implementation of an exposure monitoring program.

OSHA's mandatory monitoring requirements were designed to establish baseline information about employee exposures. Only under the "best of circumstances [will] all questions regarding employee exposure be answered."[46] For example, if exposures for all employees are truly controlled or better, the application of OSHA's mandatory requirements almost certainly will result in the employer's concluding that exposures are acceptable. However, low exposures collected on a single day or across several days do not automatically guarantee the employer that the workplace is currently or will continue to remain in compliance with a TWA PEL. Even poorly-controlled work environments often have a majority of exposures less than the PEL. The employer should be aware that in such circumstances strict application of the minimalistic mandatory requirements for exposure monitoring often lead the mistaken conclusion that exposures, in general, are acceptable.

National Institute for Occupational Safety and Health

NIOSH was created by the 1970 OSHAct primarily to "develop and establish recommended occupational safety and health standards."[22] Since then NIOSH has developed and issued over 100 "criteria documents" recommending new or revised exposure limits. These limits are called recommended exposure limits (RELs). They are not legal limits but recommendations to OSHA and occasionally the Mine Safety and Health Administration (MSHA). With one exception (radon), NIOSH TWA

RELs are defined as upper limits for single-shift exposures. Most of NIOSH's early RELs were health-based; that is, set so that the overwhelming majority of exposed workers are protected, without regard to feasibility. According to NIOSH's current policy, RELs "will be based on risk evaluations using human or animal health effects data, and on an assessment of what levels can be feasibly achieved by engineering controls and measured by analytical techniques. To the extent feasible, NIOSH will project not only a no-effect exposure, but also exposure levels at which there may be residual risks. This policy applies to all workplace hazards, including carcinogens."[111]

NIOSH's criteria document on respirable coal mine dust[13] illustrates a risk assessment process similar to that recommended by the NRC.[12] NIOSH considered epidemiology, sampling and analytic feasibility, and technologic feasibility before issuing a recommendation. NIOSH determined that a long-term average exposure of 0.5 mg/m³ was both reasonably consistent with a target significant risk level and feasible. NIOSH also determined, using estimates of within-occupation variability for underground coal mining, that the 95th percentile daily exposure (i.e., single-shift TWA) for a miner whose long-term average exposure is 0.5 mg/m³ will be approximately 1 mg/m³. Therefore, for purposes of risk management, NIOSH[13] recommended an upper limit of 1 mg/m³ for each single-shift TWA. NIOSH recognized that the underground mining environment can be highly variable and recommended, as part of a proper risk management program, that exposures be monitored on a regular basis:

(1) Exposure sampling should be periodic and should occur frequently enough that a significant and deleterious change in the contaminant generation process or the exposure controls is not permitted to persist.

(2) The objective of an effective exposure sampling strategy is to periodically obtain sufficient, valid, and representative exposure estimates so that the work environment is reliably classified as either acceptable or unacceptable.

NIOSH cautioned that this REL may not be sufficiently protective to prevent all occupational respiratory disease among coal miners exposed for a working lifetime and therefore recommended additional measures to reduce the risk of disease: participation of miners in medical screening and surveillance programs, development and application of improved dust control techniques, use of personal protective equipment as an interim measure if exposures cannot be adequately controlled, and routine monitoring of exposures. NIOSH provided sufficient information so that, in principle, either the indirect or direct between-shift control model could be used to develop a statistically rigorous exposure assessment strategy; that is, both long-term and daily risk management goals are clearly stated. However, NIOSH's other recommendations in the document for exposure sampling and data interpretation are consistent with the commonly applied indirect control model.

Corporate and Other Occupational Exposure Levels

Only a relative handful of the tens of thousands of substances and mixtures encountered in industrial operations have OELs. Many corporations that produce or use chemicals without OELs find themselves compelled by both ethical and liability considerations to develop corporate occupational exposure limits.[10,11] (Industrial hygienists should review Harris[112] for a discussion of professional ethics and the use of new toxicologic and epidemiologic information.) Paustenbach[10] recommends that companies that set corporate OELs accept three propositions: (1) OELs are needed whenever employees are exposed to toxic agents; (2) the company should fully document the rationale for establishing a corporate OEL; and (3) "tentative" corporate

OELs should be set even if adequate toxicologic and epidemiologic data are not available.

Producers of specialty chemicals, byproducts, intermediate chemicals, and pharmaceuticals[113] regularly set internal or corporate OELs. The process is usually-multidisciplinary, involving industrial hygienists, toxicologists, physicians, and epidemiologists. Once the corporate OEL is set by the corporate risk assessors, the plant risk manager or industrial hygienist should treat it like any legal or authoritative OEL and effectively manage employee risks by controlling exposures to the extent required.

A PHILOSOPHY FOR OCCUPATIONAL EXPOSURE MANAGEMENT

Management by a physician of a patient's risk of cholesterol-related diseases is analogous to the practice of exposure management by an industrial hygienist. We are all familiar with the often encountered target upper limit for total blood cholesterol of 200 mg/dl. This limit was developed using population-based studies and represents a target average value that cholesterol risk managers at the National Institutes of Health would like to see for the U.S. population.[114] However, for purposes of individual risk management, the NIH recommends that each individual maintain total blood cholesterol below 200 mg/dl. As the cholesterol risk manager for a specific patient, a physician is concerned primarily with that patient's current exposure to excessive cholesterol. The physician has little knowledge of how well a patient's cholesterol levels were managed by previous health care providers, nor can the physician predict the quality of care provided by the responsible physician in the future. What the physician can do, however, is to ensure that during the time that the patient is under his or her care, the risks associated with elevated cholesterol levels are properly managed, i.e., minimized. The physician does so through the use of proper and regular tests, comparison of each cholesterol measurement with a target value corresponding to an acceptable level of risk, and regular issuance of sound advice based on the current measurement. Assuming that the patient visits the physician once per year, the goal of the physician is to ensure that the cholesterol level of each patient is less than or equal to the target value for each year of observation. Given the recommendations of authoritative organizations such as the NIH, it would be inappropriate, in fact wrong, for the physician to average a current high cholesterol measurement with low past measurements and compare the average with the target value. The current high value indicates that a change of some sort has occurred and needs attention.[115]

Like the personal physician, the plant industrial hygienist is responsible for the proper management of the risk experienced by each employee. The industrial hygienist usually has little knowledge of how well risk was managed in the past when others were responsible. Past exposure data are usually sparse at best and almost certainly unavailable for employees with work histories elsewhere. In any case, exposures in the distant past have little predictive value regarding future exposures. In addition, the industrial hygienist cannot predict how well others will manage the exposures of the employee after the industrial hygienist leaves or the employee moves to other jobs or worksites. What the industrial hygienist can do, however, is to act as the steward of each employee's good health by ensuring that each employee's current risk is properly managed during the time that the industrial hygienist is employed by the company and the employee is in his or her sphere of responsibility. Consequently, current exposure data have the best predictive value regarding the continued quality of risk management for an employee or group of similarly exposed employees. As in the cholesterol example above, a current high exposure measurement suggests that a change of some sort has occurred and should be investigated (see the earlier discussion of interpretation of single overexposures).

CURRENT TRENDS

Several current trends have the potential to affect the practice of industrial hygiene:

- Development of hybrid exposure assessment strategies
- Development of occupational exposure databases
- Increased capability to collect exposure data
- Increased use of formal statistical tests
- Statistically defined OELs
- Generic "performance-based" exposure assessment standards

It has long been recognized that data collected solely for the purpose of determining compliance usually reflect the exposures of the maximum risk employees within each exposure group. Such data may present occupational epidemiologists with a distorted picture of the exposure experience of each exposure group. Many researchers are promoting the routine collection of surveillance exposure data from all occupations in addition to the measurements typically collected to determine current compliance.[28,36,116] Because the shape of an exposure-response curve is most contentious at the low end, such data could be extremely useful in determining the often critical low exposure cells in the epidemiologist's job-exposure matrix. Hybrid exposure sampling strategies—that is, strategies that permit the collection of exposure information for compliance and surveillance or research purposes—should become more common in the future and eventually lead to more accurate exposure-response analyses.

Farsighted researchers are envisioning occupational exposure databases that cover a multitude of substances and span across companies and industries.[117,118] Such databases could be used to generate research hypotheses, to evaluate the efficacy of different types of controls, and to provide accurate industrywide exposure data for trade organizations and standards-setting organizations, among other uses.

The current state-of-the-art exposure measurement model is as follows: *For purposes of measuring worker exposure across a single shift it is sufficient to place a reasonably accurate exposure measuring device on the worker, within the worker's breathing zone, and have it operate for nearly the full shift.* Two trends during the 1960s led to this model: (1) the movement from area to personal exposure measurements and (2) the move from short-term (i.e., less than 30 minutes) to full-shift (or nearly full-shift) sampling.[48] These trends resulted primarily from the development of battery-powered personal sampling pumps. For particulate substances the development of sensitive analytic balances and improved filtration materials permitted industrial hygienists to shift from measuring particles per unit volume to measuring particulate mass per unit volume. During the 1970s a major concern on the part of NIOSH and OSHA was to ensure that reasonably accurate sampling and analyticl methods were available for measuring the substances regulated by OSHA. Because of the efforts of NIOSH, OSHA, and many company and private laboratories, the majority of regulated substances now have sampling and analytic methods with coefficients of variation less than 0.1. However, even imperfect or imprecise measures of exposure, such those for asbestos, crystalline silica, cotton dust, or coal tar pitch volatiles and coke oven emissions, can be used effectively for risk management.

Since the early 1970s the improvements have been important, but subtle: improvements in the reliability of sampling pumps and analytic method sensitivity and development of automated analytic techniques. Researchers have recently developed data acquisition systems suited for task analysis or the process of determining which task (i.e., component of a job) or work practice contributes most to the worker's overall exposure.[119] The increased use of direct reading instruments coupled with data storage devices, the development of electronic sensors for specific chemicals, and the increased availability of passive dosimeters provide industrial hygienists the means to characterize more accurately exposures for a larger percentage of the workforce and may eventually lead to the inexpensive and accurate characterization of within-shift and between-shift exposure profiles for nearly all workers.[120]

In the 1960s and well into the 1970s data analysis often consisted of the comparison of one or several TWA estimates with the TWA OEL.[40,48,81,83,85] Consequently, formal statistical tests were used in a compliance context to determine whether a single TWA was significantly above or below the TWA OEL. Employers determined the acceptability of a work environment by collecting one or several measurements from one or more maximum risk employees and applying simple decision rules.[40] As the quantity of data increased, industrial hygienists have adopted ever more sophisticated and statistically defensible data analysis procedures,[36,44,47,48,55,71,121] although the need for simple decision rules remains.[47,49,52,55]

The AIHA[122] recently issued a white paper on generic exposure assessment standards and recommended that OSHA issue "clear statistical definitions of overexposure." Stated differently and in a more positive manner, OSHA should issue a clear statistical definition of compliance. As previously discussed, NIOSH recently took a step in this direction in a criteria document about respirable coal mine dust by recommending a single-shift limit and indicating the long-term mean exposure that should result when the single-shift limit is met on the majority of work shifts for each individual coal miner.[13] It would be helpful if regulatory agencies and authoritative bodies would state clearly both proximate and long-range goals of an OEL. In this manner the industrial hygienist could acquire a clear understanding of the logic underlying the OEL and an appreciation for the range in which current exposures should fall for a work environment to be considered currently controlled for each worker and the range in which individual long-term average exposures should fall so that the long-range goal of the OEL is truly realized.

In 1988 OSHA[123] issued an "advanced notice of proposed rulemaking" regarding a proposal to issue a "generic exposure assessment standard." This standard would apply to the majority of PELs, which have no specific requirements for exposure sampling strategies and data interpretation. OSHA anticipates that the generic standard will be performance-based; that is, it will set out broad goals and leave it to individual companies to design exposure sampling strategies and decision logics that are consistent with the performance goals yet tailored for specific work environments. To date there has been little progress toward a final standard, even though this announcement led to considerable interest and activity.[122,124,125]

NOTES

1. Monson RR: Occupational Epidemiology, 2nd ed. Boca Rotan, FL, CRC Press, 1990, p 244.
2. Burke TA: The proper role of epidemiology in regulatory risk assessment: Reaction from a regulator's perspective. In Graham JD (ed): The Role of Epidemiology in Regulatory Risk Assessment. 1995.
3. Industrial hygienist means a professional qualified by education, training, and experience to anticipate, recognize, evaluate, and develop controls for occupational health hazards.[68]

4. Many of the concepts and observations in this chapter can be generally applied to irritants, acutely toxic substances, and substances that are not usually considered chronic disease agents but have (TWA) OELs as control limits.

5. Paustenbach DJ: Occupational exposure limits: Their critical role in preventive medicine and risk management [editorial]. Am Ind Hyg Assoc J 51:A332–A336, 1990.

6. OSHA's single substance, 6b standards and NIOSH's RELs consist additionally of minimal exposure monitoring, exposure control, respiratory protection, and medical monitoring requirements and recommendations, respectively. The combination of an occupational exposure limit with these additional requirements can enhance the level of protection afforded the individual workers.[7,68] However, such complete standards are usually not recommended by nonregulatory risk assessors.

7. OSHA (Occupational Safety and Health Administration): Occupational exposure to benzene: Final rule. Fed Reg 52(176):34460–34578, 1987.

8. The number of measurements collected during a single shift can vary from a single, full-shift measurement to several consecutive, partial-shift measurements as long as the TWA is accurately estimated.

9. Finkel AM: Commentary: Who's exaggerating? Discover May:48–54, 1996.

10. Paustenbach DJ: Occupational exposure limits, pharmacokinetics, and unusual work schedules. In Harris RL, Cralley LJ, Cralley LV (eds): Patty's Industrial Hygiene and Toxicology. 3rd ed, volume 3. New York, John Wiley & Sons, 1994.

11. Paustenbach D, Langner R: Corporate occupational exposure limits: The current state of affairs. Am Ind Hyg Assoc J 47:809–818, 1986.

12. National Research Council : Risk Assessment in the Federal Government: Managing the Process. Washington, DC, National Academy Press, 1983.

13. National Institute for Occupational Safety and Health: Criteria for a Recommended Standard— Occupational Exposure to Respirable Coal Mine Dust. Washington, DC, National Institute for Occupational Safety and Health, DHHS (NIOSH) publication no. 95-106, 1995.

14. This refers to the ability to measure accurately concentrations of respirable coal mine dust at or near the REL.

15. Paustenbach DJ: Health risk assessment and the practice of industrial hygiene. Am Ind Hyg Assoc J 51:339–351, 1990.

16. Leung H, Paustenbach DJ: Assessing health risks in the workplace: A study of 2,3,7,8-tetra-chlorodibenzo-p-dioxin. In Paustenbach DJ (ed): The Risk Assessment of Environmental and Human Health Hazards: A Textbook of Case Studies. New York, Wiley-Interscience, 1989.

17. Hallenbeck WH: Quantitative Risk Assessment for Environmental and Occupational Health. 2nd ed. Ann Arbor, MI, Lewis Publishers, 1993.

18. Some industrial hygienists believe that they should not be classified as risk managers but instead as risk assessors. This is because, in most cases, the prerogative to implement or augment controls resides solely with the plant manager. My view is that industrial hygienists should be considered not only part of a company's occupational exposure risk management program but also an integral, critical part. A "risk assessment," as the term is commonly used in government and academia when considering occupational exposures, typically involves the determination, based on an analysis of exposure and health effects data from a cohort, of the probability of an adverse outcome given a specific level of working lifetime average or cumulative exposure. It is difficult, if not impossible, to determine this probability for any specific employee.

19. McMahan S, Meyer J: Communication of risk information to workers and managers: Do industrial hygienists differ in their communication techniques. Am Ind Hyg Assoc J 57:186–190, 1996.

20. Adkins CE, et al: Letter to the editor. Appl Occup Environ Hygiene 5:748–750, 1990.

21. Roach SA: A most rational basis for air sampling programmes. Ann Occup Hyg 20:65–84, 1977.

22. Occupational Safety and Health Act of 1970 (OSHAct): Public Law 91-596, 1970.

23. Federal Mine Safety and Health Act of 1977 (FMSHAct): Public Law 91-173, 1977.

24. "Acceptable risk" or "de minimis" risk for occupational risk factors has yet to be quantified.

25. Occupational Safety and Health Administration: Updating permissible exposure limits (PELs) for air contaminants; Meeting. Fed Reg 61:1947–1950, 1996.

26. Alavanja MCR, Brown C, Spirtas R, Gomez M: Risk assessment for carcinogens: A comparison of approaches of the ACGIH and EPA. Appl Occup Environ Hygiene 5:510–517, 1990.

27. Peak exposures or sustained periods of high exposures may be important in the etiology of many occupational chronic diseases. However, exposure histories are nearly always incomplete. Consequently, the epidemiologist by default uses the estimates of long-term exposure in exposure-response analyses.

28. Park CN, Hawkins NC: Cancer risk assessment. In Cralley LJ, Cralley LV, Bus JS (eds): Patty's Industrial Hygiene and Toxicology. 3rd ed, vol 3. New York, John Wiley & Sons,1995.

29. Drinker P , Hatch T: Industrial Dust—Hygienic Significance, Measurement, and Control. 2nd ed. New York, McGraw-Hill, 1954.

30. Roach SA: A more rational basis for air sampling programs. Am Ind Hyg Assoc J 27:1–12, 1966.

31. Roach SA: Health Risks from Hazardous Substances at Work—Assessment, Evaluation, and Control. New York, Pergamon Press,1992.

32. Tebbens BD, Spear RC: Quality control of work environments. Am Ind Hyg Assoc J 32:546–551, 1971.

33. Esmen NA: A distribution-free double-sampling method for exposure assessment. Appl Occup Environ Hygiene 7:613–621, 1992.

34. An "observation period" or "sample period"[52] is some arbitrary but manageable period, typically no more than a year.[36,52] Longer observation intervals are justified only when exposures have been demonstrated to be "minimal" (i.e., only infrequently exceed one-tenth of the TWA OEL)[31] and the processes that generate and control exposures are reasonably stable. The frequency of periodic monitoring for work environments that are nominally in compliance varies, depending on the exposure history of the work environment, the type of controls in place (e.g., total or partial enclosure, local or general exhaust ventilation), and the likelihood of significant change since the last evaluation (largely a judgment call).[31,36,52,53] After a baseline evaluation periodic evaluations should occur at least yearly. If, after several years, a consistent history of well-controlled exposures or better can be demonstrated, the employer may be justified in reducing the number of measurements collected and/or the frequency of sampling (for example, to once every two or three years, depending on the circumstances).

35. Rappaport SM, Selvin S, Roach SA: A strategy for assessing exposures with reference to multiple limits. Appl Ind Hygiene 3:310–315, 1988.

36. Hawkins NC, Norwood SK, Rock JC (eds): A Strategy for Occupational Exposure Assessment. Fairview, VA, American Industrial Hygiene Association, 1991.

37. Often an exposure assessment strategy will have multiple purposes. Exposures may also be collected to evaluate point sources of contaminants, to determine the efficacy of controls, or for research (epidemiologic) purposes.[29,47,116,121]

38. An exposure monitoring program or exposure assessment strategy is composed of two parts: an exposure sampling strategy and a decision logic. The exposure sampling strategy specifies the process for selecting whom to monitor, when to monitor, how many TWA measurements to collect, and how often to repeat this process. The decision logic specifies the procedure for interpreting the exposure data and deciding whether or not the work environment is currently acceptable or unacceptable.

39. "Significant" exposures are usually interpreted to be those above one-tenth of the OEL.[31,48,71]

40. Leidel NA, Busch KA, Lynch JR: Occupational Exposure Sampling Strategy Manual. National Institute for Occupational Safety and Health publication no. 77-173 (available from the National Technical Information Service, publication no. PB274792), 1977.

41. The decision logic was simple: If the first measurement is less than half the PEL, conclude that the work environment is acceptable for the exposure group represented by the MRE. If the first measurement is above the PEL, conclude that the work environment is unacceptable and take corrective action. Otherwise, collect additional measurements at specified intervals until either two consecutive measurements are less than half the PEL (and conclude that the exposures are acceptable) or any single measurement is above the PEL (and conclude that exposures are unacceptable and take appropriate actions to reduce exposures).

42. Tuggle RM: The NIOSH decision scheme. Am Ind Hyg Assoc J 42:493–498, 1981.

43. Rappaport SM: The rules of the game: An analysis of OSHA's enforcement strategy. Am J Ind Med 6:291–303, 1984.

44. Rappaport SM: Interpreting levels of exposures to chemical agents. In Harris RL, Cralley LJ, Cralley LV (eds): Patty's Industrial Hygiene and Toxicology. 3rd ed, vol 3. New York, John Wiley & Sons, 1994.

45. OSHA frequently uses the term "representative employees" in its standards for specific substances [6(b) standards]. If there are known or readily discernable differences in the exposure potential of the employees in an exposure group, the "representative employee" can be considered equivalent to NIOSH's concept of the "maximum risk employee."[7,46] Otherwise, a random sampling strategy should be devised so that there is a high likelihood that the higher exposed employees are represented in the sample.

46. Occupational Safety and Health Administration: Code of Federal Regulations 29, Part 1910.1048 Formaldehyde (Appendices A and B), 1994.[46]

47. Guest IG, Cherrie JW, Gardner RJ, Money CD: Sampling Strategies for Airborne Contaminants in the Workplace. British Occupational Hygiene Society Technical Guide No. 11 (ISBN 0 948237 14 7). Leeds, H and H Scientific Consultants, 1993.

48. Ayer HE: Occupational air sampling strategies. In Hering SV (ed): Air Sampling Instruments for Evaluation of Atmospheric Contaminants. 7th ed. Cincinnati, American Conference of Governmental Industrial Hygienists,1989.

49. Lynch JR: Measurement of worker exposure. In Harris RL, Cralley LJ, Cralley LV (eds): Patty's Industrial Hygiene and Toxicology. 3rd ed, vol 3. New York, John Wiley & Sons, 1994.

50. Corn M, Esmen NA: Workplace exposure zones for classification of employee exposures to physical and chemical agents. Am Ind Hyg Assoc J 40:47–57, 1979.

51. Esmen NA: Mathematical basis for an efficient sampling strategy. In Marple VA, Liu BYU (eds): Aerosols in the Mining and Industrial Work Environment. Vol I. 1983.

52. Still KR, Wells B: Quantitative industrial hygiene programs: Workplace monitoring. Appl Ind Hygiene 4:F14–F17, 1989.

53. Corn M: Sampling strategies for prospective surveillance: Overview and future directions. In Industrial Hygiene Science Series—Advances in Air Sampling. Ann Arbor, MI, Lewis Publishers, 1988.

54. The Committee allows that the industrial hygienist may select the "most exposed worker" when determining whether an HEG is in compliance with a government standard.

55. CEN (Comité Européen de Normalisation): Workplace atmospheres—Guidance for the assessment of exposure by inhalation of chemical agents for comparison with limit values and measurement strategy. European Standard EN 689, effective no later than Aug 1995 (Feb 1995).

56. "[I]f an individual exposure is less than half or greater than twice the arithmetic mean [for the HEG], the relevant work factors should be closely re-examined to determine whether the assumption of homogeneity was correct."[55]

57. Kromhout H, Symanski E, and Rappaport SM: A comprehensive evaluation of within- and between-worker components of occupational exposure to chemical agents. Ann Occup Hyg 37:253-270, 1993.

58. Rappaport SM, Kromhout H,Symanski E: Variation of exposure between workers in homogeneous exposure groups. Am Ind Hyg Assoc J 54:654–662, 1993.

59. Such data include repeat measurements randomly collected from a random sample of workers within each exposure group, which then could be analyzed using ANOVA techniques.

60. Efficiency refers to the ability to come to a decision, right or wrong, with a limited number of measurements.

61. Tuggle RM: Assessment of occupational exposure using one-sided tolerance limits. Am Ind Hyg Assoc J 43:338–346, 1982.

62. Any LTA OEL should have a corresponding TWA OEL to prevent abuse of the LTA OEL concept. For example, it is inappropriate to expose workers to 12 times the LTA OEL for 1 month followed by 11 months of zero exposure.

63. Roach[31] recommended a similar goal: "A [reasonably homogeneous] job-exposure group which is within 0.1–1.0 x exposure limit band but yields results consistently below one-third the exposure limit could be sampled at a reduced frequency, namely once every two months" (p 327).

64. Roach SA, Rappaport SM: But they are not thresholds: A critical analysis of the documentation of threshold limit values. Am J Ind Med 17:727–753, 1990.

65. The effective OEL, or citation value, is the OEL plus an allowance for sampling and analytical error (SAE). SAE is calculated using the total coefficient of variation (CVT) for the sampling and analytical method. For a typical CVT of 0.1 the allowance is easily calculated: SAE = (1.645 • CVT • OEL).

66. Spear RC, Selvin S, Schulman J,Francis M: Benzene exposure in the petroleum refining industry. Appl Ind Hygiene 2:155–163, 1987.

67. Rappaport SM, Lyles RH, Kupper LL: An exposure-assessment strategy accounting for within- and between-worker sources of variability. Ann Occup Hyg 39:469–495, 1995.

68. Occupational Safety and Health Administration: Occupational exposure to asbestos; final rule. Fed Reg 59:40964–41158 (p 41058), 1994.

69. The AIHA Exposure Assessment Strategies Committee monograph[36] was directed at persuading industrial hygienists to collect sufficient measurements for each homogeneous exposure group (HEG) so that the underlying parameters of the group exposure distribution are reliably estimated. These parameter estimates are then used in various statistical procedures to assess the acceptability of the exposure distribution for the HEG.

70. Cope RF, Pancamo BP, Rinehart WE, Haar GLT: Personnel monitoring for tetraalkyl lead in the workplace. Am Ind Hyg Assoc J 40:372–379, 1979.

71. Rock JC: Occupational air sampling strategies. In Cohen BS, Hering SV (eds): Air Sampling Instruments for Evaluation of Atmospheric Contaminants. 8th ed. Cincinnati, American Conference of Governmental Industrial Hygienists, 1995.

72. Nicas M, Simmons BP, Spear RC: Environmental versus analytical variability in exposure measurements. Am Ind Hyg Assoc J 52:553–557, 1991.

73. The survey notes should be evaluated for unusual occurrences (e.g., spills, temporary control equipment breakdowns) that are unlikely to recur or for systematic changes in the work environment (e.g., increased production level, process changes, decreased efficiency of the control equipment, introduction of new or untrained workers, changes in work practices).

74. In the preamble to the 1987 benzene revised PEL,[7] OSHA recommended that exposure data more than 1 year old be given little or no weight in evaluating the current exposure management practices. In the preamble to the 1992 cadmium revised PEL, OSHA stated that when using "historic monitoring" results to meet the "initial monitoring" requirements of the new standard, the employer must meet two conditions: (1) the historic exposure conditions must be similar to current conditions and the measurement method must conform to the requirements of the standard, and (2) monitoring must have been conducted "within 12 months prior to the publication date of this standard" (Fed Reg 57(178):42337, Sept 14, 1992).

75. Ziem GE, Castleman BI: Threshold limit values: Historical perspectives and current practice. J Occup Med 31:910–918, 1989.

76. Castleman BI, Ziem GE: American Conference of Governmental Industrial Hygienists: Low threshold credibility. Am J Ind Med 26:133–143, 1994.

77. American Conference of Governmental Industrial Hygienists: Threshold Limit Values: A more balanced appraisal. Appl Occup Environ Hygiene 5:340–344, 1990.

78. Corn M: Regulations, standards, and occupational hygiene within the U.S.A. in the 1980s. Ann Occup Hyg 27:91–105, 1983.

79. Corn M: Historical perspective on approaches to estimation of inhalation risk by air sampling. Am J Ind Med 21:113–123, 1992.

80. Stokinger HE: Threshold Limit Values. Dangerous Properties of Industrial Materials Report. May/June pp 8–13, 1981.

81. Stokinger HE: Threshold limits and maximum acceptable concentrations: Their definition and interpretation. Am Ind Hyg Assoc J 23:45–47, 1962 (see also a nearly identical article in Arch Environ Health 4:115–117, 1962).

82. Stokinger HE: Modus operandi of threshold limits committee of ACGIH. In Transactions of the Twenty-sixth Annual Meeting of the American Conference of Governmental Industrial Hygienists 26:23–29, 1964.

83. Stokinger HE: Industrial air standards—theory and practice. J Occup Med 15:429–431, 1973.

84. Stokinger HE: Intended use and application of the TLVs. In Transactions of the Thirty-third Annual Meeting of the American Conference of Governmental Industrial Hygienists, 33:113–116, 1971.

85. Roach SA, Baier EJ, Ayer HE, Harris RL: Testing compliance with threshold limit values for respirable dusts. Am Ind Hyg Assoc J 28:543–553, 1967.

86. Readers should be aware, when reading these references, that in the 1960s and early 1970s the usual practice was to use several short-term, partial shift measurements to estimate a single TWA.[48,85]

87. American Conference of Governmental Industrial Hygienists: Threshold Limit Values for Air-borne Contaminants for 1968, Recommended and Intended Values, 1968.

88. Nearly identical wording has been included in the introduction of every TLV booklet since 1968, including the current 1995–1996 booklet.

89. Stokinger HE: Current problems of setting occupational exposure standards. Arch Environ Health 19:277–280, 1969.

90. In 1969 and 1971 Stokinger lamented the fact that occasionally the "factory inspector" and "legal profession" interpreted high short-term measurements (i.e., partial shift, the common type of measurement prior to the 1970s) as evidence that the TWA TLV had been breached or as "proof or disproof of an existing disease or physical condition." Stokinger noted that such short-term measurements were best compared to ceiling values and the then newly developed short-term limits and not to the TWA TLVs.

91. American Conference of Governmental Industrial Hygienists: 1995–1996 Threshold Limit Values (TLVs) for Chemical Substances and Physical Agents and Biological Exposure Indices (BEIs). ACGIH, Cincinnati, 1995.

92. Stokinger also mentioned that TLVs should not be used as a measure of "relative index of toxicity." The strength of the data for each TLV vary, the site and mode of action vary, and, most importantly, the actual risk depends on the likelihood and severity of exposure. (It also may be assumed that the exposure-response curves for different substances will have different shapes or slopes.)

93. Brief RS , Scala RA: Occupational exposure limits for novel work schedules. Am Ind Hyg Assoc J 36:467–469, 1975.

94. American Conference of Governmental Industrial Hygienists: Documentation of the Threshold Limit Values and Biological Exposure Indices. 6th ed. ACGIH, Cincinnati, 1991.

95. Consider your response if your physician announced that your blood cholesterol was 400 mg/dl but that you should not be concerned because the average across all the patients that day was equal to or less than the goal of 200 mg/dl.

96. Occupational Safety and Health Administration: Occupational exposure to lead; final standard. Fed Reg 43(220):52952–53014, 1978.

97. Paull JM: The origin and basis of threshold limit values. Am J Ind Med 5:227–238, 1984.

98. ACGIH also recommends "ceiling" limits for fast-acting substances. A TLV-C represents "the concentration that should not be exceeded during any part of the working exposure." Exposures should be measured using an "instantaneous" direct reading instrument or averaged over a period not longer than 15 minutes.[91]

99. American Conference of Governmental Industrial Hygienists: Documentation of the Threshold Limit Values for Substances in Workroom Air. 3rd ed. ACGIH, Cincinnati, 1971.

100. Within-shift excursion factors make little or no sense if the TWA TLV is truly an upper limit for the long-term, lifetime average exposure of each worker.

101. Silva P: TLVs to protect "nearly all workers." Appl Occup Environ Hygiene 1:49–53, 1986.

102. American Industrial Hygiene Association: Workplace environmental exposure level guides. Am Ind Hyg Assoc J 55:71–72, 1994.

103. American Industrial Hygiene Association: AIHA WEEL Committee Charter, May 11, 1994.

104. U.S. Supreme Court: *Industrial Union Department, AFL-CIO v. American Petroleum Institute et al.*, case nos. 78-911, 78-1036. Supreme Court Reporter 100:2871, 1980.

105. Asbestos, vinyl chloride, inorganic arsenic, lead, benzene, coke oven emissions, cotton dust, 1,2-dibromo-3-chloropropane, acrylonitrile, ethylene oxide, and formaldehyde.

106. de la Cruz PL, Sarvadi DG: OSHA PELs: Where do we go from here? Am Ind Hyg Assoc J 55:894–900, 1994.

107. Nicholson WJ, Landrigan PJ: Quantitative assessment of lives lost due to delay in the regulation of occupational exposure to benzene. Environ Health Perspect 82:185–188, 1989.

108. Imagine, if you will, the excuses that could be made if speed limits were legally defined as "65 mph and under, 95% of the time" or "65 mph, on average." Enforcement would be difficult indeed.

109. Occupational Safety and Health Administration: OSHA Technical Manual (OTM), Directive TED 1.15, September 22, 1995.

110. Historical measurements will not be comparable to OSHA's full-shift compliance measurements if the measurements represent grab-samples or short-term exposures; were collected from substantially different shifts, processes, operations, or occupations; or process changes have occurred.

111. National Institute for Occupational Safety and Health: NIOSH Recommended Exposure Limit Policy, May 24, 1996.

112. Harris RL: Information, risk, and professional ethics. Am Ind Hyg Assoc J 47:67–71, 1986.

113. Naumann BD, et al.: Performance-based exposure control limits for pharmaceutical active ingredients. Am Ind Hyg Assoc J 57:33–42, 1996.

114. National Institutes of Health: Detection, Evaluation, and Treatment of High Blood Cholesterol in Adults (Adult Treatment Panel II). NIH publication no. 93-3095, 1993.

115. There is one aspect of cholesterol risk management that does not easily translate to the workplace. The NIH recommends that physicians encourage patients with a record of high cholesterol to reduce their cholesterol level considerably below the target value to balance the excessive exposures. With the exception of coal miners (who can be transferred to low dust areas based on evidence that pneumoconiosis has developed) and lead workers (who are transferred to low lead areas on the basis of excessive blood lead levels), this concept is not usually practiced by occupational health risk managers.

116. Harris RL: Guideline for Collection of Industrial Hygiene Exposure Assessment Data for Epidemiologic Use. Prepared for the Chemical Manufacturers Association, 1993.

117. Gomez MR, Rawls G: Conference on occupational exposure databases: A report and look at the future. Appl Occup Environ Hygiene 10:238–243, 1995.

118. Lippmann M: Exposure data needs in risk assessment and risk management: database information needs. Appl Occup Environ Hygiene 10:244–250, 1995.

119. Gressel MG, Heitbrink WA (eds): Analyzing Workplace Exposures Using Direct Reading Instruments and Video Exposure Monitoring Techniques. National Institute for Occupational Safety and Health publication no. 92-104, 1992.

120. Bierbaum PJ, Doemeny LJ, Smith JP, Abell MT: U.S. approach to air sampling of workplace contaminants: Current basis and future options. Appl Occup Environ Hygiene 8:247–250, 1993.

121. Leidel NA, Busch KA: Statistical design and data analysis requirements. In Harris RL, Cralley LJ, Cralley LV (eds): Patty's Industrial Hygiene and Toxicology. 3rd ed, vol 3. New York, John Wiley & Sons, 1994.

122. American Industrial Hygiene Association American Industrial Hygiene Association white paper: A generic exposure assessment standard. Am Ind Hyg Assoc J 55:1009–1012, 1994.

123. Occupational Safety and Health Administration: Generic standard for exposure monitoring—Advance notice of proposed rulemaking. Fed Reg 53:37591–37598, 1988.

124. Organization Resources Counselors, Inc.: A Proposed Generic Workplace Exposure Assessment Standard. Washington, DC, Organization Resources Counselors, Inc., 1992.

125. In a sense the current legal requirements for exposure assessments are performance standards. They represent minimalistic strategies and leave considerable room for voluntary improvement and enhancement. OSHA all but stated this in Appendix B of the 1992 final standard for formaldehyde.[46]

INDEX

Entries in **boldface type** indicate complete chapters.